Quick Look Nursing:
Pathophysiology

QUICK LOOK NURSING

Pathophysiology

Eileen M. Crutchlow, EdD, APRN-C

Associate Professor of Nursing
Southern Connecticut State University
New Haven, Connecticut
Family Nurse Practitioner
Bridgeport Community Health Center
Bridgeport, Connecticut

Pamela J. Dudac, MS, MSN, APRN-C

Assistant Professor of Nursing
Fairfield University
Fairfield, Connecticut

Suzanne MacAvoy, EdD, APRN-C

Professor of Nursing
Fairfield University
Fairfield, Connecticut
Family Nurse Practitioner
Bridgeport Community Health Center
Bridgeport, Connecticut

Bernadette R. Madara, EdD, APRN-CS

Associate Professor of Nursing
Southern Connecticut State University
New Haven, Connecticut

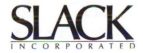

SLACK
INCORPORATED

An innovative information, education and management company
6900 Grove Road • Thorofare, NJ 08086

**For constant updates and weblinks to the book, please visit
www.slackbooks.com/pathophysiology.**

Copyright © 2002 by SLACK Incorporated

Original illustrations by Barbara Minnick.

The procedures and practices described in this book should be implemented in a manner consistent with the professional standards set for the circumstances that apply in each specific situation. Every effort has been made to confirm the accuracy of the information presented and to correctly relate generally accepted practices. The author, editor, and publisher cannot accept responsibility for errors or exclusions or for the outcome of the application of the material presented herein. There is no expressed or implied warranty of this book or information imparted by it.

The work SLACK publishes is peer reviewed. Prior to publication, recognized leaders in the field, educators, and clinicians provide important feedback on the concepts and content that we publish. We welcome feedback on this work.

Library of Congress Cataloging-in-Publication Data

Pathophysiology / Eileen M. Crutchlow ... [et al.].
   p. ; cm. – (Quick look nursing)
Includes bibliographical references and index.
  ISBN 1-55642-565-1 (alk. paper)
  1. Physiology, Pathological. 2. Nursing.
  [DNLM: 1. Disease–Nurses' Instruction. 2. Diagnostic Techniques and Procedures–Nurses' Instruction.
  QZ 140 P2942 2002] I. Crutchlow, Eileen M. II. Series.
  RB113 .P3573 2002
  616.07–dc21

                       2002007740

Printed in the United States of America.

Published by: SLACK Incorporated
               6900 Grove Road
               Thorofare, NJ 08086 USA
               Telephone: 856-848-1000
               Fax: 856-853-5991
               www.slackbooks.com

Contact SLACK Incorporated for more information about other books in this field or about the availability of our books from distributors outside the United States.

Last digit is print number: 10 9 8 7 6 5 4 3 2 1

Dedication

We dedicate this book to our students, who have challenged and inspired us.

Contents

Part IX   Renal System

Bernadette R. Madara, EdD, APRN-CS

Part X   Orthopedics

Suzanne MacAvoy, EdD, APRN-C

About the Authors

Eileen M. Crutchlow is a tenured professor at Southern Connecticut State University (SCSU) and has been involved in the education of graduate, undergraduate, and RN-BSN nursing students for most of her professional career. She began teaching at Fairfield University where she met Pamela Dudac and Suzanne MacAvoy, co-authors of this book, and later moved to Albertus Magnus College in New Haven to begin an RN-BSN program. She went to SCSU to help begin its graduate programs. She and Bernadette Madara continue to teach there together. In organizing this book, Eileen looked to known, experienced colleagues who were able to develop a well-written book that would serve the needs of students and practicing nurses.

Eileen has always maintained a clinical practice and has worked in a variety of settings including intensive care, coronary care, home care, and long-term care. In 1995, she graduated from Pace University in Pleasantville, NY as a family nurse practitioner (FNP) and since that time has maintained a practice as an FNP at Bridgeport Community Health Center. There she has served a variety of roles including managing a school-based health center and an off-site community clinic. She is currently based in the pediatric clinic where she oversees the health component of a comprehensive screening for children entering the foster care system. She also runs the center's Reach Out and Read Program.

Eileen is from New Jersey. Originally a diploma graduate from St. Mary's Hospital School of Nursing in Passaic, NJ, she completed her BSN at Seton Hall University in South Orange, NJ. Her first master's degree was earned at The Catholic University of America, Washington, DC in medical surgical nursing. A second was in family primary care from Pace University. Her doctorate was earned at Teachers College, Columbia University in New York City.

Eileen currently resides in Connecticut with her daughters Kara and Aruna.

Pamela J. Dudac is an assistant professor of nursing at Fairfield University with areas of interest in health assessment, adult health, and cardiovascular nursing. She has also held teaching positions at Columbia University and the University of Maine at Portland. She has practiced in adult acute care settings and until recently, she practiced as an adult nurse practitioner in the Homeless Department of Southwest Community Health Center in Bridgeport, CT. She is a parish nurse. She holds a bachelor of arts degree from Manhattanville College, a master of science degree in biology from Fordham University, a master of science in nursing degree from the New York Medical College, and certification as an adult nurse practitioner from The University of Rochester. She is currently interested in developing a nursing practice with Southeast Asian immigrants.

She is an intercultural (Phillipine) adoptive parent. Her most relaxing moments are on the ski slopes at Okemo Mountain, VT.

Suzanne MacAvoy began teaching nursing 34 years ago after spending 3 years in clinical practice in various roles. Her master's degree is in medical/surgical nursing and her doctorate is in curriculum and instruction from Teachers College, Columbia University. The majority of her teaching experience has been in the area of adult health and nursing research, although she has recently begun teaching a course in primary care of special populations, in the graduate program. Sue also teaches a course in homelessness in the peace and justice minor at the University and a nursing elective entitled Health in Rural Appalachia, which offers a 1-week immersion experience in eastern Kentucky.

Two years ago Sue returned to school, completing a family nurse practitioner certificate program. In addition to full-time teaching, Sue works 1 day a week at an inner city pediatric clinic in the asthma program.

In addition to teaching and scholarship in the aforementioned areas, Sue has been actively involved in the Mission Volunteer Program through Campus Ministry and leads groups of students, yearly, in 2-week immersion experiences in Latin America and the Caribbean. She has presented several papers on social juustice initiatives, as a consequence of these activities. She is a member of several professional nursing and advanced practice nursing organizations.

Bernadette R. Madara is a tenured associate professor at Southern Connecticut State University. She received her BSN from St. Anselm College in Manchester, NH; her MA from the University of Tulsa, OK; her MSN from Sacred Heart University in Fairfield, CT; and her doctorate from Teacher's College, Columbia University. Her clinical experience and certification are in adult health nursing.

Bernadette has taught in a variety of nursing education programs including licensed practical nurse programs in Connecticut and Oklahoma, and diploma and associate degree nursing programs in Connecticut. She currently teaches at both the undergraduate and graduate levels at SCSU. Her areas of interest related to undergraduate coursework include pharmacology, pathophysiology, adult health, and research. On the graduate level she has taught family nursing and the role of the nurse educator.

Preface

This book is intended for undergraduate students and registered nurses entering a new area of practice. It is intended to be a quick reference rather than a full pathophysiology text. Each part includes an overview of the body system's anatomy and physiology and common laboratory and diagnostic tests pertinent to that system. Chapters address commonly occurring problems and are organized to include an overview, physiology, and goals of treatment. References for each section are included at the end of the book. We trust that you will find this book useful.

For constant updates and weblinks to the book, please visit www.slackbooks.com/pathophysiology.

PART I
Fluid and Electrolyte Balance

Suzanne MacAvoy, EdD, APRN-C

1 Fluid Balance

Definitions

- Osmosis—Movement of H_2O across a semipermeable membrane.
- Diffusion—Movement of solutes across a semipermeable membrane.
- Active transport—Movement of molecules by a protein transporter across a membrane against a concentration gradient and requiring an expenditure of energy.
- Facilitated diffusion—Movement of molecules by a protein transporter across a membrane without an expenditure of energy.
- Osmolality—Concentration of molecules by weight of water.
- Osmotic (oncotic) pressure—Overall osmotic effect of colloids.
- Hydrostatic pressure—Mechanical force of water against cellular membranes.
- Edema—Accumulation of fluid within the interstitial spaces.

Movement of Water Across Cell Membranes

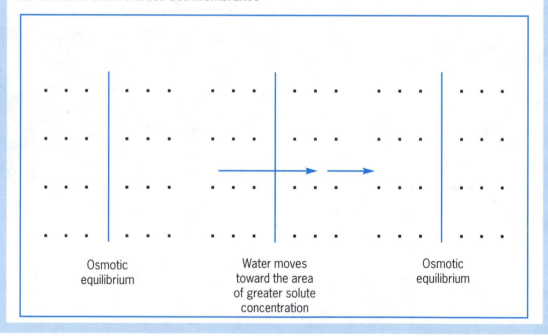

Osmotic equilibrium

Water moves toward the area of greater solute concentration

Osmotic equilibrium

Introduction

Fluids are distributed in various compartments in the body, with movement back and forth to maintain homeostasis. This movement is a result of variations in hydrostatic pressure and osmotic forces, especially in interstitial and intravascular compartments. The fluid environment serves as the medium for exchange and distribution of electrolytes and nutrients and elimination of waste products from cellular metabolism.

Distribution

The three main fluid compartments are *intracellular* (within cells); *extracellular*, including interstitial (between cells); and *intravascular* (blood plasma).

Other extracellular compartments include those areas of the body containing smaller amounts of fluid such as lymphatic, synovial, cerebrospinal, pericardial, and others. These smaller compartments are important in particular diseases or conditions but less so in terms of overall fluid and electrolyte balance and maintenance of homeostasis.

The percentage of total body water varies with age and amount of body fat. The more body fat present, the less water present. Infants have a proportionally larger percent of total body water, which makes them particularly vulnerable to fluid shifts and dehydration. Their rapid metabolic rate, greater body surface area, and immature renal function also contribute to their susceptibility to fluid imbalances. The elderly have proportionally smaller percentages of body water due to higher amounts of body fat, less lean tissue, and reduced ability of organ systems to compensate to maintain homeostasis. These variations are particularly important during periods of illness or stress, making the elderly especially vulnerable to dehydration, electrolyte imbalance, and system dysfunction.

Daily fluid intake varies from person to person within a range of 2,400 to 3,200 ml with roughly two thirds obtained by drinking and one third obtained through food and water of oxidation (300 to 400 ml). Daily output balances intake in roughly the same proportions—two thirds through urine and one third through insensible losses. It is important to take insensible losses into account during periods of illness, as these may be significantly increased (diarrhea, ventilator-assisted breathing, diaphoresis, fever).

Fluid Movement

Movement of water between the intracellular and extracellular fluid compartments is primarily affected by osmotic forces. Since water moves freely across cell membranes (i.e., toward the side with the greatest solute or particle concentration), an equilibrium ordinarily exists between compartments. Sodium (Na+) is the most abundant extracellular ion and is responsible for maintaining osmotic balance in that compartment. Potassium (K+) performs the same role in the intracellular compartment. The osmotic force of intracellular proteins and active transport of ions out of the cell are additional forces contributing to this process.

Plasma proteins play an important role in maintaining osmolality through plasma oncotic pressure in the intravascular compartment. These osmotic forces are balanced by hydrostatic pressure in the vascular compartment. Forces that favor movement of water out of the capillary and into the interstitial compartment are vascular hydrostatic pressure and interstitial fluid osmotic pressure. Forces that favor movement of water into the capillary from the interstitial compartment are interstitial hydrostatic pressure and vascular (plasma) osmotic pressure. The major forces for this filtration process are within the capillary because plasma proteins do not readily cross the capillary membrane. Under normal circumstances, hydrostatic pressure exceeds capillary oncotic pressure at the arterial end of the capillary, causing water to move into the interstitial space. Consequently, hydrostatic pressure is lower than capillary oncotic pressure at the venous end of the capillary. This causes fluid to be reabsorbed back into the vascular system. Changes in capillary membrane permeability may alter this process by allowing plasma proteins to enter the interstitial space. Water will follow and edema results.

Fluid volume imbalances (i.e., deficits or excesses) that occur may involve either changes in volume only or changes in volume and concentration. The causes of these differ, as will lab values, and effect the treatment prescribed. The nurse's role in assessing and educating the patient and monitoring the effectiveness of management is crucial. See p. 4 for manifestations of fluid volume deficit (dehydration) and fluid volume overload (circulatory overload).

Edema

Edema is a problem of fluid distribution, not necessarily one of fluid overload. It results when forces favoring movement of fluid from the vascular (or lymphatic) compartment exceed those retaining fluid within that compartment. The most common mechanisms causing edema are increased hydrostatic pressure, decreased plasma oncotic pressure, increased capillary membrane permeability, and lymphatic obstruction. Any condition that increases blood volume or that causes venous or lymphatic obstruction can cause edema (e.g., tumors, advanced pregnancy, tight clothing, and Na and H_2O retention). Conditions that cause inflammation increase capillary permeability and cause edema (e.g., tissue injury, infection, and allergies). Any condition that either prevents the formation of plasma proteins, particularly albumin (e.g., cirrhosis), or causes their loss (e.g., chronic renal failure) will cause edema. In all of these situations, the balance between hydrostatic and oncotic pressures in capillaries and interstitial fluid has been altered. It is not uncommon for more than one condition to coexist. It is important to understand the basic pathophysiologic processes involved so that nursing assessment will be thorough and various measures can be instituted to alleviate the edema.

It is also important for nurses to understand the consequences of edema in a particular organ system or part of the body because pressure from edema can impair tissue perfusion, leading to hypoxia and decreased transport of nutrients and waste products. One way to do this is to first, recall the anatomical structures and characteristics of involved tissues/organs; second, recall the physiological

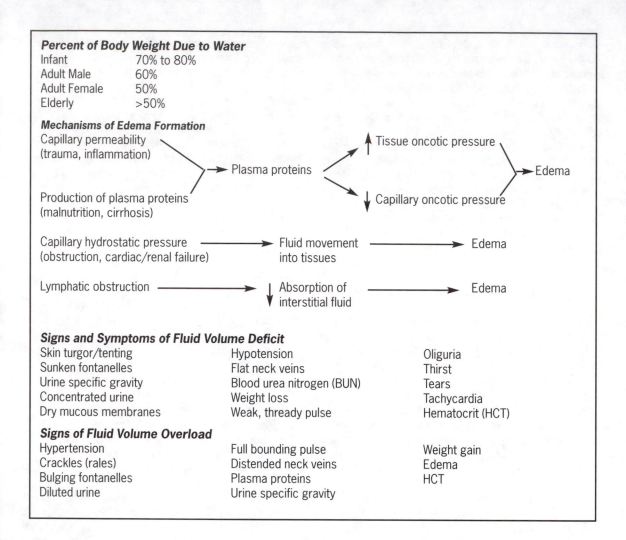

Percent of Body Weight Due to Water

Infant	70% to 80%
Adult Male	60%
Adult Female	50%
Elderly	>50%

Mechanisms of Edema Formation

Capillary permeability (trauma, inflammation)

Production of plasma proteins (malnutrition, cirrhosis)

→ Plasma proteins →

↑ Tissue oncotic pressure

↓ Capillary oncotic pressure

→ Edema

Capillary hydrostatic pressure (obstruction, cardiac/renal failure) → Fluid movement into tissues → Edema

Lymphatic obstruction → ↓ Absorption of interstitial fluid → Edema

Signs and Symptoms of Fluid Volume Deficit

Skin turgor/tenting	Hypotension	Oliguria
Sunken fontanelles	Flat neck veins	Thirst
Urine specific gravity	Blood urea nitrogen (BUN)	Tears
Concentrated urine	Weight loss	Tachycardia
Dry mucous membranes	Weak, thready pulse	Hematocrit (HCT)

Signs of Fluid Volume Overload

Hypertension	Full bounding pulse	Weight gain
Crackles (rales)	Distended neck veins	Edema
Bulging fontanelles	Plasma proteins	HCT
Diluted urine	Urine specific gravity	

processes/functions of the organ system or area of the body; and third, visualize the consequences of the presence of fluid (and resultant pressure) on that organ system, tissue or area of the body. For example, fluid accumulation in the brain is life threatening because the bony skull is hard and cannot expand (except in infants). Therefore, any intracranial pressure buildup from even small amounts of fluid will cause compression of the softer tissue, the brain. On the other hand, fluid accumulation in the abdomen (i.e., ascites) may not create observable abdominal distention until two or more liters are present. This is because there is room in the abdominal cavity for greater amounts of fluid to collect before tissue/organ compression causes physiological disturbances.

A term often used in clinical situations is *third spacing*, which means that fluid is leaving one compartment and moving elsewhere. Ordinarily it has not left the body but has become sequestered and is unavailable for use in maintaining fluid balance. When this occurs, signs of dehydration may be present. Third spacing is used in describing large fluid shifts. Common examples are postoperative patients and persons with significant burns. When large amounts of fluid move from the vascular space into the interstitial space, to be followed in a few days with a reverse fluid shift, care must be taken to avoid circulatory overload while attempting to compensate for the initial reduced circulating volume.

Edema is often referred to as either *pitting* or *brawny*. Pitting edema is that which can be compressed by finger pressure, resulting in a "dent" in the subcutaneous tissue. Brawny edema is firm and noncompressible. It accompanies tissue injury and the fluid includes clotting factors, hence its character.

Management

The goal of management is to reduce or eliminate the edema, thereby preventing (further) tissue injury. Determining the cause or causes is essential. Treatment may be supportive (e.g., positioning, use of compression stockings) or therapeutic (e.g., use of diuretics, dietary Na restrictions).

Electrolyte Balance: Part I

2

Normal Serum Values of Major Electrolytes*

Na	135 to 145 mEq/L	Mg	1.8 to 2.4 mEq/L
Cl	104 to 110 mEq/L	PO_4	2.5 to 4.5 mg/dl
K	3.5 to 5 mEq/L	Albumin	3.5 to 5.5 mg/dl
Ca	4.5 to 5.5 mEq/L	Urine specific gravity	1.010 to 1.030

*There are slight variations in published normal values; use those of the lab with which you are affiliated.

Definitions

- Isotonic—Same concentration (osmolality) of solute as body fluid.
- Hypertonic—Higher concentration of solute than body fluid.
- Hypotonic—Lower concentration of solute than body fluid.
- Osmosis—Movement of water across a semipermeable membrane from low solute concentration to higher solute concentration.
- Diffusion—Continuous movement of particles among each other in a gas or liquid.
- Filtration—Movement of water and dissolved substances from an area of high pressure to one of lower pressure.
- Chvostek's sign—Tapping over facial nerve results in twitching of nose and/or lip.
- Trousseau's sign—Restricting arterial blood flow (via blood pressure cuff) for 5 minutes results in contraction of hand and/or fingers.
- Hypernatremia—Increased sodium.
- Hyponatremia—Decreased sodium.

Sodium, Chloride, and Water Balance

The balance of sodium (Na) and water is closely related because of the osmotic relationship between the two. Water balance is regulated by the antidiuretic hormone (ADH) from the posterior pituitary and Na is regulated by aldosterone from the adrenal cortex.

Thirst is experienced when water loss equals 2% or more of body weight or when there is an increase in osmolality. *Osmolality* can be increased by either a reduction in water or an increase in Na. *Osmoreceptors* are located in the hypothalamus and are stimulated by increases in osmolality and decreases in blood volume. Drinking increases blood volume and decreases osmolality. Osmoreceptor stimulation also causes an increased release of ADH. ADH increases renal tubular permeability to water and

increases its reabsorption, causing increased concentration of urine. If fluid (blood) volume is decreased, centrally located volume and pressure sensitive receptors (baroreceptors) are stimulated, which also stimulates the release of ADH.

Na is the most powerful cation in extracellular fluid (ECF), and chloride is the most powerful ECF anion. In addition to its primary role in maintenance of osmolality, Na also helps to maintain neuromuscular irritability, acid base balance, various cellular chemical reactions, and membrane transport. Chloride neutralizes the positive charge of Na and is passively transported along with the active transport of Na. Bicarbonate is the other major ECF anion and its concentration varies inversely with that of chloride.

Na concentrations are regulated by the kidneys via aldosterone, a mineralocorticoid synthesized and secreted by the adrenal cortex, and atrial natriuretic factor (ANF), a natriuretic hormone from the atrial muscle of the heart. These affect tubular reabsorption of Na. (Note: The former increases it and the latter decreases it). When Na is conserved, potassium is lost. ANF is released when there is an increase in atrial pressure. There is a similar hormone in the left ventricle of the brain, which is called *brain natriuretic peptide* (BNP), that is released in response to increases in blood volume and causes natriuresis, vasodilation, and inhibition of aldosterone.

Aldosterone secretion is also influenced by blood volume (increased with decreased renal perfusion). In addition, the renin-angiotensin system is stimulated by reductions in blood volume and renal perfusion. Activation of this system causes an increase in aldosterone release (increased Na and H_2O reabsorption) and vasoconstriction, both of which serve to increase circulating blood volume and improve renal perfusion.

Alterations in Sodium, Chloride, and Water Balance

Alterations in sodium and water balance are closely linked (i.e., sodium imbalances can develop because of water imbalances and vice versa). Usually, these changes are discussed in terms of *tonicity*. Some authors use the terms *tonicity* and *osmolality* interchangeably.

Isotonic alterations occur when changes in both solutes and water are proportionally the same as body fluids (e.g., blood loss, severe wound drainage, excessive administration of intravenous [IV] normal saline). *Isotonic losses* produce the classic signs of *dehydration* or fluid volume deficit. *Isotonic excesses* are usually iatrogenic (excessive IV fluid administration, glucocorticoid administration), and signs of fluid volume excess (circulatory overload) become evident.

Hypertonic alterations develop when there is excess solute concentration (increased osmolality). *Hypernatremia* is usually caused by an excess of Na or a deficit of H_2O. When this occurs, water is drawn out of the cells, causing cellular dehydration. This hypertonicity can lead to symptoms of hypervolemia if the causative agent is increased Na or ingestion of $NaHCO_3$, or hypovolemia if the causative agent is decreased H_2O (e.g., fever or diabetes insipidus). *Hyperchloremia* accompanies hypernatremia or a deficit in bicarbonate (metabolic acidosis). There are no specific symptoms.

Hypotonic alterations occur with a deficiency of Na (i.e., hyponatremia) or an excess of water. The loss of osmotic pressure in the ECF causes movement of water into the cell (i.e., intracellular edema). This hypotonicity can lead to signs of hypovolemia if the causative agent is a decrease in Na, or signs of hypervolemia if the causative agent is excess water. *Hyponatremia* is usually caused by extrarenal losses (e.g., vomiting, nasogastric [NG] drainage) or by iatrogenic causes (e.g., diuretics, excessive enemas). Hyponatremia interferes with cellular depolarization and repolarization, resulting in nonspecific clinical manifestations of headache, malaise, lethargy, confusion, and apprehension. *Hypochloremia* also accompanies hyponatremia or elevated bicarbonate levels. Hyponatremia is not uncommon in high risk groups (i.e., elderly and infants/children) and should be suspected if there is an unexplained change in mental status or lethargy.

Management

The goal of management is to normalize fluid and electrolyte levels, prevent complications of imbalances, and treat the underlying cause.

Electrolyte Balance: Part II

Definitions
- Hyperkalemia—Increased potassium.
- Hypokalemia—Decreased potassium.
- Hypermagnesemia—Increased magnesium.
- Hypomagnesemia—Decreased magnesium.
- Hypercalcemia—Increased calcium.
- Hypocalcemia—Decreased calcium.

Isotonic IV Solutions
D5NS
NS (0.9%)
Ringer's lactate
Lipids

Hypotonic IV Solutions
D5W
0.45% saline (half strength)

Hypertonic IV Solutions
3% saline
TPN

Common Chemical Symbols

Na	Sodium	Fe	Iron
K	Potassium	Mg	Magnesium
P	Phosphorus	SO_4	Sulfate
PO_4	Phosphate	NH_3	Ammonia
Cl	Chloride	NH_4	Ammonium
HCl	Hydrochloric acid	OH	Hydroxide
H	Hydrogen	Ca	Calcium
O	Oxygen	CO_2	Carbon dioxide
HCO_3	Bicarbonate	H_2CO_3	Carbonic acid

Dietary Intake of Electrolytes

	Average Daily	Minimal Requirement
Na	5 to 6 gm	500 mg
K	40 to 150 mEq	40 mEq

Alterations in Potassium, Calcium, and Phosphate

Potassium

Potassium (K) is the major intracellular electrolyte (cation). The balance between intracellular and extracellular K levels is maintained by an active transport system. K's primary role is in maintaining the resting potential of cell membranes, which allows for transmission and conduction of nerve impulses, maintenance of cardiac rhythm, and skeletal and smooth muscle contraction. It also plays a role in glycogenesis. Most K is located in the small intestine with a moderate amount in gastric secretions and lesser amounts in other body fluids.

K is excreted by the kidneys via passive transport, which occurs as Na is reabsorbed, and is related to the concentration gradient between the plasma and the distal tubular cells. Therefore, any mechanism or condition that influences this gradient will influence K excretion (e.g., renal blood flow, dietary intake, and changes in pH). Mechanisms for tubular conservation of K are weak.

During states of acid-base imbalance, K+ and H+ will shift back and forth, in an inverse relationship, across the cell membrane in order to maintain a healthy balance of these cations. In other words, when there is excess H+ in the extracellular fluid (ECF) during states of acidosis, H+ will cross into the cell, causing K+ to leave, which results in hyperkalemia. Conversely, when there is a deficit of H+ in the ECF during states of alkalosis, H+ will leave the cell, causing K+ to enter the cell, which results in hypokalemia. Renal excretion will be affected in these conditions to either conserve or eliminate K as necessary.

Aldosterone also plays a role in K balance because it is released when K levels are high. This causes renal conservation of Na and excretion of K. Insulin facilitates the passage of K into liver and muscle cells. This fact should be recalled when patients are receiving insulin for management of diabetes, particularly if they have other disorders that might be influenced by this mechanism.

Hypokalemia

Serum hypokalemia can result from either loss of K from the body or shifts of K into the cell from alkalosis or insulin administration. It is difficult to measure the amount of total body K since only serum K is available for such determinations. Total body losses may be present and not reflected in the serum level (due to the body's maintenance of the balance between ECF and intracellular fluid [ICF] levels and its passive excretion by the kidneys). Therefore, extreme care must be taken by physicians and others to monitor patient status in regard to this electrolyte. Dietary deficiencies are rare under normal circumstances but may become important if intake is severely restricted or occurs in the presence of certain comorbidities or medication use (most diuretics). Since K is not stored in the body, daily intake is essential. This becomes important if patients are to take nothing by mouth (NPO) for longer than a few days. The two most common causes of hypokalemia are diarrhea and losses from diuretics. Diarrhea can cause the loss of 100 to 200 mEq of K/day. Vomiting or nasogastric (NG) tube drainage can result in hypokalemia primarily due to the kidneys response to blood volume depletion and metabolic alkalosis. Other causes of hypokalemia include renal disease and certain antibiotics.

Hypokalemia affects carbohydrate metabolism and renal function, as well as neuromuscular and cardiac function. The latter two are most obvious with a decrease in neuromuscular excitability (due to hyperpolarization of the cell membrane), which manifests as skeletal and smooth muscle atony (ileus, abdominal distention; nausea and vomiting; and weakness) as well as cardiac dysrhythmias due to delayed ventricular repolarization (bradyrhythmias, reflecting delayed repolarization). Hypokalemia increases the risk of digitalis toxicity. Acute losses create more symptoms than gradual losses.

Management

The goal of management is to prevent and/or replace losses and treat underlying conditions. Dietary supplementation may be indicated. Because intravenous (IV) K is so irritating, concentrations greater than 40 mEq should not be used. The usual dilution is 20 to 40 mEq/L. Care must be taken to avoid administration that is too rapid. The maximum K replacement is 40 to 80 mEq with 20 mEq daily commonly prescribed for maintenance.

Hyperkalemia

Hyperkalemia is relatively uncommon and is most likely to be caused by accidental ingestion, iatrogenesis, extensive cellular destruction or changes in cell membrane permeability, acidosis, or renal failure. Early manifestations would be those related to increased neuromuscular irritability (due to hypopolarization of the cell membrane) such as restlessness, intestinal cramping, diarrhea, and electrocardiogram (EKG) changes. Severe hyperkalemia can cause some of the same manifestations as deficiency states (i.e., bradyrhythmias and muscle weakness) because the cell is not able to repolarize. Because of the overlap between the roles of calcium and K on membrane potentials, manifestations of hyperkalemia may also be influenced by calcium levels.

Management

The goal of management is to normalize K levels by treating the causative disease or condition, preventing its accumulation, or enhancing its excretion through the use of exchange resins (i.e., sodium polystyrene sulfonate), other medications, or by dialysis.

Calcium

The amount of calcium (Ca) circulating in the blood is small; approximately two fifths of that is in ionized form and available for physiologic functions. Ca is the main element in bones and teeth. It plays an important role in blood clotting, hormone secretion, receptor function, nerve transmission, and muscular contraction. Phosphate (P) is also found in the bone with small amounts in circulation in the form of phospholipids and others. It plays an important role in cellular metabolism and acts as a buffer in acid-base balance. These two ions have an inverse relationship to each other.

The balance between Ca and P is mediated by the parathyroid hormone (PTH), vitamin D, and calcitonin (a thyroid hormone), which regulate their absorption (from gastrointestinal [GI], bone, and renal), deposition, and excretion. PTH is released in response to low serum Ca levels and causes renal reabsorption of Ca and excretion of P. It also stimulates renal activation of vitamin D, which increases GI absorption, renal reabsorption, and bone absorption of Ca. These hormones also regulate the exchange of Ca and P between the bones and the serum. Low levels of Ca and P cause bone resorption (via osteoclasts) thereby releasing more Ca and P into the circulation. Calcitonin is secreted to prevent Ca levels from becoming too high by stimulating osteoblasts, which causes formation of new bone and decreases serum Ca levels. The amount of ionized versus bound serum Ca is influenced by pH. Acidosis causes increases in serum Ca, while alkalosis causes decreases.

Hypocalcemia

Hypocalcemia occurs when ionized Ca drops below 4 mg/dl. This can occur from decreased GI absorption, decreased dietary intake, multiple blood transfusions (citrate, used to prevent clotting in the bag, binds with Ca), pancreatitis (an increase in free fatty acids binds Ca), vitamin D deficiency, removal of the parathyroid glands, alkalosis, and hypoalbuminemia (decreases bound Ca levels).

Manifestations are primarily related to neuromuscular excitability due to a decrease in membrane threshold potential (e.g., confusion, paresthesias, muscle spasms, and hyperreflexia). Two clinical signs often assessed are Chvostek's and Trousseau's signs (see p. 6). Severe signs are convulsions, tetany, EKG changes (prolonged QT), increased bowel sounds, and cramps.

Hypercalcemia

Hypercalcemia exists when levels rise above 12 mg/dl and is most commonly caused by hyperparathyroidism; bone metastasis with breast, prostate, and cervical cancer (many tumors produce PTH); sarcoidosis (increases vitamin D levels); and excess vitamin D. Symptoms are related to loss of cell membrane excitability and often are nonspecific, including weakness, fatigue, anorexia, nausea, constipation, renal stones, and EKG changes (shortened QT, bradyrhythmia).

Management

The goal of management in both of these conditions is to identify and treat the underlying pathology. With hypocalcemia, oral Ca supplements or IV Ca gluconate may be used. Phosphate intake may be reduced if indicated. Oral PO_4 preparations or other medications may be used with hypercalcemia.

Phosphorus

Phosphate is an important component of adenosine triphosphate (ATP), which is the major source of energy for many cellular processes.

Hypophosphatemia

Hypophosphatemia occurs when levels drop below 1 to 2 mg/dl and is usually caused by phosphate deficiency due to renal excretion (hyperparathyroidism) or intestinal malabsorption. Vitamin D deficiency, Mg or Al antacids, or alcohol (ETOH) abuse can also be causes. Manifestations include paresthesia, malaise, diminished reflexes, muscle weakness, and confusion.

Hyperphosphatemia

Hyperphosphatemia occurs with blood levels >4.5 mg/dl and is usually associated with endogenous or exogenous phosphorus intake, renal failure, cellular destruction (PO_4 is an intracellular ion), or hyperparathyroidism (from increased P reabsorption). There may be deposition of Ca and P in soft tissue. Clinical manifestations are similar to those of hypocalcemia.

Management

The goal of management in both of these conditions is to identify and treat the underlying pathology. AlOH binds to PO_4 and causes intestinal excretion. Dialysis will be used for renal failure.

Magnesium

Mg++ is an intracellular ion stored in muscle and bone with 30% stored in the cells. A very small amount is in the serum. It is regulated by the kidneys and plays an important role in the release of acetylcholine at neuromuscular junctions affecting neuromuscular excitability. *Hypomagnesemia* occurs at values of <1.5 mEq/L and results in increased excitability and tetany (similar to signs of Ca deficits). Chronic alcoholism is a major risk factor for hypomagnesemia, which may also be accompanied by hypokalemia. *Hypermagnesemia* (>2.5 mEq/L) is rare and is caused by renal failure or excess intake through cathartics and antacids, especially in the elderly. Signs are those related to decreased neuromuscular excitability. The goal of management is to treat the cause and normalize values. IV administration of $MgSO_4$ may be required with hypomagnesemia.

4 Acid-Base Balance

Common Causes of Respiratory Acidosis
- Chronic obstructive pulmonary disease
- Pneumonia
- Severe asthma
- Hypoventilation (thoracic surgery and others)
- Central nervous system depression (drugs, injury)

Common Causes of Metabolic Acidosis
- Ketoacidosis (diabetes mellitus, starvation)
- Renal failure
- Diarrhea
- Tissue anoxia (cardiac arrest and others)
- Intestinal decompression

Signs and Symptoms of Acidosis

Metabolic
Headache
Lethargy
Kussmaul's respiration
Anorexia
Nausea/vomiting
Diarrhea
Abdominal discomfort

Respiratory
Restlessness
Apprehension
Headache
Lethargy
Muscle twitching
Tremors
Convulsions/coma

Signs and Symptoms of Alkalosis

Metabolic
Weakness
Muscle cramps
Hyperreflexia
Confusion
Slow/shallow respiration
Tingling of the fingers/toes
Dysrhythmias
Coma/death

Respiratory
Dizziness
Confusion
Paresthesias
Convulsions
Coma

pH of Selected Body Fluids

Gastric	1.0 to 3.0		Cerebrospinal fluid	7.32
Urine	5.0 to 6.0		Blood	7.35 to 7.45
Bile	7.6 to 8.6		Pancreatic	7.1 to 8.2

Maintenance of acid-base balance is critical for life and health and is achieved through various buffer systems and compensatory mechanisms of the lungs and kidneys.

Hydrogen Ions and pH

Hydrogen ions maintain membrane integrity and speed of enzymatic reactions. Their concentration is expressed as pH. The higher the number of H+, the more acidic the solution. The more acidic the solution, the lower the pH. Conversely, the lower the number of H+, the more basic the solution (higher pH). Acids are produced as a by-product when protein, carbohydrate, and fat metabolize.

The respiratory and renal systems have primary responsibility for maintaining pH within a normal range. The lungs excrete volatile acids (carbonic acid) by eliminating carbon dioxide (CO_2), while the kidneys excrete nonvolatile acids (e.g., sulfuric, phosphoric, and organic) by regulating bicarbonate. Buffer systems assist in this process.

Buffer Systems

Buffers absorb excess acid (H+) or excess base (OH-) without a significant change in pH. They work as pairs, each containing a weak acid and a weak base. The *carbonic acid-bicarbonate buffer system* is the most important extracellular buffer system. Hemoglobin is an important buffer in erythrocytes. Phosphorus and protein are the primary intracellular buffers. Most buffer systems disassociate rapidly in response to changes in pH. The carbonic acid-bicarbonate buffer system acts in both the lungs and the kidneys. As the $PaCO_2$ increases in the blood, more carbonic acid is formed. This increase is compensated for by the lungs blowing off CO_2 and by the kidneys either reabsorbing bicarbonate or producing more. The respiratory response begins within minutes or hours. The renal response occurs within hours or days. Conversely, if the ratio between bicarbonate (HCO_3) and carbonic acid (H_2CO_3) shifts toward the basic side, H+ will be conserved or produced by the kidneys and the lungs will retain CO_2 (allowing more carbonic acid to be formed). The lungs respond similarly to changes in nonvolatile acid levels, which compensates for it. This response takes a little longer. When the body is adequately compensating for changes in pH, the pH of the blood will be normal but there will be variations in the levels of HCO_3 or $PaCO_2$ and other blood chemistry values. This compensation may also be reflected in changes in respiratory rate and depth and pH of the urine. The elderly respond less quickly to changes in pH.

Proteins carry negative charges and are buffers for H+. Hemoglobin is an excellent intracellular buffer because it binds readily with H+ and CO_2. In addition, the kidney regulates amounts of phosphate and ammonia in response to changes in the pH of the blood, which allows H+ to be excreted in the urine. These systems work in conjunction with the hydrogen ion and bicarbonate renal mechanisms previously described to effect a normal pH and maintain homeostasis. Shifts in ions (e.g., K+ and H+) in acidosis or alkalosis also assist in buffering. In acidosis, H+ cannot be excreted without another cation being retained. Since potassium (K) is the ion retained, hyperkalemia develops in acidosis. Additionally, when excess H+ moves into the cell, K leaves, which further contributes to hyperkalemia. The reverse happens with alkalosis, resulting in hypokalemia. Calcium is also affected by serum pH. More calcium is bound with serum proteins in an alkalotic state; therefore, hypocalcemia accompanies alkalosis and hypercalcemia accompanies acidosis.

Acid-Base Imbalances

Imbalances can be manifested as either acidosis or alkalosis and may be of respiratory, metabolic, or mixed origin. Acidosis is the result of either a loss of base or excess acid; alkalosis is the result of either excess base or loss of acid. Imbalances of respiratory origin will be compensated for by the kidneys; imbalances of metabolic origin will be compensated for by the lungs and/or the kidneys (if they are not the cause of the problem).

In *metabolic acidosis* either noncarbonic acids increase or bicarbonates decrease. The body compensates by increasing the respiratory rate, thereby blowing off CO_2 and lowering the amount of carbonic acid. In addition, the kidneys excrete H+ by binding it with ammonia or phosphate. If acidosis is severe, the buffers may not be able to compensate effectively. Severe acidosis can decrease ventricular contraction and is life threatening. Uncompensated metabolic acidosis exists with a pH <7.35 and a HCO_3 <23 mEq/L.

Metabolic alkalosis is usually the result of excess loss of acid (e.g., vomiting, gastric suctioning) or ingestion of excessive bicarbonate. When the acid loss is accompanied by loss of fluids and electrolytes, renal compensatory mechanisms are not effective because the kidneys are also trying to compensate for the lost fluids and electrolytes. These two mechanisms work at cross-purposes, the end result of which is excretion of H+ (to balance the loss of K+), reabsorption of HCO_3 (to balance the loss of chloride), and a worsening of the alkalosis. Correction can be achieved if extracellular volume is expanded with intravenous (IV) sodium chloride (NaCl) and K, thereby allowing the kidney to use its buffers to correct the alkalosis. Metabolic alkalosis also inhibits the respiratory center and decreases the rate and depth of respirations, causing CO_2 retention and consequent formation of carbonic acid. Clinical manifestations will vary depending on the cause. Metabolic alkalosis exists when the pH is >7.45 and the HCO_3 is >26 mEq/L. If compensated, the $PaCO_2$ may be >40 mmHg and the K and chloride (Cl) may be below normal.

Respiratory acidosis occurs when ventilation is depressed, causing CO_2 retention and consequent increases in carbonic acid, resulting in acidosis. If it is acute, renal compensatory mechanisms are inadequate because they take time to work. Hemoglobin buffers help and, depending on the cause, there may be an (initial) increase in respiratory rate. Lab values in acute uncompensated respiratory acidosis will show slightly lowered pH, increased $PaCO_2$, and normal or slightly increased HCO_3 (due to delayed renal response). Chronic respiratory acidosis is adequately compensated for by the kidneys and the lab values will indicate normal pH, elevated $PaCO_2$, and elevated HCO_3. Clinical manifestations will depend on acuity of onset and severity. The respiratory center gradually adapts to prolonged elevations of CO_2 so the respiratory rate, although initially increased, may be normal or depressed. Cyanosis will not occur unless there is also hypoxemia.

Respiratory alkalosis occurs with alveolar hyperventilation and excessive loss of CO_2. Common causes include high altitude, hysteria, early salicylate poisoning, hypermetabolic states, congestive heart failure, and others. Improper use of ventilators can cause iatrogenic respiratory alkalosis. Cellular buffers provide immediate response although these are not very effective. Renal buffers, however, are effective. Lab values show a pH >7.45, a $PaCO_2$ of <38 mmHg, and a normal HCO_3; if compensated, the pH is normal and the HCO_3 decreased.

Management

The goal of management in all four conditions is to return the pH to normal as rapidly and as safely as possible and to treat the underlying cause so recurrences are prevented. Each condition has additional treatment options. Severe metabolic acidosis may be treated with $NaHCO_3$ administration. Metabolic alkalosis will be treated with IV administration of sodium, chloride, and potassium to replace volume and electrolytes. Respiratory acidosis is treated by trying to restore normal ventilation; mechanical ventilation may be required. Oxygen must be administered with care so as not to further depress the respiratory center. Treatment in respiratory alkalosis varies depending on the cause. With hysteria, breathing into and exhaling from a paper bag helps to restore CO_2 levels.

1. Which of the following groups is most at risk for fluid volume deficits?

(A) School-aged children

(B) Infants

(C) Middle-aged women

(D) Athletes

2. Which of the following is the best example of third spacing?

(A) Edema following a sprain

(B) Rales

(C) Pedal edema

(D) Ascites

3. Which of the following conditions will increase fluid needs?

(A) Anorexia

(B) Hypertension

(C) Renal failure

(D) Fever

4. Which of the following is most likely to result in edema?

(A) Low albumin levels

(B) Low hemoglobin levels

(C) Decreased blood volume

(D) Decreased hydrostatic pressure

5. What is a common consequence of hypokalemia?

(A) Tetany

(B) Ileus

(C) Thirst

(D) Paresthesias

6. You just received the lab reports on your patients and you notice that Mrs. T. has a K level of 5.2. What would you do?

(A) Nothing; it's within the normal range.

(B) Suggest use of a K supplement to her doctor.

(C) It's at the bottom of the normal range; suggest dietary modifications.

(D) It's elevated; report it to her doctor.

7. Which of the following is the major intracellular ion?

(A) Na

(B) K

(C) Cl

(D) HCO_3

8. What is a common sign of hyponatremia?

(A) Confusion

(B) Diarrhea

(C) Muscle spasms

(D) Insomnia

9. What often accompanies acidosis?

(A) Hypokalemia

(B) Hyperkalemia

(C) Hypocalcemia

(D) Hypercalcemia

10. Someone with emphysema is at risk for what?

(A) Respiratory acidosis

(B) Respiratory alkalosis

(C) Metabolic acidosis

(D) Metabolic alkalosis

11. What is the kidneys' role in maintaining acid-base balance?

(A) Excrete or conserve bicarbonate

(B) Regulate carbon dioxide levels

(C) Influence respiratory rate

(D) Increase or decrease renal output

12. Someone with vomiting is at risk for what?

(A) Respiratory acidosis

(B) Respiratory alkalosis

(C) Metabolic acidosis

(D) Metabolic alkalosis

PART I ANSWERS

1. The correct answer is B.

The greater the proportion of body water, the greater the risk. Choices A, C, and D are at no particular risk. Athletes may be more so if doing strenuous exercise in high temperature environments and if not replacing their fluids periodically.

2. The correct answer is D.

When large amounts of fluid become sequestered in a body compartment and therefore are unavailable for body processes, it is referred to as third spacing. Choices A, B, and C are not examples of third spacing, which ordinarily refers to large fluid shifts.

3. The correct answer is D.

Fever increases metabolism and, therefore, increases fluid needs.. Choices A, B, and C do not increase fluid needs.

4. The correct answer is A.

An important function of albumin is to maintain osmotic pressure. Choices B, C, and D do not cause edema.

5. The correct answer is B.

Ileus results from the decreased peristalsis that is a consequence of reduced neuromuscular function and is one of the earlier clinical signs of hypokalemia. Tetany results from hypocalcemia, thirst is associated with hypernatremia, and paresthesias sometimes occur with respiratory alkalosis.

6. The correct answer is D.

It is important to report even small variations in potassium outside the normals for your institution due to the importance of this electrolyte in cardiac function. The other choices are incorrect because although normals vary from lab to lab, the commonly accepted normal range is from 3.5 to 5.

7. The correct answer is B.

Potassium is the major intracellular ion. Sodium is the major extracellular ion. Although important, neither choice C or D is considered to be a major ion.

8. The correct answer is A.

Confusion often occurs early and is especially important to watch for in the elderly. The other choices are incorrect because diarrhea occurs with hyperkalemia, muscle spasms occur with hypocalcemia, and insomnia is not relevant.

9. The correct answer is B.

In acidosis, as hydrogen enters the cell, it causes potassium to leave, resulting in hyperkalemia. The other choices are incorrect because hypokalemia results in muscle weakness, atony, and EKG changes; hypocalcemia causes tetany, and hypercalcemia causes muscle weakness and renal stones.

10. The correct answer is A.

Decreased ventilation causes CO_2 retention, resulting in an increase in carbonic acid and respiratory acidosis. The other choices are incorrect because respiratory alkalosis occurs with increased exhalation of CO_2 and metabolic acidosis and metabolic alkalosis both have metabolic etiologies.

11. The correct answer is A.

Bicarbonate-carbonic acid is the major buffer system. The other choices are incorrect because the lungs regulate carbon dioxide levels, the central nervous system influences respiratory rate, and an increase or decrease in renal output is a function of the glomerular filtration rate and overall kidney function.

12. The correct answer is D.

Metabolic alkalosis occurs because there is loss of gastric acid. The other choices are incorrect because respiratory acidosis is due to CO_2 retention, respiratory alkalosis is due to loss of CO_2 and metabolic acidosis is due to excess acid or loss of base.

PART II

Immune Disorders

Bernadette R. Madara, EdD, ARPN-CS

Immune Response

5

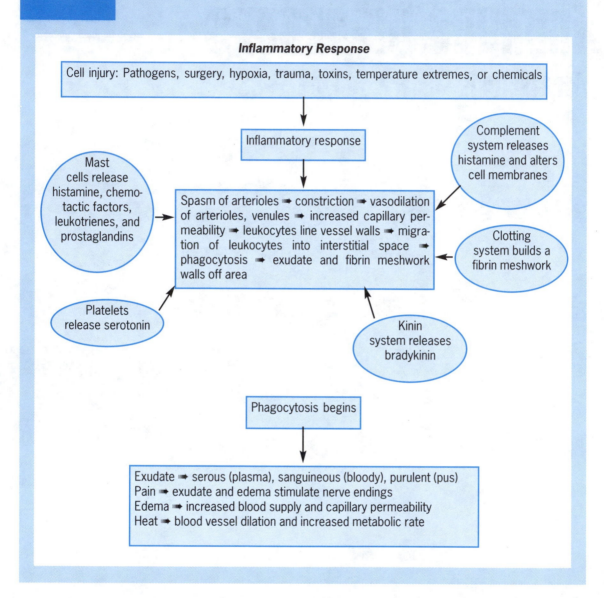

Inflammatory Response

Cell injury: Pathogens, surgery, hypoxia, trauma, toxins, temperature extremes, or chemicals

Inflammatory response

Complement system releases histamine and alters cell membranes

Mast cells release histamine, chemotactic factors, leukotrienes, and prostaglandins

Spasm of arterioles ➡ constriction ➡ vasodilation of arterioles, venules ➡ increased capillary permeability ➡ leukocytes line vessel walls ➡ migration of leukocytes into interstitial space ➡ phagocytosis ➡ exudate and fibrin meshwork walls off area

Clotting system builds a fibrin meshwork

Platelets release serotonin

Kinin system releases bradykinin

Phagocytosis begins

Exudate ➡ serous (plasma), sanguineous (bloody), purulent (pus)
Pain ➡ exudate and edema stimulate nerve endings
Edema ➡ increased blood supply and capillary permeability
Heat ➡ blood vessel dilation and increased metabolic rate

Overview of Inflammation

Immune system functions include protecting the body against invasion by foreign substances including microorganisms such as bacteria, maintaining homeostasis by removing damaged cells, and destroying tumor cells. Inflammation is not synonymous with infection, although the two terms are often erroneously used interchangeably. Colonization (i.e., the presence of microorganisms without cellular injury) alone does not produce inflammation—cell injury initiates the inflammatory process.

Any cellular injury will produce a nonspecific inflammatory response that is generally local but can also be systemic. Infection is only one activity that causes cell injury and inflammation. Other ways a cell can be injured include surgery, hypoxia, trauma, exposure to

18

toxins, or temperature extremes. Regardless of the mechanism of injury, the result is the same—inflammation. When the immune system is overactive, damage to the body from the inflammatory response can occur such as in autoimmune diseases and hypersensitivity reactions or allergies. By contrast, a weak immune system will lead to opportunistic infections, and possibly sepsis and malignant disease.

Inflammatory Response

The inflammatory response, indicated by the suffix "itis," begins immediately after cell injury when arterioles in the region briefly go into spasm and constrict in order to limit bleeding and the extent of the injury. This vasoconstriction is immediately followed by arteriolar and venular vasodilation, which brings increased blood flow to the injured area in an attempt to dilute toxins and provide the area with neutrophils, monocytes, nutrients, and oxygen. As capillary permeability increases, leukocytes line the vessel walls in preparation for emigration into the surrounding tissue. At the same time leukocytes are lining the vessel walls, endothelial cells lining the capillaries and venules react to biochemical mediators that cause these tiny vessels to retract. This retraction makes space for the leukocytes to emigrate, a process by which leukocytes migrate into the interstitial space in order to begin the process of phagocytosis or the engulfing and digesting of bacteria in order to clean up cellular debris. Also during this time, fibrinogen transforms into fibrin, which is used to wall off the injured area so that bacteria/toxins are contained, a meshwork for new cells to use in the healing process is formed, and blood clotting begins if blood vessels have been damaged.

Mast Cells and Chemical Mediators

The cells mainly responsible for the inflammatory response are called *mast cells*. In response to cell injury caused by mechanical factors such as surgery, chemical irritants such as toxins, or IgE hypersensitivity reactions, mast cells activate the inflammatory response by immediately releasing their granular content into the injured area along with chemical mediators including histamine, neutrophil chemotactic factor, and eosinophil chemotactic factor of anaphylaxis. As part of this initial response, platelets release serotonin. Temporary blood vessel dilation and increased permeability are caused by histamine and serotonin, while neutrophils and eosinophils, which are phagocytes, are attracted to the area by the release of neutrophil and eosinophil chemotactic factors.

Other chemical mediators synthesized by mast cells are leukotrienes (slow-reacting substances of anaphylaxis) and prostaglandins. Leukotrienes are acidic, sulfur-containing lipids released from the mast cell membrane that produce a slower and more prolonged inflammatory response by creating reactions that mirror the action of histamine.

Prostaglandins have many functions. They can either cause actions similar to histamine, inhibit the inflammatory response, produce fever and pain, or promote platelet aggregation. The enzyme cyclooxygenase is necessary for the production of prostaglandins. If this enzyme is blocked, as occurs with nonsteroidal anti-inflammatory drugs (NSAIDs) and aspirin (ASA) use, the inflammatory response is blunted.

Plasma Protein System

The complement system, the clotting system, and the kinin system are also important mediators of the inflammatory response. Each system contains proenzymes that produce a cascade of events when activated, much like a row of dominoes falling after the first domino is pushed. Plasma enzymes rapidly inactivate many of the mediators of the inflammatory response in order to prevent wide-spread, uncontrolled tissue damage.

The complement system is made up of about 20 different plasma proteins that remain inactive until stimulated by cell injury, by-products from invading bacteria, or an antigen-antibody reaction. Once activated, these proteins aid in the inflammatory process by causing the release of histamine from mast cells and basophils, altering cell membranes so lysis can occur and coating the surface of cells so that phagocytosis can occur.

The clotting system (cascade), through a chain reaction, is responsible for building a fibrin meshwork that traps exudates, microorganisms, and foreign material at the site of cellular injury. The clotting cascade can be activated by the intrinsic pathway, which reacts to vascular injury, or the extrinsic pathway, which reacts to chemical mediators released from damaged endothelial cells. Regardless of the mechanism of activation, the end result is a fibrin clot. The infection is contained, phagocytosis is more easily accomplished, and bleeding is controlled because of this fibrin meshwork.

Bradykinin, which is part of the final plasma protein system—the kinin system—is responsible for many actions that are similar to the actions produced by histamine and prostaglandin. Some of these actions include increasing vascular permeability and induction of pain.

Acute Inflammatory Response

Acute inflammation produces fever, leukocytosis, and an increase in plasma proteins. Interleukin I, a substance produced by neutrophils and macrophages that acts on the hypothalamus, is primarily responsible for fever production. Fever has both beneficial and harmful effects. While a fever can create an environment that kills some microorganisms, it can also make the host more sensitive to endotoxins produced by some bacteria. The process by which the number of circulating white blood cells is increased is called *leukocytosis*.

Chronic Inflammatory Response

If the inflammatory response lasts weeks or longer, it is termed *chronic*. Chronic inflammation can occur because the acute inflammatory process was unsuccessful at repairing cellular damage, chemical irritants persisted, or the invading microorganism was difficult to kill. The inflammatory response will continue as long as the invading bacteria are present.

Granuloma formation is a classic sign of chronic inflammation. A granuloma is formed when giant cells (fused macrophages) engulf large foreign particles. The granuloma is encased by a collagen network and may eventually calcify. Inside the granuloma the debris decays and forms a liquid that eventually diffuses out of the granuloma, leaving just the thick-walled casing.

Signs and Symptoms of the Inflammatory Response

Regardless of the cause, the signs and symptoms of the inflammatory response are similar: an exudate is formed; pain, heat, and swelling are present; and it is hoped that healing will begin. The exudate is comprised of plasma, blood cells, and products of phagocytosis. The exudate dilutes toxins produced by dying cells and bacteria, transports plasma (proteins and white blood cells [WBCs]) to the injured area, and carries away cellular debris.

Serous exudate is a watery fluid made of plasma. If the inflammation continues, then the exudate becomes thick and clotted and is called *fibrinous exudate*. Bacterial infections commonly lead to *purulent* (suppurative) *exudate*, which is composed of leukocytes, pus, and dead cells. The accumulation of exudate causes swelling and pain as nerve fibers are stimulated by chemical mediators such as prostaglandins and bradykinin. Warmth of the inflamed area is caused by an increased blood supply to the area.

6 Infectious Microorganisms

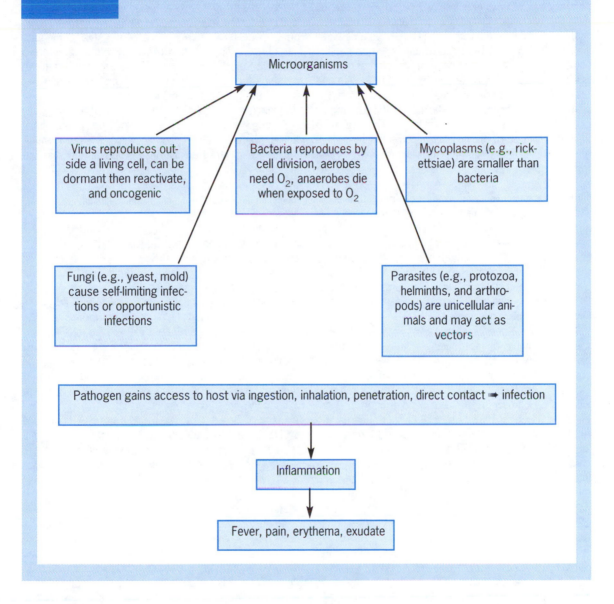

Overview

Many microorganisms live on the internal and external exposed surfaces of the human body without causing harm. When the normal balance of microorganisms is disrupted or the body is subjected to noncolonized virulent microorganisms that cause injury or pathologic changes, an infection results. Viruses, bacteria, mycoplasms, fungi, parasites, rickettsiae, and chlamydiae are some of the common organisms associated with the infectious process.

Pathology

Viruses are the smallest pathogens, can reproduce outside of a living cell, and are composed of a protein coat that surrounds a nucleic acid core of either ribonucleic acid (RNA) or deoxyribonucleic acid (DNA).

Some viruses (e.g., herpes virus) are continually shed from the infected cell's surface, while others cause the host cell's death during replication. A virus may remain dormant after host cell invasion only to replicate and produce symptoms of the disease months or years after the initial infection. Some retroviruses that belong to the oncogenic group are capable of transforming normal cells into malignant cells during their replication process.

Bacteria contain both RNA and DNA, have a rigid cell wall, and reproduce by cell division. Spore production allows survival in a latent state until growing conditions are favorable. Aerobes require oxygen for growth and metabolism, while anaerobes die when exposed to oxygen. The shape of the cell wall identifies the bacteria as coccus (i.e., spherical), spirillum (i.e., helical), or bacillus (i.e., elongated). Some bacteria have flagella, which are whip-like appendages that allow them to move through blood and lymph fluid. Gram-positive bacteria acquire a purple stain when exposed to a basic dye, while gram-negative bacteria do not accept the stain.

A special class of bacteria called *spirochetes* is an anaerobic, gram-negative rod capable of movement by filaments that cover the entire cell wall. Spirochetes can cause human infection through contact with infected animals or contaminated surroundings (leptospira/Weil's syndrome), through the bite of an arthropod vector (Borrelia/Lyme disease), or person-to-person contact (*Treponema pallidum*/syphilis).

Mycoplasms, one third smaller in size than bacteria, are also capable of reproducing independently. Unlike bacteria they do not have a rigid cell wall. Some are capable of causing pneumonia. Typhus and Rocky Mountain spotted fever are caused by rickettsiae, which are microorganisms that depend upon the host cell for nutrients, multiply by cell division, and have a rigid cell wall. Human infection is caused through the bite of an infected arthropod.

Most fungi, which include yeast and molds, cause infections that are self-limiting and involve the skin and subcutaneous membranes, but they can also cause opportunistic infections. Some of the illnesses associated with fungi are athlete's foot and candida infections.

Parasites include protozoa, helminths, and arthropods. Protozoa are minute unicellular animals responsible for diseases such as malaria and amebic dysentery. Transmission of protozoa may be from human to human, by arthropod vector, or through contaminated water or food. Helminths are worm-like parasites that are transmitted through the ingestion of fertilized eggs or larva penetration of the skin. The infection can involve many organ systems. Helminth infections are most common in developing countries.

Parasitic arthropod vectors include ticks, mosquitoes, and biting flies, as well as localized tissue inflammation from burrowing ectoparasites such as mites, lice, and chiggers. Ectoparasites are transmitted as immature or mature arthropods or eggs through contact with infected clothing, bedding, or grooming articles such as hair brushes.

Pathology of Infection

The *chain of infection* includes virulence of the pathogen, transmission to the host, and entry into the host. Once these conditions are met, the pathogens can cause an infection. *Virulence of a pathogen* refers to its disease-causing potential. Transmission from the reservoir (i.e., where the pathogen lives) to the host can occur through direct or indirect contact, airborne droplets (tuberculosis [TB]), or a vector (Lyme disease).

Pathogens gain access to the body through inhalation, ingestion, direct contact, and penetration. A healthy respiratory tract contains functional cilia that sweep invading microorganisms and dust away from the lungs, while coughing removes invaders from the lower respiratory tract. Enzymes, naturally occurring antibiotics in respiratory secretions, and alveolar macrophages mitigate most respiratory tract pathogens. Influenza, pneumonia, and the common cold result when these natural defenses are rendered ineffective by smoking, respiratory diseases, or an ineffective immune system.

Ingestion of contaminated food or water is responsible for introducing a wide variety of pathogens into the body, including those responsible for hepatitis A, food poisoning, and cholera. Normally, low gastric pH, enzymes, peristalsis, and intestinal flora protect the body from ingested pathogens. Medications that reduce gastric acid increase the chance of an infection caused by ingested pathogens.

Some pathogens can live for hours or weeks on hard surfaces such as bedrails and tables and are transmitted easily. Direct contact is also responsible for sexually transmitted diseases and for infections passed from mother to child during childbirth, which may cause severe congenital defects involving the neurological system in newborns.

Any break in the skin or mucosal surface leaves the body open to infection. These breaks may result from dry, chapped skin; scratches; burns; bites; intravenous (IV) drug use; surgery; trauma; or medical procedures. Antibiotic therapy may result in the development of a superimposed infection as the balance of the body's normal flora is disrupted. For example, a fungal infection is likely to develop if a patient is taking three antibiotics.

Signs and Symptoms of Infection

The clinical signs and symptoms of an infection can be specific to the site, such as nausea, vomiting, and diarrhea for a gastrointestinal (GI) infection, or reflective of the general inflammatory process, such as fever, malaise, and myalgia. The signs and symptoms presented provide a picture of the struggle between the pathogen and immune system.

Fever, pain, erythema (i.e., redness), swelling, and exudate formation are classic signs of an infection in otherwise healthy adults. Infection in the elderly and immunocompromised patients may be represented by a normal or low-grade temperature, malaise, changes in mental status, weakness, fatigue, and weight loss.

Fever is generally considered harmless, and in fact may be beneficial, producing enhanced movement of macrophages, stimulation of interferon production, T cell activation, and destruction of some pathogens, if the body temperature does not rise above 104 °F in otherwise healthy adults. Rectal temperatures above 100.4 °F generally indicate serious illness in children 1 to 36 months and elevations of 2 °F above baseline (around 97.6 °F) in the elderly require immediate medical attention as does a mild fever in immunocompromised patients, such as those on oral prednisone or with bone marrow suppression.

The four stages of a fever are a prodromal period, a chill, a flush, and finally defervescence. The patient may complain of headache, fatigue, malaise, and aches and pains during the prodromal stage. These vague symptoms are followed by vasoconstriction, which results in pallor and a feeling of being cold. The chill stage produces shaking, which increases the metabolic rate and body temperature. The third stage produces cutaneous vasodilation, resulting in a feeling of warmth and flushing. The final stage, defervescence, produces diaphoresis. During a fever, the patient's respiratory and heart rates also increase and dehydration may develop because of diaphoresis and tachypnea. Delirium and confusion may result during a fever, especially in the elderly, because of a reduced supply of oxygen to the brain.

An explanation of the inflammatory process is presented in Chapter 5.

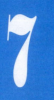

Leukocytes

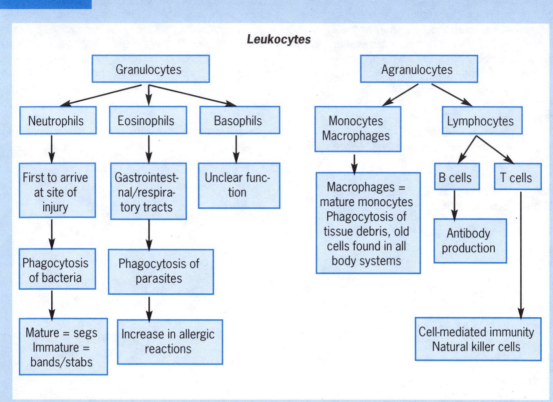

Leukocytes

Granulocytes
- Neutrophils
  - First to arrive at site of injury
  - Phagocytosis of bacteria
  - Mature = segs Immature = bands/stabs
- Eosinophils
  - Gastrointestnal/respiratory tracts
  - Phagocytosis of parasites
  - Increase in allergic reactions
- Basophils
  - Unclear function

Agranulocytes
- Monocytes Macrophages
  - Macrophages = mature monocytes Phagocytosis of tissue debris, old cells found in all body systems
- Lymphocytes
  - B cells
    - Antibody production
  - T cells
    - Cell-mediated immunity Natural killer cells

Overview

Leukocytes (i.e., white blood cells [WBCs]) have specific functions concerned with the inflammatory process, namely to defend the body against infection and to clean up the by-products of inflammation and infection. They travel via the circulatory system to the site of inflammation or infection by responding to chemical signals released by damaged cells. The total leukocyte count in a healthy adult is between 5,000 and 10,000/mm³ of blood. Leukocytes are divided into phagocytic granulocytes (i.e., neutrophils, eosinophils, and basophils) and agranulocytes (i.e., phagocytic monocytes, phagocytic macrophages, and immunocytic lymphocytes). Colony-stimulating factors produced by endothelial cells, fibroblasts, and lymphocytes are responsible for the production, maturation, and function of leukocytes.

All leukocytes come from stem cells in the bone marrow. Granulocytes are released from the bone mar-row as mature cells, while agranulocytes are released as immature cells. Leukocyte production is increased in response to biological triggers such as infection, strenuous exercise, fever, stress, and tachycardia, as well as psychological triggers such as pain and anxiety.

Pathophysiology

Granulocytes are leukocytes that contain cytoplasmic granules, which contain enzymes and multilobar nuclei. The enzymes in granulocytes have several functions, including killing invading microorganisms, cleaning up the resulting debris, and releasing chemical mediators involved in the inflammatory process. The three types of granulocytes are neutrophils, eosinophils, and basophils.

Neutrophils, which are also called *polymorphonuclear leukocytes*, make up approximately 55% of the total WBC count and are the first to arrive at the site of cell injury, generally within 90 minutes. They remain the primary leukocytes at the inflammatory site until the monocytes/macrophages arrive and take over 6 to 12 hours after the initial injury. Neutrophils have a short life span of approximately 48 hours and are charged with the phagocytosis of bacteria and small particles of debris. Hydrogen peroxide and hypochloric acid, which are highly toxic and damaging to cells, are produced during the phagocytic process. Each neutrophil is capable of ingesting up to 20 bacteria before it becomes inactive and dies. As dead neutrophils are phagocytized by monocytes, they release enzymes that help prepare the site for healing. Mature neutrophils are called *segs* while immature neutrophils are called *bands* or *stabs* and are released from the bone marrow when the inflammatory response is activated.

Eosinophils, which make up 1% to 3% of the total WBC count, are found mainly in the gastrointestinal (GI) and respiratory tracts where they protect the body from parasitic infections by secreting toxic enzymes that destroy the invader. Eosinophils live approximately 30 minutes (when circulating) to 12 days (in tissue). Eosinophils also increase in response to an allergic reaction.

Basophils are not phagocytic and account for between 0.3% and 0.5% of the WBC count. Basophils contain substances also found in mast cells, such as bradykinin, serotonin, histamine, as well as heparin and leukotrienes, and are involved in an allergic response or stress although their function is unclear.

Agranulocytes, which are WBCs that do not contain lysosomal granules, include monocytes, macrophages, and lymphocytes. Monocytes and macrophages are called the *mononuclear phagocyte system*, formerly known as the *reticuloendothelial system*. Monocytes, or macrophages that have matured, are the largest WBC and account for 3% to 8% of the WBC count. Their function is one of phagocytosis of tissue debris and large particles such as some parasites, whole red blood cells (RBCs), and dead neutrophils. If the foreign matter cannot be phagocytized, the macrophages simply encapsulate it. Monocytes circulate for approximately 48 hours after being released by the bone marrow, then migrate into tissue where they mature into macrophages and live for months to years. Macrophages in the liver sinusoids are called *Kupffer's cells* and are a main defense against bloodborne pathogens. Macrophages are termed *histiocytes* in connective tissue, *alveolar macrophages* in the lung, and *microglia* in the nervous system. Mesangial cells are *macrophages* in the kidney, *osteoclasts* in the bone, *Langerhans' cells* in the skin, and *dendritic cells* in lymphoid tissue.

Lymphocytes comprise 20% to 30% of the WBC count and include B cells, which are involved with antibody production; T cells, which are involved with cell-mediated immunity; and natural killer cells. Natural killer cells act as surveillance agents. They are cytotoxic cells that do not need prior sensitization to attack foreign cells or cancer cells and are found in the spleen, lymph nodes, bone marrow, and blood. B cells and T cells are discussed in Chapter 8.

Lymphoid Organs

The thymus gland and the bone marrow are called *primary lymphoid organs*, while the spleen, lymph nodes, tonsils, and Peyer's patches in the small intestine are called *secondary lymphoid organs*. Lymphoid tissue in the spleen, which contains macrophages and lymphocytes that filter and clean the blood, is called *splenic pulp*. White splenic pulp initially filters blood entering the spleen and is constructed of masses of lymphoid tissue that form clumps around arterioles in the spleen. Red splenic pulp is the site of residence of macrophages that digest old cells, pathogens, and debris. Red pulp macrophages are responsible for the breakdown of old red blood cells and the liberation/recycling of heme (from hemoglobin). From the red pulp, blood enters the venous sinuses and then the portal circulation.

Lymph Nodes and Fluid

Lymph nodes, which are clustered in the inguinal, axillary, and cervical areas of the body, group around lymphatic veins that collect lymph (i.e., interstitial fluid). Lymphocytes, monocytes, and macrophages develop and function in the lymph nodes. The function of these cells is to clean the lymph of pathogens and foreign matter. During the infectious process, the lymph nodes enlarge and become tender as they increase the production of macrophages.

Phagocytosis

The process of phagocytosis (i.e., ingestion of foreign particles by leukocytes) is initiated by chemical mediators that guide leukocytes to the area of pathogen invasion. The pathogens are first coated with complement or antibody so that they can be identified as foreign. Receptors on leukocytes bind to the coated pathogen, then the leukocyte extends pseudopodia around the pathogen, totally engulfing it. The engulfed pathogen is called a *phagosome*. Intracellular cytoplasmic lysosomes then bind to the phagosome to create a phagolysosome. Once this process is complete, granulocytes release their contents, including oxygen radicals and lysosomal enzymes that digest the invading organism.

8 Antigens, Antibodies, and Immunity

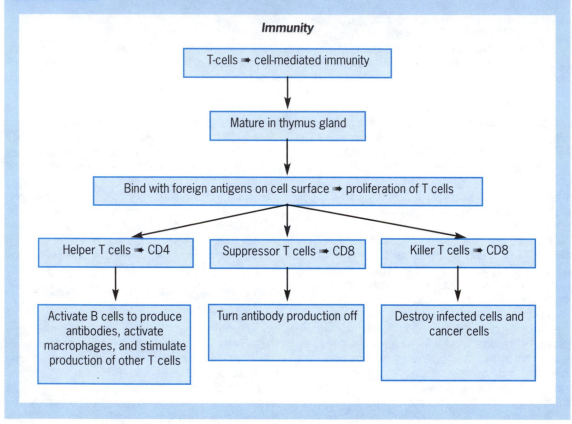

Immunity

T-cells ➡ cell-mediated immunity

⬇

Mature in thymus gland

⬇

Bind with foreign antigens on cell surface ➡ proliferation of T cells

Helper T cells ➡ CD4	Suppressor T cells ➡ CD8	Killer T cells ➡ CD8
Activate B cells to produce antibodies, activate macrophages, and stimulate production of other T cells	Turn antibody production off	Destroy infected cells and cancer cells

Overview

An antigen is any substance recognized as foreign by the immune system and is, therefore, capable of producing an immune response. Antigens may be proteins, polysaccharides, polypeptides, nucleic acids, or substances such as pollen or bee and snake venom. Cells and tissues, including red blood cells, also contain antigens that the body recognizes as "self" or "nonself." The major histocompatibility complex (MHC) is a large cluster of genes located on chromosome 6 and the process by which the body codes its own antigens. Human leukocyte antigens (HLA) are part of our individual genetic makeup and the closer the HLA types are matched, the less chance of organ or tissue transplant rejection. If the immune system mistakes its own antigens as foreign, an autoimmune response results.

Pathophysiology

T cells and B cells are produced in the bone marrow and thymus gland. These cells interact with antigens as they circulate between body fluid and peripheral lymphoid tissue (e.g., tonsils, lymph nodes, spleen, intestinal lymphoid tissue) to either destroy the invading substance (T cell function) or produce antibodies (B cell function).

T Cell Function

There are two major types of T cells: regulator cells, including helper T cells and suppressor T cells, and effector cells or killer T cells. The function of helper T cells is to activate B cells to produce antibodies, while the suppressor T cells turn the antibody production off. Cytotoxic T cells are capable of destroying cells infected with viruses by releasing lymphokines that destroy cell walls.

T cells mature in the thymus gland and are the largest group of lymphocytes, making up approximately 60% to 70% of the total lymphocyte count. Cell-mediated immunity is the responsibility of the T cells and macrophages and is concerned with protecting the body against viruses and cancer cells. These cells are also responsible for delayed hypersensitivity and transplant rejections.

T cells are activated when they bind with foreign antigens on the surface of a cell. These cell-surface antigens may occur naturally (e.g., when a virus invades a host cell or on transplant tissue). Cell-surface antigens may also occur when a foreign substance enters the body, is engulfed by macrophages that then move the antigen fragments to the macrophage's receptor sites, and then presents the antigen to the T cell. Once activated by a specific antigen, the T cell divides and multiplies to form killer T cells and helper T cells. Killer T cells destroy foreign antigen cells. Some killer T cells become memory killer T cells. These memory killer T cells "remember" a specific antigen so that upon subsequent exposure, activation of cell-mediated immunity is rapid.

Helper T cells have several functions including stimulating the production of other T cells, activating macrophages, helping killer T cells, and activating B cells to produce antibodies against the offending antigen. Suppressor T cells turn off the immune response by stopping the activity of B cells and T cells.

Proteins on the surface of the T cells called *the cluster of differentiation antigen* or *CD antigen* enable the cells to be identified. Killer T cells and suppressor T cells both have the CD8 marker (CD8 cells), while helper T cells have the CD4 marker (CD4 cells).

B Cell Function

Humoral immunity (antibody-mediated immunity) is controlled by B lymphocytes, which eliminate bacteria, neutralize toxins produced by bacteria, prevent viral reinfection, and produce an immediate allergic response. B cells, which mature in the bone marrow, differentiate into memory cells or immunoglobulin-secreting (antibody) cells. Each B cell has receptor sites for a specific antigen or antigens and when it encounters the antigen(s) the B cell activates and multiplies into either an antibody-producing cell or a memory cell. Although antibody-producing B cells live only 24 hours, they produce millions of antibody molecules before they die.

When an antigen is first introduced into the body it takes between 48 and 72 hours for the antigen to be recognized as foreign and antibody production by B cells to begin. Subsequent exposures to the antigen produce a quick response because B memory cells "remember" the antigen as foreign and antibody production is rapid. This response is termed *humoral immunity*.

When the body makes its own antibodies, the person is said to have *acquired active immunity*. Active immunity generally provides long, in some cases life-long, immunity. Antibody production may be the result of exposure to a specific bacteria or virus or the result of immunization with a small amount of killed or weakened (attenuated) organism or toxin. Examples of active immunity acquired by vaccine include hepatitis B, poliomyelitis, and *Haemophilus influenza*.

Passive immunity is obtained when a person receives antibodies made outside the body by another person, animal, or recombinant deoxyribonucleic acid (DNA). Examples of passive immunity include the transfer of antibodies from mother to fetus across the placenta or through breastfeeding and gamma globulin vaccinations. Passive immunity is short-lived but effective in preventing illness after exposure to snake or rat toxins and diseases such as hepatitis A and varicella.

Antibody Classifications

There are five classes of immunoglobulins (antibodies): IgG, IgA, IgM, IgE, and IgD. IgG, gamma globulin, is the most common of the immunoglobulins and the only one to cross the placenta. It prevents systemic infections from bacteria, viruses, and damage from toxins and is used to provide passive immunity. IgA is found in saliva; tears; and gastrointestinal (GI), bronchial, prostatic, and vaginal secretions and is responsible for protecting these areas against local viral and bacterial infections. IgM activates complement and is the first antibody formed when B cells initially encounter an antigen. IgE binds to mast cells and causes the release of histamine and other mediators of an allergic reaction including anaphylaxis. The role of IgD is unclear, but it may be responsible for binding the antigen to the surface of the B cell, allowing for B cell activation.

Hypersensitivity Reaction

Hypersensitivity reaction is an excessive immune response. This reaction may be immediate (within 30 minutes of exposure) or delayed, taking several days to develop. Hypersensitivity reactions occur because of activation of IgE and the release of inflammatory chemicals, including histamine and prostaglandins by mast cells and basophils. IgE-secreting B cells are numerous in the skin, lungs, and GI tract. Activation of these B cells accounts for the signs and symptoms of allergic reactions, which include edema, increased mucous production, coughing, wheezing, laryngeal edema, vomiting, hives, redness, itching of the skin, and vascular collapse and shock in severe reactions.

Anaphylaxis is a severe, life-threatening systemic response to an antigen. Anaphylactoid reactions, which produce anaphylaxis-like reactions, do not involve IgE antibodies. The exact cause of these reactions is

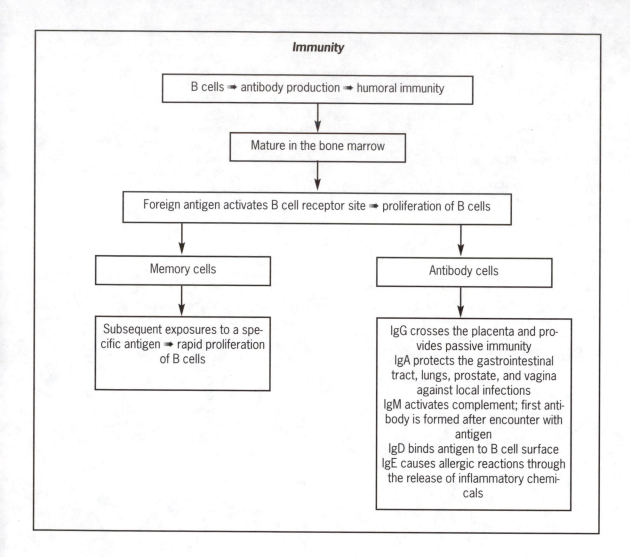

Immunity

B cells ➡ antibody production ➡ humoral immunity

↓

Mature in the bone marrow

↓

Foreign antigen activates B cell receptor site ➡ proliferation of B cells

↓ ↓

Memory cells   Antibody cells

↓ ↓

Subsequent exposures to a specific antigen ➡ rapid proliferation of B cells

IgG crosses the placenta and provides passive immunity
IgA protects the gastrointestinal tract, lungs, prostate, and vagina against local infections
IgM activates complement; first antibody is formed after encounter with antigen
IgD binds antigen to B cell surface
IgE causes allergic reactions through the release of inflammatory chemicals

unknown. Substances that can produce an anaphylactoid reaction include diagnostic radiographs (contrast medium) used for some x-rays, drugs, and foods.

Delayed hypersensitivity is a local T cell mediated response to an offending allergen that occurs within 3 days of exposure and may involve a skin irritant such as poison ivy, lotions, tape, jewelry, or clothing. Memory T cells account for the increased severity of reactions on subsequent exposure. Purified protein derivative (PPD) testing relies on a delayed hypersensitivity reaction.

Lyme Disease and Systemic Lupus Erythematosus

9

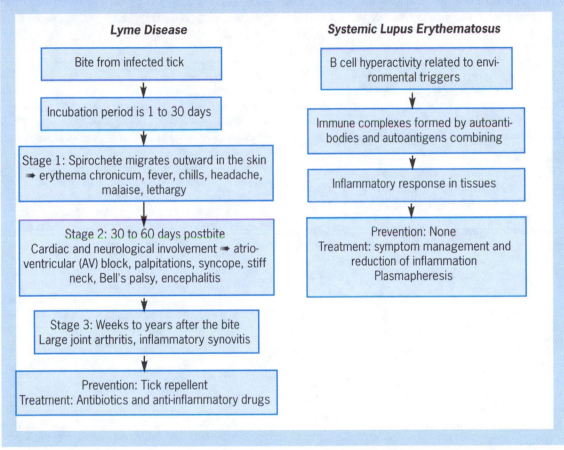

Lyme Disease

Bite from infected tick

↓

Incubation period is 1 to 30 days

↓

Stage 1: Spirochete migrates outward in the skin ➡ erythema chronicum, fever, chills, headache, malaise, lethargy

↓

Stage 2: 30 to 60 days postbite
Cardiac and neurological involvement ➡ atrioventricular (AV) block, palpitations, syncope, stiff neck, Bell's palsy, encephalitis

↓

Stage 3: Weeks to years after the bite
Large joint arthritis, inflammatory synovitis

↓

Prevention: Tick repellent
Treatment: Antibiotics and anti-inflammatory drugs

Systemic Lupus Erythematosus

B cell hyperactivity related to environmental triggers

↓

Immune complexes formed by autoantibodies and autoantigens combining

↓

Inflammatory response in tissues

↓

Prevention: None
Treatment: symptom management and reduction of inflammation
Plasmapheresis

Lyme Disease

Overview

Lyme disease was first identified in 1975 in Lyme, Connecticut. Some deer and small mammals such as mice carry Ixodidae ticks, which act as a reservoir for the spirochete *Borrelia burgdorferi* and cause Lyme disease in humans. Lyme disease is the most common tickborne illness in the United States. If bitten by an infected tick that remains attached to the skin for at least 24 hours, the spirochete is transmitted and produces endotoxins that cause an inflammatory process involving the skin, musculoskeletal system, and central nervous system. This spirochete may remain localized at the site of the tick bite or may invade any tissue, accounting for the variety and severity of symptoms presented.

Pathophysiology

There are three stages of infection with Lyme disease. After an incubation period of 1 to 30 days, stage one occurs when the spirochete migrates outward in the skin, resulting in the appearance of erythema chronicum migrans, the characteristic "bull's eye" rash some infected people develop. This expanding rash has a clear center at the site of the bite surrounded by a red ring and may reach a diameter of 50 cm. During this stage, the spirochete may also spread to other sites by way of the lymph or blood. Other symptoms of the initial infection include fever and chills, headache, malaise, and lethargy. If the infection is undetected or untreated, the disease becomes chronic and cardiac and neurological involvement occurs 2 to 3 months after the bite as part of the second stage of the disease. Symptoms of this stage of the infection include severe AV block, palpitations, syncope, stiff neck, photophobia, Bell's palsy, fatigue, encephalitis, and radiculoneuritis (i.e., inflammation of spinal nerves producing pain and increased sensation) that can last 6 months or longer. If untreated, approximately 70% of people infected with Lyme disease develop arthritis primarily of large joints as part of the third stage of the disease within weeks to years after the initial infection. Arthritis associated with Lyme disease may be in the form of arthralgia or, in 10% of people, a chronic, inflammatory synovitis. The third stage of the disease is thought to be the result of treatment failure, relapses caused by persistent infection, or possibly an autoimmune reaction to the spirochete.

Cultures of the organism from tissue and blood confirm the diagnosis. The enzyme-linked immunosorbent assay (ELISA) can detect antibodies within 2 to 4 weeks after the appearance of the rash. The presence of the characteristic rash is also used to make the diagnosis.

Management

Prevention of Lyme disease involves avoiding tick-infested areas, using tick repellent, covering exposed skin, and checking for and removing ticks as soon as possible. Deer ticks are very small and hard to detect.

Treatment includes the use of antibiotics such as tetracycline, doxycycline, amoxicillin, cefuroxime, and erythromycin for 2 weeks for a stage one infection to 3 to 4 weeks for stages two and three infection. Anti-inflammatory drugs may also be used.

Systemic Lupus Erythematosus

Overview

Systemic lupus erythematosus (SLE) is a chronic, multisystem, inflammatory disease of unknown cause affecting approximately 500,000 people in the United States. This is a disease that mainly affects young adult women with more African Americans, Hispanics, and Asians affected more than Caucasians.

Pathophysiology

The pathology of SLE includes hyperactivity of B cells, which is thought to be triggered by environmental (e.g., hair dyes, hydralazine), hormonal (e.g., estrogen), genetic (e.g., familial tendency), and/or viral factors. In response to triggers, B cells produce a multitude of autoantibodies and autoantigens. These autoantibodies and autoantigens combine to form immune complexes against the body's own tissues such as nucleic acids, red blood cells (RBCs), platelets, coagulation proteins, and lymphocytes. It is postulated that hyperactivity of helper T cells and a diminished response of suppressor T cell function set the stage for the B cells to over produce, leading to hypergammaglobulinemia. The depositing of immune complexes in body tissues, such as the kidneys, brain, heart, lung, spleen, gastrointestinal (GI) tract, skin, peritoneum, and musculoskeletal system, sets up an inflammatory response leading to tissue destruction in these areas.

People with SLE have periods of remission and exacerbations of the disease, and the signs and symptoms depend upon which body system(s) are involved. SLE can affect the body in many ways. Polyarthritis, for example, affects approximately 90% of people with SLE. Hand deformity and loss of function and femoral head avascular necrosis may also occur. Skin manifestations include the characteristic "butterfly" (malar) rash on the cheeks and bridge of the nose and sensitivity to ultraviolet (UV) light. Discoid SLE, which may be the only symptom, manifests itself as chronic cutaneous lesions on the head, scalp, and neck.

If SLE involves the renal system, glomerulonephritis and nephrotic syndrome may develop, leading to leg, abdominal, and eye edema and hypertension because the damaged kidneys are unable to effectively regulate fluid balance. Pleural effusion and/or pleuritis signals pulmonary involvement. Pericarditis occurs in approximately 40% of people with SLE. Up to 75% of people with SLE will have neurological involvement ranging from seizures and psychosis to depression. Anemia and thrombocytopenia are indicative of hematologic involvement. GI involvement leads to anorexia, nausea and vomiting, intestinal ischemia, and pancreatitis. Buccal and esophageal ulcerations are also possible.

A positive antinuclear antibody (ANA), which detects autoantibodies, is present in 95% to 98% of people with SLE. When the cell is stained and examined under a UV microscope, a distinctive nuclear pattern is revealed. Other test results that may be abnormal during active SLE include an elevated sedimentation rate (ESR), decreased serum complement level, decreased RBCs, white blood cells (WBCs), platelets, hematuria, and proteinuria.

Management

There is no way to prevent SLE; however, close medical surveillance is recommended for people in high risk groups such as those of Hispanic, Asian, and African American descent and those with family members who have SLE.

Treatment is directed at symptom management and reduction of inflammation. Nonsteroidal anti-inflammatory drugs are used to control inflammation, while antimalarial drugs control musculoskeletal and cutaneous symptoms. Corticosteroids are used to treat severe and/or acute symptoms. The use of sunscreen lotions is also advised. Recently, low dose Cytoxan (Bristol-Myers Squibb, New York, NY) and prednisone therapy have been used in order to control symptoms and avoid the necessity of high dose corticosteroid use. Some patients may also benefit from plasmapheresis, a process similar to dialysis that removes antibodies from plasma, but this process is no more effective than conventional medication. Because exposure to the sun and ingestion of alfalfa sprouts has been implicated in exacerbations of SLE, avoidance of these factors is recommended for people with the disease.

10 Acquired Immunodeficiency Syndrome

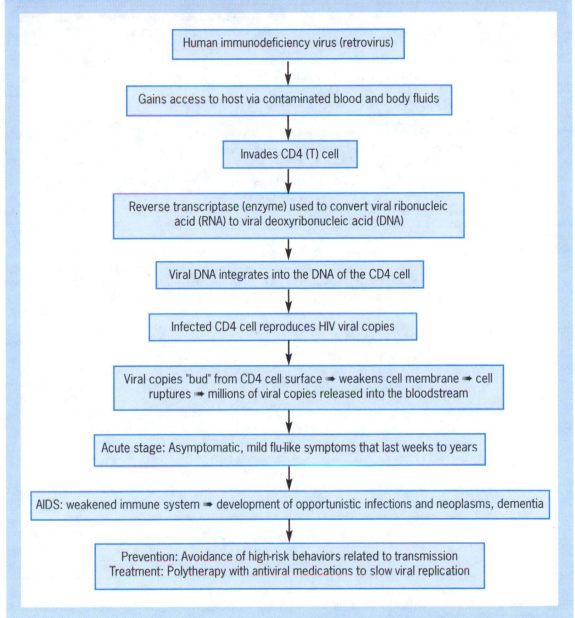

Human immunodeficiency virus (retrovirus)

↓

Gains access to host via contaminated blood and body fluids

↓

Invades CD4 (T) cell

↓

Reverse transcriptase (enzyme) used to convert viral ribonucleic acid (RNA) to viral deoxyribonucleic acid (DNA)

↓

Viral DNA integrates into the DNA of the CD4 cell

↓

Infected CD4 cell reproduces HIV viral copies

↓

Viral copies "bud" from CD4 cell surface ➡ weakens cell membrane ➡ cell ruptures ➡ millions of viral copies released into the bloodstream

↓

Acute stage: Asymptomatic, mild flu-like symptoms that last weeks to years

↓

AIDS: weakened immune system ➡ development of opportunistic infections and neoplasms, dementia

↓

Prevention: Avoidance of high-risk behaviors related to transmission
Treatment: Polytherapy with antiviral medications to slow viral replication

Overview

Acquired immunodeficiency syndrome (AIDS) is a result of cell-mediated (T cell) immune system failure caused by the proliferation of the human immunodeficiency virus (HIV), which replicates by invading T cells, thus weakening the immune system. Since it was first identified in 1984, HIV has reached pandemic proportions, currently infecting approximately 10 million people worldwide. It is the second leading cause of death in the 24 to 44 age group in the United States. HIV is transmitted through direct contact with infected blood, blood products, and body fluids, including breast milk, vaginal/cervical secretions, and semen. It is also found in the cerebrospinal fluid (CSF) and saliva of infected individuals. Two major types of the virus account for the majority of HIV infection: HIV-1 is found in most areas of the world and HIV-2 is found primarily in West African nations.

Pathophysiology

As a retrovirus, HIV carries its genetic code for reproduction in its ribonucleic acid (RNA). Once inside the CD4 cell it uses an enzyme called *reverse transcriptase* to convert this viral RNA to deoxyribonucleic acid (DNA). The viral DNA is then integrated into the CD4 cell's DNA. As the infected CD4 cell reproduces, it inadvertently produces viral copies. As the virus replicates inside the CD4 cell, it buds from the CD4 cell surface, destroying the cell membrane and releasing millions of viral copies into the bloodstream.

The plasma viral load, or number of viral particles per mm of blood, is an indicator of clinical progression of the disease. A viral load below 10,000 copies per mm signals control of the disease and a low probability of disease progression. In contrast, a viral load above 100,000 copies per mm signals a poor prognosis and a high likelihood that the disease will progress rapidly. The aim of antiviral therapy is to reduce the viral load to a level at which the body's immune system can keep the virus in check. Treatment failure is indicated by a rising viral load even in the absence of symptoms.

In the acute stage of the disease process, the infected person is asymptomatic except for short-lived (2 weeks or less) mild flu-like symptoms. During the asymptomatic phase of the infection, which may last a few weeks or 8 to 10 years depending upon the strength of the person's immune system and the amount of virus transmitted during infection, the body's T cells are numerous enough to keep the virus in control and the person remains symptom free, although he or she is still able to transmit the virus to others. During the persistent generalized lymphadenopathy stage, the person presents with several enlarged extra inguinal lymph nodes.

Eventually, the number of viral cells will greatly outnumber healthy T cells, resulting in a weakened immune system and the development of opportunistic infections, neurological disease, and neoplasms characteristic of AIDS. The term *AIDS* is applied when a person is infected with HIV and has a CD4 cell count of less than $200/mm^3$. Illnesses associated with AIDS include Kaposi's sarcoma, wasting syndrome, and opportunistic infections such as candidiasis. Opportunistic infections and neoplasms develop because the immune system is not strong enough to kill malignant cells or bacteria and viruses.

The AIDS disorders that occur include AIDS dementia complex, neoplasms, and opportunistic infections including *Pneumocystis carinii*, tuberculosis (TB), candidiasis, mycobacterium avium complex, and other infections. Dementia affects over 50% of people with AIDS and is caused by direct effects of the virus on brain tissue. Opportunistic infections develop because the body is unable to keep commonly occurring organisms, including fungi, bacteria, and parasites, in check. Neoplasms, including Kaposi's sarcoma, lymphomas, and cervical cancer in women, develop because the body's surveillance system is damaged.

Diagnostic Tests

The enzyme-linked immunoabsorbent assay (ELISA) and Western blot tests are used to detect the presence of HIV antibodies (seroconversion) in blood and blood products. Because ELISA and Western blot test for antibodies and not viral antigens, they cannot detect the earliest stage of the infection prior to antibody formation; however, they are sensitive enough to detect 99.5% of HIV infected blood samples 12 weeks after initial infection. The Western blot test is used to confirm positive ELISA results. For persons in high risk groups, a negative ELISA will be followed by the more antibody-sensitive Western blot test. If the ELISA is negative and the Western blot is positive, the results are highly suggestive of HIV infection. False positive results can occur in persons with conditions such as autoimmune disease, syphilis, leukemia, lymphoma, or alcohol abuse (ETOH). False negative tests will occur prior to antibody formation and in the end-stage of the disease.

OraSure HIV-1 (OraSure Technologies, Bethlehem, PA) allows for HIV testing using an oral fluid specimen instead of a blood sample. Although it is highly accurate and convenient to use, it is not as accurate as blood testing. If someone in a high risk group has a negative test result using an oral fluid specimen, the test is repeated or a blood sample is tested instead.

The immune-complex-dissociated *p24* assay is a test available in some research laboratories that detects the *p24* antigen, which is an indication of active HIV replication, within 2 to 6 weeks of HIV infection. It is used to confirm HIV infection prior to seroconversion (HIV antibody production) and to monitor the effectiveness of antiretroviral therapy.

Lymphocyte immunophenotyping is a test to determine the number of serum CD4 cells. A recent viral illness and immunosuppressive drugs will decrease lymphocyte counts, while steroids can increase the counts. Laboratories are now capable of determining HIV viral load or the number of HIV viral particles in blood. By evaluating both the CD4 count and viral load, the likelihood of appropriate antiretroviral therapy is increased.

Management

Current research is directed at developing a vaccine against the virus. Until a safe, effective vaccine is developed, prevention of HIV infection includes actions taken to avoid direct contact with blood and blood products, semen, vaginal secretions, and breast milk of infected individuals. Educational programs concerned with explaining how the virus is transmitted are vital to stopping the spread of the disease. Because HIV infection continues to carry a stigma in many parts of the world, discussion of HIV and its modes of transmission must be culturally sensitive. Screening of donated blood and blood products for HIV is a routine practice in the United States; however, an infected blood donation prior to seroconversion is possible because the tests detect antibodies and not the actual virus. For that reason, autologous transfusion is suggested for planned procedures that may require a blood transfusion .

Pharmacological approaches to HIV treatment include polytherapy to interrupt the replication process at different stages and slow the progression of the disease and chemotherapy to treat opportunistic infections and neoplasms. None of the antiviral medications kills the virus and because the virus mutates readily if a dose of medication is skipped, adherence to the prescribed medication regime is essential. Opportunistic infections are treated as they develop. HIV infection remains fatal, although both the quantity and quality of life has been vastly improved for people with the disease because of advances in pharmacotherapy.

PART II QUESTIONS

1. What causes Lyme disease?

(A) Spirochete

(B) Virus

(C) Parasite

(D) Helminth

2. When conducting a community education program related to Lyme disease, the nurse stresses that if left untreated, Lyme disease result in which of the following?

(A) Respiratory failure

(B) Acute renal failure

(C) Cardiac dysrhythmias

(D) Permanent skin lesions

3. Systemic lupus erythematosus is the result of what?

(A) Lack of helper T cells

(B) Hyperactivity of killer T cells

(C) Hypoactivity of B cells

(D) Hyperactivity of B cells

4. What increases the risk of contacting gastrointestinal infections?

(A) Smoking

(B) Using antacids

(C) Taking H2 blockers

(D) Eating a spicy diet

5. Which of the following statements about a fever is correct?

(A) A fever is generally harmful.

(B) Oral prednisone masks a fever.

(C) A fever suppresses the action of macrophages.

(D) A rectal fever of 99.6 °F in children and the elderly indicates serious infection.

6. What is the most accurate test to detect HIV infection currently on the market?

(A) Elisa

(B) OraSure

(C) Western blot

(D) B cell analysis

7. Which of the following statements about HIV is true?

(A) HIV infects CD8 T cells.

(B) HIV uses reverse transcriptase to convert its RNA to DNA.

(C) HIV infections can be completely eradicated by the use of antivirals.

(D) HIV infection initially causes pronounced signs and symptoms.

8. What is the role of histamine in the inflammatory process?

(A) Causes vasoconstriction to limit bleeding

(B) Coats pathogens for easier phagocytosis

(C) Promotes hyperthermia

(D) Increases capillary permeability

9. Which of the following statements about chronic inflammation is true?

(A) It lasts 5 to 7 days.

(B) It results in granuloma formation.

(C) It results from viral infections.

(D) It produces copious amounts of serous exudate.

10. Which of the following is true about granulocytes?

(A) They produce antibodies.

(B) They include killer T cells.

(C) They contain enzymes capable of killing bacteria.

(D) They arrive at the site of cell injury in approximately 24 hours.

11. Which of the following is true about macrophages?

(A) They are primarily responsible for debris clean-up at the inflammatory site.

(B) They are responsible for producing allergic reactions.

(C) They live approximately 120 days.

(D) They are immature monocytes.

12. Which of the following statements about B cells is correct?

(A) B cells provide cell-mediated immunity.

(B) B cells produce antibodies.

(C) B cells release histamine.

(D) B cells live approximately 3 months.

13. Which of the following statements about suppressor T cells is true?

(A) They turn off antibody production.

(B) They mature in the bone marrow.

(C) They are the most numerous type of T cell.

(D) They release lymphokines that destroy pathogen cell walls.

14. What is the antibody classified as IgE responsible for?

(A) Passive immunity

(B) Protecting the lungs from infection

(C) Activating complement

(D) Allergic reactions

PART II ANSWERS

1. The correct answer is A.

Lyme disease is caused by the spirochete *Borrelia burgdorferi*, which is carried by ticks.

2. The correct answer is C.

Untreated Lyme disease will result in severe AV block 2 to 3 months after infection.

3. The correct answer is D.

SLE is an autoimmune disease caused by overactive B cells.

4. The correct answer is B.

Antacids change the pH of gastric contents, a natural protection against pathogens.

5. The correct answer is B.

Immunosuppressed patients will have a low grade fever even during a serious infectious process.

6. The correct answer is C.

The Western blot is the most sensitive test to detect HIV antibodies.

7. The correct answer is B.

As a retrovirus, HIV carries its genetic code in RNA, which must be converted to DNA.

8. The correct answer is D.

Histamine promotes capillary permeability, allowing leukocytes to emigrate to the injured area.

9. The correct answer is B.

A granuloma results from fused macrophages, which engulf large foreign particles and are a classic sign of chronic inflammation.

10. The correct answer is C.

Granulocytes include neutrophils, which are the first leukocytes to arrive at the site of injury and capable of bactericidal action.

11. The correct answer is A.

Macrophages are highly efficient at phagocytosis. They live for years in tissue and are mature monocytes.

12. The correct answer is C.

B cells have many functions, including antibody production.

13. The correct answer is A.

Suppressor T cells, which mature in the thymus gland, stop antibody production.

14. The correct answer is D.

IgE binds to mast cells and causes histamine release and other mediators of allergic reactions.

PART III

Anemias

Eileen M. Crutchlow, EdD, APRN-C

11 Common Anemias

Classification of Anemias

By Etiology

I. Decreased red blood cell (RBC) production
   a. Deficiency of dietary agents
   b. Bone marrow failure
   c. Decreased erythropoiesis
II. Increased RBC destruction
   a. Hemolysis
   b. Hemorrhage

By Cell Morphology

I. Determined according to mean corpuscular hemoglobin concentration (MCHC) and mean corpuscular volume (MCV)
   a. Cytic refers to the size of the cell
   b. Chromic refers to the color of the cell
II. Normocytic or normochromic anemia: MCHC 31 to 35; MCV 85 to 100 (RBCs are normal in size and appearance)
   a. Acute bleeding
   b. Bone marrow failure
   c. Hemolysis
   d. Anemia of chronic disease
III. Microcytic anemia or hypochromic microcytic anemia: MCHC <30; MCV <85 (RBCs are small and pale)
   a. Iron deficiency
   b. Thalassemia
   c. Sideroblastic anemia
   d. Anemia of chronic disease
IV. Macrocytic anemia or normochromic macrocytic anemia: MCHC 31 to 35; MCV >100 (RBCs are large and normal color)
   a. Vitamin B_{12} deficiency
   b. Folate deficiency
   c. Aplastic anemia
   d. Lead poisoning
   e. Liver disease

Overview

Anemias are common disorders with numerous causes. Some anemias can be easily treated and some have lifelong, life-threatening consequences. They are considered to be symptomatic of an underlying disease process rather than an illness in their own right, but all present with a deficiency in the number of red blood cells (RBCs) and hemoglobin content. Symptoms depend on the cause and rapidity with which the anemia develops.

Pathophysiology

Blood is composed of plasma (55%) and cells (45%). Cells include leukocytes, RBCs, and platelets. RBCs comprise one half of the total number of cells. RBCs are made in the bone marrow in response to a low oxygen level in arterial blood, which triggers the kidneys to produce the hormone erythropoietin. Erythropoietin stimulates the development of RBCs, which must pass through several stages before they enter the blood stream. Initially, a large, poorly differentiated cell called a *proerythrocyte* develops. The proerythrocyte contains no hemoglobin but is programmed, under the influence of the erythropoietin, to pass on the capacity to produce it. When proerythrocytes divide, they produce cells much smaller than themselves called *erythroblasts*. An erythroblast contains a nucleus that shrinks as the cell's cytoplasm fills with hemoglobin (Hgb) synthesized from the endoplasmic reticulum. When the cell is about 80% filled with Hgb, its nucleus is expelled and the cell is sent into the general circulation to complete its development. The newly developed, immature RBC is called a *reticulocyte*. Mature RBCs live about 120 days but cannot reproduce because they have no nucleus. When they wear out, they are sent to the spleen to be reduced to their component parts for recycling. For the process to occur as described there must be a normal stem cell pool in the bone marrow, sufficient caloric intake, and adequate supplies of erythropoietin, iron, folate, and vitamin B_{12}.

Anemia is defined as a reduction below established limits of the amount of Hgb or volume of red blood cells (hematocrit [Hct]) in a sample of peripheral venous blood. Anemias can be classified by etiology or by cell morphology (see p. 38).

Iron Deficiency Anemia

This is the most common anemia in the world with an estimated 20 million individuals affected by it in the United States alone. It is most commonly seen in women of childbearing age, children <2 years old, and the elderly. It occurs when the amount of iron available to make Hgb, which is the oxygen carrying component of RBCs, is affected by either excessive demand for new RBCs or an inadequate supply to make Hgb.

Iron is ingested from two food sources: heme is from animal sources and is broken down in the duodenum as iron then attached to a transport molecule, transferrin, for distribution via the blood stream to the bone marrow and other blood manufacturing sites as needed; trivalent and divalent iron are from plant sources and require an acid gastric environment to make them soluble for entry into the small intestine where they are absorbed via the brush borders.

Eighty percent of the body's iron is found in Hgb. The rest is stored in the liver as ferritin and is transported via transferrin to the bone marrow to make RBCs as needed. Men store about 1,000 mg and women 600 mg of iron. These iron stores are depleted before erythropoiesis is affected. Without sufficient iron, RBCs are small and contain less Hgb, producing a pale colored cell. These small, pale cells cannot carry enough oxygen from the lungs to the tissues so less energy is released from cells. Every cell in the body is affected and the individual becomes tired, weak, and apathetic. Children deprived of iron are restless and irritable; adults appear unmotivated, are less physically active, and have trouble concentrating and doing physical work.

Iron deficiency anemia in young people is most often a nutritional problem. A diet with too little food or not enough of the right kind of food (i.e., one high in fats and refined sugars) offers too little iron to maintain stores. Excessive nutritional demands are another cause. Men normally need 10 mg of iron daily, childbearing women, 15 mg daily. People absorb only 10% to 15% of the dietary iron available to them but that amount varies according to the body's need and ability to alter absorption. Those with gastrointestinal (GI) disorders may absorb as little as 2%; a growing child may take up to 35%. In pregnancy about 3 mg of iron is lost daily as the placenta takes most of the dietary iron for the developing fetus. Menstruating women loose 0.3 to 0.5 mg daily. Newborns rely on iron stores that last for about 6 months then they must begin to rely on dietary sources. It is common for an anemia to develop sometime after 6 months of age. Between the ages of 1 and 3, 9% of children have iron deficiency and 3% have iron deficiency anemia.

Bleeding is the most common cause of iron deficiency anemia in men, menstruating women, and the elderly. In women a heavy menstrual flow or abnormal uterine bleeding commonly results in an iron deficiency anemia. Bleeding, usually from the GI tract, either as an acute hemorrhage or a slow chronic bleed such as occurs when taking nonsteroidal anti-inflammatory drugs (NSAIDs) or with many GI disorders (i.e. peptic ulcer disease [PUD], gastritis, inflammatory bowel disease, or a malignancy) will have an iron deficiency anemia as a symptom. It also occurs postgastrectomy or with parasites as is common in developing countries.

Symptoms of iron deficiency anemia are not usually noted until after all iron stores are depleted and the Hgb falls to <10. All patients will demonstrate signs with a Hgb <7. The elderly may complain of angina, but all anemics will be weak, dizzy, lightheaded, have shortness of breath on exertion, palpitations, a lack of endurance, and pale conjunctiva.

Management

The cause for the anemia must be determined and the underlying problem corrected. Diet must include iron rich foods, and iron supplements (see p. 40) are usually given. Patients should avoid foods that bind iron and should take vitamin C to help absorb the iron. The response to therapy is measured by the reticulocyte count, which should rise by the tenth day after treatment is initiated; the Hgb should approach normal in 6 to 8 weeks. Treatment is continued for 4 to 6 months because the iron stores must also be replenished.

Red Blood Cell Terminology

	Normal	Increased	Decreased
Volume	Normocytic	Macrocytic	Microcytic
Hemoglobin	Normochromic	Hyperchromic	Hypochromic

Iron Rich Foods

Meat	Spinach	Navy beans
Fish	Parsley	Lima beans
Oysters	Sauerkraut	Kidney beans
Poultry	Peaches	Soy beans
Beef liver	Black-eyed peas	Green beans

Consume vitamin C in same meal to maximize absorption. Teas and foods and/or drugs containing calcium will decrease absorption.

Folic Acid Rich Foods

Brewers yeast	Spinach	Pinto beans
Beef liver	Asparagus	Navy beans
Parsley	Turnip greens	Black eyed peas
Beets	Broccoli	Lima beans

Common Iron Preparations

Optimally 50 to 60 mg/d of elemental iron should be taken daily until serum ferritin levels exceed 50 ug/L.

Preparation	Elemental Iron/Tablet	Dosing/Day
Ferrous sulfate (most economical)	65 mg	325 mg/three to four times a day
Ferrous gluconate	37 mg	320 mg/three to four times a day
Ferrous fumarate	106 mg	325 mg/two to three times a day
Ferrous fumarate	66 mg	200 mg/three to four times a day

Anemia of Chronic Disease

This second leading cause of anemia that is commonly found with many chronic illnesses (i.e., chronic renal or liver disease, tuberculosis [TB], human immunodeficiency virus [HIV], rheumatoid arthritis) results from the body's inability to use iron stores and get the iron into the Hgb. Several problems associated with having a chronic disease state precipitate development of this anemia (e.g., depression, poor appetite, polypharmacy, shortened RBC survival from drug therapy, excessive radiation, or mechanical trauma [i.e., artificial heart valves]).

Management

Management is directed at the underlying illness and includes adequate caloric intake, good nutrition, and nutritional and iron supplements as needed.

12 Thalassemia, Sickle Cell Anemia, and Pernicious Anemia

Common Laboratory Tests Associated with Anemias

- Blood indices—Tests done to determine the characteristics of red blood cells (RBCs) and their hemoglobin; help determine the type of anemia present; consist of mean corpuscular volume (MCV) (volume of the RBC), MCH (weight of hemoglobin in each RBC), mean corpuscular hemoglobin concentration (MCHC) (amount of hemoglobin in a cell compared to its size), RBC, hemoglobin, and hematocrit.

- Complete blood count (CBC)—Broad spectrum test evaluating different cellular components of blood, including hemoglobin, hematocrit, RBCs, and blood cell indices. Normal values vary by age and sex.

- Fetal hemoglobin (HbF)—Fetal hemoglobin is present during fetal development and remains up to 6 months of age; test can differentiate between thalassemia and other disorders.

- Hematocrit (Hct)—Percentage of RBCs in a volume of whole blood; ratio of RBCs to whole blood.

- Hemoglobin (Hgb)—The oxygen carrying component of RBCs made up of two amino acids: heme and globin.

- Hemoglobin electrophoresis—Process by which hemolyzed RBCs are matched against standards for >350 varieties of hemoglobin to identify normal and abnormal types; HbS is present in sickle cell anemia and increased amounts of HbA2 are diagnostic for thalassemia.

- Mean corpuscular volume (MCV)—The average size of the RBCs.

- Mean corpuscular hemoglobin concentration (MVHC)—The amount of hemoglobin contained in RBCs.

- Red blood cell (RBC)—Formed in the red bone marrow; lives about 120 days; transports oxygen to tissues bound to the hemoglobin inside the cell; passes through multiple developmental stages as it matures; mature cells have no nucleus.

- Red cell distribution width (RDW)—Determines the relative size and variability of RBCs.

- RBC morphology—Examination of RBCs under a microscope to compare their size, shape, color, developmental stage, structure, and content.

- Reticulocyte count—A measure of bone marrow function and its ability to produce new RBCs.

- Schilling test—Measures 24 hour urinary excretion of an oral dose of a radiolabeled substance to determine if intrinsic factor needed for vitamin B_{12} absorption is present.

- Serum ferritin—Index of body's store of iron.

- Sickle cell test—Screening test used to identify HbS responsible for RBCs assuming a sickle shape when under reduced oxygen tension.

- Total iron binding capacity (TIBC)—The maximum amount of iron that can be bound to transferrin.

- Transferrin—A glycoprotein that transports iron from the intestine to the liver for storage and from the liver to sites engaged in hemoglobin synthesis.

Vitamin B_{12} Rich Foods
Animal sources of all types: beef, poultry, shellfish

Eggs	Cheese	Milk

Overview

Each of these anemias is due to some type of genetic disorder affecting the production of red blood cells (RBCs). Thalassemias may be of the alpha or beta, major or minor types and are found predominately in people of Italian or Greek descent. Sickle cell anemias are found in 1:500 African Americans with 8% having the sickle cell trait. Both have asymptomatic carrier states and active states that can be fatal. Pernicious anemia is actually an autoimmune disorder found in adults over 60 with a strong familial tendency for developing it.

Thalassemia

Pathophysiology

Thalassemia is an anemia of defective hemoglobin synthesis. Hemoglobin is normally synthesized by a combination of two alpha chains located on chromosome 16 and two beta chains found on chromosome 11. Alpha thalassemias are due to a genetic defect that causes the alpha chains to be too short. Beta thalassemias are due to a mutation of the chromosome, resulting in reduced or absent beta chain synthesis. An individual heterozygous for the thalassemia gene will have a condition called *thalassemia minor*, which produces a mild, chronic, hemolytic anemia with microcytic and hypochromic RBCs. A person with thalassemia minor tends to produce extra RBCs to compensate for the anemia. If two people, each having thalassemia minor, pass the defective gene onto their offspring, the child will have thalassemia major. Children born with this disorder are usually normal at birth but develop a severe anemia during the first year of life that requires blood transfusions. They experience growth failure, developmental problems, hepatosplenomegaly, jaundice, and bony deformities. The transfusions produce an overload of iron, which causes heart failure, cirrhosis, and endocrinopathies that, in turn, cause the child's death.

Management

Those with thalassemia minor will have a chronic hemolytic anemia but require no treatment except in times of great or prolonged stress. Patients should be aware of their status and receive genetic counseling. Those with thalassemia major should have a regular transfusion schedule and folate supplements. A persistently enlarged spleen may be removed. Deferoxamine is routinely given as an iron chleating agent. Children who have not yet experienced an episode of iron overload with resulting organ toxicity may be candidates for an allogenic bone marrow transplant.

Sickle Cell Anemia

Pathophysiology

Sickle cell anemia is a genetic defect occurring at the sixth amino acid position on the beta chain of the hemoglobin molecule. As a result, neither the hemoglobin molecule nor the RBCs form properly. When oxygen tension is reduced, as occurs in the venous system, RBCs sickle, assuming a crescent shape. The sickle cells clump in capillaries and arterioles, obstructing blood flow and depriving tissues of oxygen. All organs, especially the heart and kidneys, are affected. Because these defective RBCs are inflexible, are odd-shaped, have a fragile cell membrane, and repeatedly go through episodes of sickling, their life span is shortened and a severe, chronic, hemolytic anemia develops. The rapid destruction of RBCs stimulates the production of reticulocytes at a rate that leaves little time for them to mature, so many nucleated reticulocytes can be seen on microscopy.

There are various types of hemoglobin and each is synthesized by a specific gene. Heterozygous carriers of the sickle cell gene are said to have *sickle cell trait*, meaning they have RBCs that contain both hemoglobin S and hemoglobin A. These individuals do not have symptoms unless engaged in vigorous exercise in a high altitude climate. *Sickle cell anemia* occurs when there is an homozygous state and the RBCs do not contain any hemoglobin A.

Newborns with sickle cell anemia are often asymptomatic with the first symptoms developing after 6 months of age. Babies are noted to be pale and may have symmetrical swelling of their hands and feet. As they grow, they have an increased susceptibility to infection, especially pneumonia, and sepsis; delayed sexual maturity; and multiorgan problems throughout childhood and adolescence. They experience a variety of crises, including vaso-occlusive or painful crisis, which is the most common and caused by tissue hypoxia and vascular occlusion, resulting in tissue necrosis and organ damage; aplastic crisis, which is caused by a severe infection, causing RBC production to be suppressed; hyperhemolytic crisis with accelerated destruction of RBCs; and sequestration crisis, which is when a large number of sickled cells collect in the spleen. Patients may complain of fever; headache; and severe pain in the arms, legs, abdomen, and back in a crisis state.

Management

Genetic counseling is essential for those with sickle cell trait but they require no other care. For those with sickle cell disease the goal is to minimize infections, minimize crisis, and manage the crises that occur with

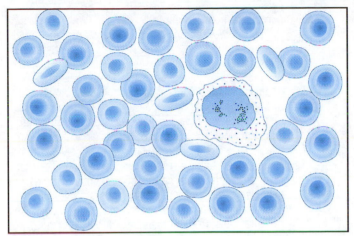

Normal blood. Note the number and consistency of the cells.

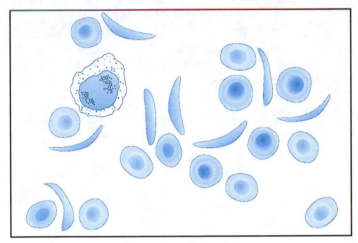

Sickle cell anemia. Note the reduced numbers of cells and abnormal shapes.

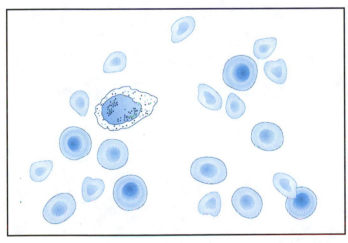

Thalassemia. Note the reduced numbers and unusual shapes.

hydration, analgesics, and bed rest. Currently, people with sickle cell disease rarely live beyond age 50.

Pernicious Anemia

Pathophysiology

Pernicious anemia is an autoimmune disease that causes autoantibodies to form against intrinsic factor and the parietal cell binding sites for vitamin B_{12}. Risk factors include vegetarian diet, gastrectomy, malabsorption syndromes, and a family history of the deficiency. Diagnosis is made from gastric analysis, Schilling test, and blood studies.

An autoimmune reaction results in atrophy of the parietal cells, leading to achlorhydria and lack of intrinsic factor. Normally, vitamin B_{12} binds with intrinsic factor in the stomach for protection from digestive enzymes. Without that protection adequate amounts cannot be absorbed in the body. Vitamin B_{12} has many important roles in the body including myelin formation, GI digestion and absorption functions, and deoxyribonucleic acid (DNA) and protein synthesis. The body stores enough vitamin B_{12} in the liver and kidney to last about 5 years so the problem has been ongoing for quite some time before symptoms develop. While all cells of the body are affected, the chief signs are neurological and hematological in nature. Patients present with neurological complaints such as problems with balance, proprioception, polyneuropathies, and maybe some cognitive changes. Blood tests show a macrocytic anemia because cells produced in the bone marrow stop maturing in the time when erythroblasts are changing into reticulocytes and the cells are large (i.e., macrocytic). They are also irregularly shaped, still contain a nucleus, and have a fragile cell membrane. They contain some hemoglobin and can bind some oxygen, but they lyse easily and need to be constantly replenished, hence the anemia. The anemia develops slowly, and patients adjust to the fatigue and chronic hypoxia. While hemoglobin levels are low, hematocrit levels may be normal because the large sized cells take up a lot of space/volume.

Management

Vitamin B_{12} is given intramuscularly (IM) daily for a week, then weekly for a month, then monthly for the rest of the person's life.

PART III QUESTIONS

1. What is the major cause of iron deficiency anemia in young people?

(A) Inadequate intake of iron

(B) GI bleeding

(C) Parasites

(D) Chronic diseases

2. What does the reticulocyte count tell you?

(A) The rate at which RBCs are being recycled and broken down

(B) The amount of iron stored in the liver

(C) The rate of RBC production

(D) The amount of transferrin available to transport iron

3. Which anemia is associated with depression, polypharmacy, and poor appetite?

(A) Iron deficiency

(B) Anemia of chronic disease

(C) Thalassemia

(D) Folic acid deficiency

4. When parents, each having the sickle cell trait, have a child and one passes on the sickle cell gene the child will:

(A) Have sickle cell disease

(B) Have sickle cell trait

(C) Have no sickle cell defect

(D) Die in utero

5. What treatment is required for pernicious anemia?

(A) Iron by mouth daily for 6 months

(B) Magnesium injections weekly for 6 months

(C) Folate supplements daily for life

(D) Vitamin B_{12} injections monthly for life

6. What will an individual with thalassemia minor experience?

(A) Premature death

(B) Mental retardation

(C) Mild, chronic hemolytic anemia

(D) Growth failure and bony deformities

7. Individuals with sickle cell anemia are susceptible to all of the following except:

(A) Infection

(B) Delayed sexual maturity

(C) Organ damage

(D) Premature aging

1. The correct answer is A.

Most often the individual either does not eat enough iron rich foods because of poor food choices or, for a time, the body requires more iron than the individual usually consumes and iron stores become depleted.

2. The correct answer is C.

New, not fully matured RBCs are called *reticulocytes*. They are produced in the bone marrow and sent into circulation. Their amount indicates how fast or slow the bone marrow is making new RBCs and is a first indicator that therapy for iron deficiency anemia is working.

3. The correct answer is B.

People with chronic illnesses, in addition to the underlying chronic condition itself, often suffer from the problems listed, making it difficult for them to take in and utilize sufficient iron to meet body requirements.

4. The correct answer is B.

This is a heterozygous situation; with only one gene passed on the child will have the trait and be essentially asymptomatic.

5. The correct answer is D.

Pernicious anemia is an autoimmune disease in which the individual can no longer absorb vitamin B_{12} from the gut and needs to have it supplemented monthly for life.

6. The correct answer is C.

Those with thalassemia minor experience a persistent mild anemia that they compensate for with increased RBC production. The other choices are all sequela of thalassemia major, which is a severe life-threatening disorder.

7. The correct answer is D.

Currently, individuals with sickle cell anemia rarely live beyond the age of 50 because of damage to major organs during childhood and adolescence and because of difficulty mounting a response to infections.

PART IV
Nervous System
Pamela J. Dudac, MS, MSN, APRN-C

13 Anatomy and Physiology of the Nervous System

Brain Anatomy and Physiology: Functions and Manifestations of Dysfunction

Brain Stem

- Medulla—Relay/crossing motor fibers; control and coordination of respiratory, vasomotor, cardiac, and reflex centers (e.g., coughing, swallowing, vomiting, gagging); cranial nerves (CN) IX, X, XI, and XII

  Signs and symptoms (S&S)—Plegia/paralysis ipsilateral; pupils dilate/fixed; decrease loss of consciousness (LOC), abnormal extensor movement; ataxic, clustered breathing, hiccups; deficits CN IX to XII, absent cough, gag

- Pons—Relay center between medulla and higher centers; respiratory center; CN V, VI, VII, and VIII

  S & S—Pinpoint pupils; semicomatose "locked-in"; abnormal extensor movement, hyperventilation, apneustic breathing (prolonged inhalation); deficits CN VI and VII

- Midbrain—Relay, contains visual and auditory reflexes; bodies for CN III and IV at level of tentorium

  S&S—Ptosis ipsilateral eyelid; pupils midposition and sluggish; LOC varies; abnormal extensor movements; hyperventilation

Cerebellum—Coordination and control of voluntary movements

S&S—Tremors, nystagmus, and ataxia

Diencephalon (superior to brainstem)

- Thalamus coordinates and regulates activity of cerebral cortex by integrating afferent input; contributes to affective expression

  S&S—Altered LOC, loss of perception, and contralateral spontaneous pain

- Hypothalamus—Integration ANS and endocrine function (tropic hormones, oxytocin, ADH); temperature; with limbic system, regulates emotional and behavioral patterns of sexual arousal, feeding, satiety, and thirst centers; diurnal rhythms/sleep

Reticular Formation—Small areas interspersed in brainstem and diencephalon

- Reticular activating system; arousal—maintains consciousness and awakens from sleep, receives incoming stimuli, and arouses the cerebral cortex

Cerebral Cortex

Analyzes sensory data; memory, learns new information, forms thoughts, and makes decisions

- Frontal lobe—Intellect, personality, recent memory, voluntary movement, motor speech

  S&S—Impaired recent memory and intellect, flat emotion, emotional lability, lack of inhibition, contralateral plegia/paresis, and expressive aphasia

- Parietal lobe—Sensory discrimination, body orientation

  S&S—Inability to discriminate sensory stimulation, body neglect, disorientation of space, inability to write

- Occipital lobe—Visual perception, visual interpretation,

  S&S—Loss of vision and loss of ability to recognize objects in opposite visual field

- Temporal lobe—Auditory receptive area, receptive speech, expressed behavior, memory

  S&S—Hearing deficits, agitation, childish behavior, and receptive aphasia (continued on pg. 50)

Neurons and the Organization of the Nervous System

The nervous system is responsible for the regulation of the activities of the body's internal organs and also for the body's ability to interact with the external environment. It regulates many activities through a complex network of structures that transmits electrical and chemical signals.

The basic structures of the nervous system, called *neurons*, are arranged into the central nervous system (CNS) (i.e., the brain and spinal cord) and the peripheral nervous system (PNS) (i.e., the somatic nervous system and the autonomic nervous system [ANS]) and includes the cranial nerves and the spinal nerves. The pathways of the PNS are divided into afferent pathways, which carry the sensory impulses toward the CNS, and efferent pathways, which innervate muscles or effector organs by carrying impulses away from the CNS. The ANS is further subdivided into the sympathetic nervous system (ANS-S) and the parasympathetic nervous system (ANS-P).

Neurons are divided into motor, sensory, and association neurons. They have three components: the body, the dendrite, and the axon. Most cell bodies are found in the CNS or organized into groups, called *ganglia*, in the PNS. Dendrites are extensions that carry electrical impulses toward the cell body and axons carry impulses away. Axons may be covered with a myelin sheath, which is a segmented layer of lipid. A thin neurilemma or sheath of Schwann underlies the myelin sheath. The myelin sheath and neurilemma have interruptions at regular intervals, which are called the *nodes of Ranvier*. Myelin insulates the axons, allowing impulses to pass quickly. Neurons use glucose for energy production. They do not store glucose nor do they need insulin for transport of glucose into the cell.

Mature nerve cells cannot divide, and injury may produce permanent loss of function. In the PNS, axon repair may occur if the neurilemma is intact.

Impulses are transmitted across synapses, which are spaces between neurons, by chemicals called *neurotransmitters*. The neurotransmitters are stored in the presynaptic neurons. The postsynaptic neurons have receptors that bind the neurotransmitters; therefore, transmission of impulses is unidirectional. Binding of the neurotransmitter changes the permeability of the postsynaptic neuron and may either excite (depolarize) or inhibit (hyperpolarize) the postsynaptic neuron (see p. 50 for a list of neurotransmitters).

The Brain

The three major divisions of the brain are the forebrain, the midbrain, and the hindbrain. The forebrain includes the cerebral hemispheres, limbic system, basal ganglia, thalamus, and hypothalamus. The cerebral cortex is composed of the following four lobes: frontal, parietal, temporal, and occipital. The midbrain, at the level of the tentorial notch, has the corpora quadrigemina (involved with movements associated with vision and hearing), part of the basal ganglia (substantia nigra), nuclei of the cranial nerves III and IV, efferent spinal tracts, and the cerebral aqueduct connecting the third and forth ventricles. The hindbrain, which is below the tentorial membrane, includes the pons, the medulla, and the cerebellum. It also has the nuclei for cranial nerves V to XII. The midbrain and hindbrain together constitute the brainstem. The reticular formation is a collection of cell bodies within the brainstem, which contains portions of vital reflexes such as cardiovascular and respiratory. It is essential for maintaining wakefulness, thus it is referred to as the *reticular activating system*. The brainstem continues as the spinal cord, which exits the skull at the foramen of Monro (see p. 48).

The brain is protected by the skull bones, meninges, cerebrospinal fluid (CSF), and four ventricles. The meninges are made up of the following three membranes: the dura mater, the arachnoid, and the pia mater. The dura mater is the double layered outer most membrane. The inner layer forms rigid plates that protect and separate brain structures. The falx cerebri separates the two hemispheres, and the tentorium cerebelli separates the cerebellum and lower brainstem from the cerebral structures. Venous sinuses are between the two layers of the dura mater.

The arachnoid membrane is the meningeal layer underlying the dura mater and the space between is the subdural space. The pia mater is the inner meninges. The subarachnoid space is between the arachnoid and the pia mater. CSF circulates in the subarachnoid space and ventricles and is formed and reabsorbed in the ventricles.

Spinal Cord

The spinal cord is also protected by the vertebrae, meninges, and CSF. It extends from the first cervical vertebra to the second lumbar vertebra. Spinal nerves that continue below that level are the cauda equina. The spinal cord functions essentially as a large cable, carrying sensory information to and motor information from the brain. It also provides neurons and synapse networks within the spinal cord that produce involuntary reflex responses to sensory stimulation.

A cross section of the spinal cord reveals an inner core of gray matter that can be divided into three regions, each with a specific functional characteristic. The posterior/dorsal horn contains interneurons and primarily afferent/sensory neurons whose cell bodies lie in the dorsal root ganglion. The lateral horn contains cell bodies involved with the ANS, and the anterior/ventral horn contains cells bodies for motor/efferent nerves that leave the spinal cord by way of spinal nerves. Ascending/sensory and descending/motor pathways/tracts are grouped into anterior, lateral, and posterior columns. The spinal tract may or may not cross to the opposite side at different levels.

- Limbic system (with hypothalamus)—Sex, rage, fear, emotions; biological rhythms; smell; and recent memory

  S & S—Loss of smell, agitation, loss of control of emotions, and loss of recent memory

- Basal ganglia—Extrapyramidal (i.e., regulation of automatic movement, balance, postural, and reflexes)

  S & S—Movement disorders (e.g., chorea), tremors (rest and intention), increased muscle tone, difficulty initiating movements, Parkinson's disease

Functions of Peripheral Adrenergic Receptor Subtypes

Receptor Subtype	Location	Response to Receptor Activation
$Alpha_1$ Epinephrine Norepinephrine	Eye	Contraction of the radial muscle of the iris causes mydriasis

Dopamine	Arterioles
	  Skin
	  Viscera
	  Mucous membranes
		Constriction

	Veins	Constriction
	Sex organs, male	Ejaculation
	Bladder neck and prostatic capsule	Contraction
$Alpha_2$* Epinephrine Norepinephrine	Presynaptic nerve terminals	Inhibition of transmitter release
$Beta_1$ Epinephrine Norepinephrine	Heart	Increased rate Increased force of contraction Increased atrial ventricular conduction velocity
Dopamine	Kidney	Renin release

$Beta_2$
Epinephrine
	Arterioles
	  Heart
	  Lung
	  Skeletal muscle
		Dilation

	Bronchi	Dilation
	Uterus	Relaxation
	Liver	Glycogenolysis
	Skeletal muscle	Enhanced contraction, glycogenolysis
Dopamine	Kidney	Dilation of kidney vasculature

*Note: $Alpha_2$ receptors in the central nervous system are postsynaptic.

Reprinted with permission from Lehne, R. A., Moore, L. A., Crosby, L. J., & Hamilton, D. (1998). *Lehne's pharmacology for nursing care* (3rd ed.). Philadelphia, PA: W. B. Saunders.

Functions of Peripheral Cholinergic Receptor Subtypes

Receptor	Subtype Location	Response to Receptor Activation
$Nicotinic_N$	All autonomic nervous system ganglia and the adrenal medulla	Stimulation of parasympathetic and sympathetic postganglionic nerves and release of epinephrine from the adrenal medulla
$Nicotinic_M$	Neuromuscular junction	Contraction of skeletal muscle

(continued)

Receptor	Subtype Location	Response to Receptor Activation
Muscarinic	All parasympathetic target organs:	
	Eye	Contraction of the ciliary muscle focuses the lens for near vision Contraction of the iris sphincter muscle causes miosis (decreased pupil diameter)
	Heart	Decreased rate
	Lung	Constriction of bronchi Promotion of secretions
	Bladder	Voiding
	GI tract	Salivation Increased gastric secretions Increased intestinal tone and motility Defecation
	Sweat glands*	Generalized sweating
	Sex organs	Erection
	Blood vessels†	Vasodilation

*Although sweating is due primarily to stimulation of muscarinic receptors by acetylcholine, the nerves that supply acetylcholine to sweat glands belong to the sympathetic nervous system rather than the parasympathetic nervous system.
†Cholinergic receptors on blood vessels are not associated with the nervous system.

Reprinted with permission from Lehne, R. A., Moore, L. A., Crosby, L. J., & Hamilton, D. (1998). *Lehne's pharmacology for nursing care* (3rd ed.). Philadelphia, PA: W. B. Saunders.

Neural circuits within the spinal cord form reflex arcs that display specific motor responses to stimuli. An afferent sensory neuron and an efferent motor neuron are needed for a reflex arc. Upper motor neurons are efferent neurons housed entirely within the CNS that influence and modify spinal reflexes. Lower motor neurons influence muscles. Their cell bodies lie in the spinal cord but their processes extend out to the PNS (see p. 48 for a diagram of tracts).

Autonomic Nervous System

The ANS regulates activity and maintains a steady state among visceral organs. Its' main functions are regulation of the heart, regulation of secretory glands (i.e., salivary, sweat, gastric, and bronchial), and regulation of the smooth muscles (i.e., bronchial, blood vessels, urogenital organs, and gastrointestinal organs). There are components of the ANS in both the CNS and PNS, afferent sensory neurons and efferent motor neurons. The two divisions of the ANS are the ANS-S (i.e., adrenergic nervous system) and the ANS-P (i.e., cholinergic nervous system). Some organs are innervated by both the ANS-S and ANS-P with opposing actions, some by both with complementary actions, and some by only one or the other.

In both the ANS-S and ANS-P there are two neurons in the pathway leading from the spinal cord, a preganglionic and postganglionic neuron. The postganglionic neurons go to the effector organ. The effector organs have receptors for the neurotransmitters released by the postganglionic neurons. The adrenal medulla is a special feature of the ANS-S. Though not a neuron itself, it functions like a postganglionic neuron, releasing epinephrine. The ANS uses four neurotransmitters: norepinephrine is released by most postganglionic sympathetic neurons; epinephrine released from the adrenal medulla; acetylcholine released from all preganglionic neurons of both the ANS-S and ANS-P, all postganglionic neurons of the ANS-P, and all motor neurons to skeletal muscles; and dopamine is released centrally and can stimulate receptors of the ANS-S. Different receptors on effector organs determine the specific activities regulated (see p. 48).

14 Altered Level of Consciousness and Increased Intracranial Pressure

Glasgow Coma Scale

Parameter	Score	Response
Eye opening	Spontaneous	4
	To voice	3
	To pain	2
	No response	1
Best verbal response	Oriented, converses	5
	Disoriented, converses	4
	Inappropriate words	3
	Incomprehensible sounds	2
	No response or intubated	1
Best motor response	Follows commands	6
	Localizes response	5
	Withdraws	4
	Abnormal flexion	3
	Abnormal extension	2
	No response	1

Highest score = 15; lowest score = 3

Terms and Descriptive Behaviors for Levels of Consciousness

- Alert—Fully awake; aware of self and environment; responds to stimuli spontaneously and appropriately.
- Confused—Disoriented to person, time, and place (progresses from time to person to place); has difficulty following commands; may be agitated or irritable; may hallucinate.
- Lethargic—Orientated to time, person, and place but sleeps often; speech and thought processes slowed.
- Obtunded—Sleeps almost but is arousable and can follow simple commands; stays awake only with persistent stimulation.
- Stuporous—Awakens only to vigorous stimulation such as shaking; responds appropriately to painful stimuli; verbal responses are incomprehensible.
- Comatose—Does not respond to environmental stimuli.
- Light coma—Arousable, no spontaneous movement; withdraws appropriately to painful stimuli; brainstem reflexes (e.g., pupillary responses, gag, and corneal reflexes) are intact.
- Coma—Unarousable; withdraws inappropriately to painful stimuli; brainstem reflexes may or may not be intact; may exhibit decerebrate or decorticate posturing.
- Deep coma—Unarousable; unresponsive to painful stimuli; absent brainstem reflexes; decerebrate posturing.

Altered Level of Consciousness

Overview

Full consciousness is a state of awareness of self and one's environment and the ability to respond optimally to the environment. Coma is the total lack of awareness and inability to respond even when vigorously stimulated. Between the two extremes, there is a full spectrum of different levels of awareness and responsiveness. Unconsciousness itself is not a diagnosis or disease but is a manifestation of various pathological processes. There are many causes of unconsciousness, some structural and some metabolic.

Pathophysiology

There are two primary components of consciousness—arousal and content. *Arousal* refers to a state of wakefulness that is a function of the upper brainstem and, in particular, the reticular activating system (RAS). *Content* refers to the ability to think, reason, feel, and react to stimuli with purpose. These activities are mediated by the cerebral hemispheres. A functioning brainstem can maintain wakefulness even without a functioning cerebrum, which is a condition referred to as *persistent vegetative state*. Disruptions in arousal, content, or both can alter the level of consciousness (LOC).

The etiology may include any condition that widely disrupts the functioning of both cerebral hemispheres or depresses or destroys the upper brainstem. Supratentorial mass lesions, such as a hematoma, interrupt consciousness by compressing and shifting cerebral contents, causing direct compression of the brainstem RAS or herniation through the falx cerebri or tentorial notch. Infratentorial mass lesions can also disrupt the RAS through compression or herniation. Metabolic problems or diffuse cerebral disorders can disturb cerebral metabolism. Among metabolic problems that disrupt consciousness are uremia, liver failure, diabetes, hypoglycemia, toxins such as alcohol, and drug overdose. Encephalitis and seizures can diffusely effect the cerebral cortex.

Complications that may result from decreased consciousness may be related to decreased mobility or loss of reflexes (e.g., asphyxiation with loss of gag reflex or corneal injury with loss of blink).

Manifestations

With full consciousness the individual is awake and spontaneously responding to stimuli in the environment in an appropriate manner. He or she is oriented and able to follow commands to move. These abilities (i.e., spontaneous eye opening, verbal and motor responses to verbal and pain stimuli) diminish with decreasing consciousness and are commonly evaluated and quantified using the Glasgow Coma Scale (see p. 52). Labels are often used to identify different LOCs; however, there is no universal agreement on the meaning of the labels. Objective descriptions of behaviors are better used to differentiate various levels of altered consciousness. See p. 52 for commonly used labels and descriptive behaviors. Bowel and bladder continence and blinking, gagging, and swallowing reflexes are lost as unconsciousness deepens.

Treatment

Primary treatment deals with the specific etiology of the unconsciousness. It is also directed at protecting the individual and maintaining body functions. Treatment may include intubation and ventilation, airway maintenance, intravenous fluid administration, feeding tube, and urinary catheterization.

Increased Intracranial Pressure

Overview

The rigid cranial cavity holds brain tissue, blood, and cerebrospinal fluid (CSF). The volume of these three components and the intracranial pressure they create are normally in equilibrium. Increased intracranial pressure (ICP) is a life-threatening situation that results from an increase in any or all of these components. Increased ICP is a common factor in many pathological conditions affecting the brain (e.g., masses, head injury, infection, vascular insults, and toxic and metabolic conditions [e.g., hypercapnia or hypoxia]). Regardless of cause, increased ICP effects cerebral blood flow, produces compression and distortion of structures, and shifts content.

Pathophysiology

A modified Monro-Kellie doctrine, which explains the relatively constant intracranial volume and pressure, hypothesizes that if the volume added to the cranial vault equals the volume removed, than the pressure remains relatively constant. Other factors that influence ICP are blood pressure, venous pressure, intrathoracic pressure, posture, temperature, and blood gases. Normal intracranial pressure is 60 to 150 mm H_2O or 0 to 15 mmHg. Nonsustained elevation fluctuations occur constantly with such things as changing position and coughing. Mechanisms such as increased absorption and decreased production of CSF, displacement into spinal subarachnoid space, and collapse of veins and sinuses that diminish blood volume compensate for elevations.

Compensatory changes have limits, however, and in sustained pathological conditions of uncontrolled increased ICP, compression of brain tissue, decreased cerebral perfusion, and cerebral herniation become major problems as the volume and pressure increase.

The brain has two compensatory mechanisms to maintain perfusion to ischemic tissues. Autoregulation is an effort to maintain blood supply by dilating vessels, thus increasing the blood flow but also allowing fluid to leak out, which increases the ICP. The other compensatory mechanism is an increased systolic blood pressure (widening the pulse pressure) to maintain cerebral perfusion pressure (CPP), which is the pressure needed to ensure perfusion. (Note: CPP equals the mean arter-

Cross section of a normal brain with intracranial shifts from supratentorial (right). (1) Herniation of the cingulate gyrus under falx cerebri. (2) Herniation of the temporal lobe into the tentorial notch. (3) Downward displacement of the brainstem through the tentorial notch. (4) Downward displacement of the brainstem through the foramen of Monroe (reprinted with permission from Smeltzer, S. C., & Bare, B. G. [1999]) *Brunner and Suddarth's textbook of medical-surgical nursing* [9th ed.]. Philadelphia, PA: Lippincott, Williams & Wilkins).

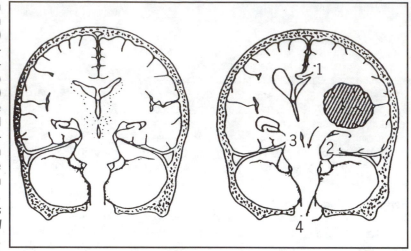

Abnormal Respiratory Patterns With Brain Dysfunction

Respiratory Pattern	Description	Area of the Brain Involved
Cheyne-Stokes	Rhythmic crescendo-decrescendo or rate and depth of respirations with brief apneic period	Bilateral hemispheres or some lesions of the cerebellum
Central neurogenic hyperventilation	Very deep and rapid respirations without apneic periods	Midbrain and pons
Apneustic	Prolonged inspiratory or expiratory pauses of 2 to 3 seconds	Mid to lower pons
Cluster breathing	Clusters of irregular, gasping respirations separated by long apneic periods	Lower pons or upper medulla
Ataxic respirations	Irregular, random pattern of deep and shallow respirations with irregular apneic periods	Medulla

Adapted from Phipps, W., Sands, J., & Marek, J. (1999). *Medical surgical nursing* (6th ed.). St. Louis, MO: C. V. Mosby Co.

ial blood pressure [MAP] minus ICP [CPP = MAP - ICP]). Normal CPP is 70 to 100 mmHg. A CPP of less than 50 mmHg causes irreversible brain dysfunction. This increase in systolic blood pressure to overcome the increased ICP is called *Cushing's reflex.*

In supratentorial lesions, as ICP increases, brain tissue is shifted down laterally under the falx cerebri or down centrally toward the tentorial notch through which it may herniate. The midbrain and upper brainstem are in this area, thus portions of RAS, bodies of some cranial nerves, including the third cranial nerve (controls pupillary function), and some portions of the respiratory centers are located here. Compression of this area can cause changes in LOC, abnormal pupillary function, and changes in respiratory pattern. Further transfer of pressure toward the brainstem, with ensuing ischemia, can interfere with vital cardiovascular and respiratory centers with slowing of the pulse and respiration. The slowing of the pulse and respirations combined with the elevation of the systolic pressure is referred to as *Cushing's triad.* Infratentorial lesions may herniate up through the tento-

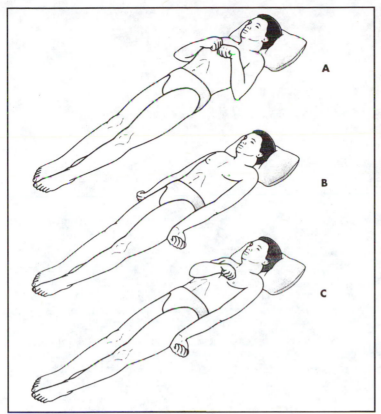

Decorticate and decerebrate posturing. (A) Decorticate response. Flexion of arms, wrists, and fingers with adduction in upper extremities. Extension, internal rotation, and plantar flexion in lower extremities. (B) Decerebrate response. All four extremities in rigid extension with hyperpronation of forearms and plantar extension of feet. (C) Decorticate response on the right side of the body and decerebrate response on the left side of the body (reprinted with permission from Phipps, W. J., Sands, J. K., & Marek, J. F. [1999]. *Medical surgical nursing: concepts and clinical practice* [6th ed.]. Philadelphia, PA: W. B. Saunders).

rium or down through the foramen magnum, compressing the respiratory centers (see above).

Two other potential complications are diabetes insipidus (DI) and syndrome of inappropriate secretion of antidiuretic hormone (SIADH) as a result of posterior pituitary dysfunction.

Manifestations

Early recognition of increased ICP is important in terms of prognosis. The manifestations of increased ICP can vary depending upon the cause, the location, and the rapidity with which it develops. Focal signs related to the location of the lesion may also be present. Manifestations include the following:

- Change in the LOC
- Changes in vital signs (Cushing's triad) including temperature regulation
- Altered respiratory pattern (see p. 54)
- Ocular signs (i.e., ipsilateral/bilateral pupillary dilation, sluggish to fixed pupil reflexes, papilledema, inability to look up, ptosis of eyelid)
- Decreased motor function including decorticate and decerebrate posturing (see above)
- Headache
- Vomiting (often projectile)
- Fluid and electrolyte disturbances, if diabetes insipidus or SIADH occurs

ICP can be directly monitored by catheters placed in brain tissue or the ventricles.

Treatment

Treatment directed at reducing the cerebral edema includes osmotic and loop diuretics and corticosteroids. Careful ventriculostomy drainage of CSF may be used in patients refractory to other methods of controlling ICP. Barbiturates or pharmacological paralyzing agents are sometimes used to reduce brain metabolism.

15 Seizures and Infections of the Nervous System

International Classification of Epileptic Seizures

I. Partial Seizures (Focal Seizures)—Initially only restricted area of one hemisphere is activated, subdivided into simple partial and complex partial. Originate from cortex.
   a. Simple Partial (consciousness is preserved, may become generalized)
      1. With motor signs—involves precentral gyrus/primary motor area; usually clonic movements
         –without "jacksonian march" focal motor activity does not extend into adjacent areas
         –with "jacksonian march" focal motor activity extend into adjacent areas, same side
         –adversive—turning of hand, eyes opposite to irritative focus
      2. With somatosensory signs (e.g., paresthesias [tingling, burning]) or special sensory symptoms (visual, hearing, gustatory, olfactory) involves postcentral gyrus/primary sensory area.
      3. With autonomic symptoms or signs (e.g., sweating, flushing, pupil dilation, abnormal epigastric sensations).
      4. With psychic symptoms (usually accompanied by impairment of consciousness) affective disturbance, illusions, hallucinations, "déjà vu".
      5. Adversive—Head, eyes turn to opposite side of irritative focus, involves frontal lobe, anterior to primary motor area, may generalize.
   b. Complex Partial (formerly Temporal Lobe or Psychomotor Seizures)—Impairment of consciousness.
      1. Simple Partial onset followed by impaired consciousness, with or without automatisms (i.e., lip smacking, grimacing, patting, picking).
      2. Impaired consciousness from the beginning with or without automatisms.
   c. Partial Seizures Secondarily Generalized—Begin in unilateral hemisphere then spread bilaterally, unconsciousness appears, generalized symptoms are produced.
II. Generalized Seizures—Begin with epileptic activity over entire cortex. Bilateral and multifocal. They originate from deep in the cortex. There is loss of consciousness and no aura.
   a. Absence seizures (formerly petit mal)—Children 4 years old till puberty; abrupt cessation of activity; momentary unconsciousness; eyes vacant and roll or stare, lips droop; sometimes mild tonic, clonic, or atonic activity; abrupt onset and termination.
   b. Myoclonic—Sudden uncontrolled shock-like jerking movement, single or successive; consciousness thought to be preserved.
   c. Tonic—Sudden sustained tone, frequently extensor or flexor posturing; may be accompanied by a shrill cry.
   d. Clonic—Repetitive, relatively symmetrical, bilateral, synchronous rhythmic jerking with diminishing frequency.
   e. Tonic-Clonic (formerly grand mal)—Occasionally prodromal period, though usually without warning
      1. Tonic phase begins with sudden loss of consciousness, brief body flexion, body stiffness, opisthotonos posture, jaw snaps shut, shrill cry as respiratory muscles stiffen, bladder and less often bowel may evacuate, apneic, pupils dilated, and unresponsive. Tonic phase lasts less than 1 minute, average 10 to 15 seconds.
      2. Clonic phase is characterized by flexion spasms of the whole body alternating with relaxation, strenuous hyperventilation, face contorted, eyes roll, excessive salivation, profuse sweating, rapid pulse, tongue may be bitten. Clonic activity subsides over about 30 seconds.

(continued on pg. 58)

Seizures

Overview

A *seizure* is a paroxysmal, uncontrolled electrical discharge of cerebral neurons that interrupts normal function. The neuronal activity may involve a restricted area of the cortex or the entire cortex. Frequently, seizures are a manifestation of a variety of underlying conditions or they may occur spontaneously without apparent cause.

Epilepsy is a condition of recurrent seizures. It is applied to conditions in which no underlying, correctable cause for the seizures is found. Seizures resulting from systemic and metabolic disturbances are not considered epileptic if the seizures cease when the underlying problem is corrected. Seizure is not a disease entity itself, rather it is a syndrome resulting from processes that affect the brain in a variety of ways.

Status epilepticus applies to seizures lasting longer than 20 minutes or the experience of subsequent seizures before the individual has fully regained consciousness from a preceding seizure. It is a medical emergency commonly due to the abrupt withdrawal of antiseizure medications. Without intervention, brain damage may occur.

More than 2 million people in the United States have epilepsy, which is one of the most common chronic neurological disorders. Seizures occur before the age of 20 in 75% of individuals. They decline through adolescence, plateau in middle age, and rise among the elderly.

Seizure disorders are on the rise probably due to improvement in obstetric and neonatal care that saves babies experiencing problems that predispose to seizures. Also, improved treatment of head injuries, tumors, and brain infections saves those whose condition often leads to seizures. The death rate for those with epilepsy is 2 to 4 times the nonepileptic population. Ten percent of the deaths are due directly to the seizure and 5% due to fatal accidents during the seizure.

Seizures have different etiologies often related to an individual's age. Seizures in infancy commonly result from birth injury or congenital defects, trauma, or infection. Idiopathic and fever-related seizures most often occur in childhood. In middle age adults, seizures commonly result from mass lesions such as trauma and tumors.

Metabolic disturbances that cause seizures include acidosis, electrolyte disturbances, hypoglycemia, hypoxia, alcohol and barbiturate withdrawal, dehydration, and water intoxication. Extra cranial disorders associated with seizures include heart, lung, liver, and kidney disease; diabetes; and hypertension. Cerebral inflammation, such as occurs with infection or injury, and structural lesions (e.g., tumors, scars) can cause seizures. Cerebrovascular disorders are a common cause of seizures in the elderly.

Pathophysiology

Normally, neurons discharge when an excitatory stimulus of sufficient magnitude alters membrane permeability, initiating an action potential. Inhibitory neurotransmitters prevent excitation. Mechanisms postulated as responsible for excessive firing of neurons in seizures include altered membrane ion channels, altered extracellular electrolytes, or imbalanced excitatory and inhibitory neurotransmitters. A genetic link has not been found for most seizures. In recurring epilepsy, abnormal neurons undergo spontaneous depolarization. The firing may spread by physiologic pathways to involve adjacent or distant areas or the whole brain.

Manifestations

Cerebral neurons control motor, sensory, autonomic, and psychic functions and are involved with conscious awareness. The clinical manifestations of a seizure will reflect the functions of the neurons that are abnormally discharging. The International Classification of Epileptic Seizures is a commonly used classification system based on location and manifestations (see pp. 56 and 58 for manifestations).

Infectious Meningitis

Overview

Meningitis is an acute inflammation of the meninges surrounding the brain and spinal cord. Infectious processes, mainly bacteria, are the most common cause though viruses and other organisms can be causative. Meningitis is classified as either aseptic or septic.

Aseptic meningitis, a noncontagious, relatively benign, self-limiting form, refers to viral meningitis or cases of meningeal irritation from causes such as blood in the subarachnoid space. *Septic meningitis*, which is also called *purulent meningitis* or *community acquired meningitis*, refers to bacterial meningitis (usually with an associated underlying encephalitis). Bacterial meningitis is contagious through droplets and is the most common and most deadly form. Individuals who acquire the organism and do not develop the disease can become carriers.

Risk factors for meningitis include extremes of age, debilitation, splenectomy, sickle cell disease, alcoholism, liver disease, upper respiratory infections, sinusitis, otitis media, pneumonia, diabetes, immunosuppression, ventricular shunt, cerebrospinal fluid (CSF) fistula, lumbar puncture, and neurosurgical procedures.

Meningitis usually occurs in fall, winter, or early spring secondary to respiratory disease.

Pathophysiology

The main viruses involved in meningitis are the mumps virus, enteroviruses, herpes viruses, and Lyme virus. Pathological organisms causing bacterial meningitis vary with age—*group B streptococci* and *Listeria* in newborns;

Neisseria meningitidis (meningococcus) in ages 2 and above; *Streptococcus pneumoniae* (pneumococcal) in ages greater than 1 month old; Staphylococcal and gram negative after surgery or trauma; and gram negative in the elderly and immunosuppressed.

Infections generally originate in three ways: through the blood stream (bacteremia) as a consequence of other infections, commonly infections of the nasopharynx, lungs, or skin; contiguous extension (e.g., otitis, sinusitis); and direct inoculation (e.g., trauma, lumbar puncture, cranial surgery). The infection then extends to the meninges, CSF, and quickly to the brain tissue, causing encephalitis. Acute inflammation causes meningeal irritation, disrupts blood-brain barrier, and, in bacterial meningitis, causes white blood cells and protein to infiltrate the CSF. Edema and obstruction can cause increased intracranial pressure (ICP), reduced cerebral blood flow, ischemia, and death.

Complications include visual or hearing impairment, seizures, paralysis, hydrocephalus, and septic shock.

Manifestations

Symptoms may include fever, a progressively worsening headache often accompanied by nausea and vomiting, stiff neck, rash (with meningococcal meningitis), somnolence or irritability, photophobia, seizures, blurred vision, numbness, and weakness.

Examination may reveal fever, decreased level of consciousness, nuchal rigidity, Brudzinski's and Kernig's signs, cranial nerve palsies, focal neurological deficits, and rashes.

Treatment

Meningitis is treated with appropriate antibiotics and antiviral agents. Management of increased ICP is crucial. Vaccinations exist for meningococcal, pneumococcal, and Haemophilus influenzae meningitis.

Encephalitis

Overview

Encephalitis is an acute febrile illness associated with inflammation of the brain parenchyma and is usually caused by viruses. There are many different viruses that can cause encephalitis, some associated with certain seasons or endemic to geographic locations. Encephalitis is a serious and sometimes fatal disease (5% to 20% mortality rate). The mortality rate is highest in encephalitis caused by the herpes simplex virus.

Pathophysiology

The most common viruses that cause encephalitis are the arthropod-borne (mosquito born) arboviruses and the herpes simplex type 1 virus. The arthropod-borne viruses occur in epidemics that vary by geographical region. Encephalitis can also be a complication of systemic viral infections such as mononucleosis, rubella, and rubeola. It can result from attenuated virus vaccines (e.g., mumps, measles, rubella vaccine [MMR]). Other less common causes are typhus, trichinosis, toxoplasmosis, schistosomiasis, and malaria. Toxoplasmosis, cytomegalovirus, and herpes simplex virus encephalitis are common opportunistic infections in acquired immunodeficiency syndrome (AIDS).

Encephalitis can range from a mild, self-limiting infection to a life-threatening disorder. Meningeal involvement occurs in all encephalitides. Large degenerative injuries are found in arthropod-borne viral hepatitis that cause widespread nerve cell degeneration, edema, and areas of necrosis.

Manifestations

Manifestations may be similar to meningitis but with a more gradual onset. The manifestations are high fever, delirium or confusion progressing to unconsciousness, seizures, cranial nerve palsies, paresis and paralysis, involuntary movements, and abnormal reflexes. Signs of increased ICP may be present.

Treatment

Treatment is supportive with control of ICP being paramount.

16 Trauma to the Nervous System

Types of Head Injury

Scalp Injuries

Abrasion, contusion, laceration, hematoma; bleed profusely, portal of entry if dura involved

Skull Fractures (with or without brain damage)

Types of Fractures

- Linear—May cross blood vessels

- Comminuted

- Depressed

- Basilar

- Open—Potential for brain infection if dura is torn

- Closed—No tear in dura

- Fractures at base of skull tend to traverse paranasal sinuses of frontal bone or middle ear, thus they may produce hemorrhage from nose, ears, and pharynx and blood may appear under conjunctiva, behind tympanic membrane, periorbital ecchymosis/edema, Battle's sign (i.e., ecchymosis over mastoid)

- Basal skull fracture suspected when cerebrospinal fluid (CSF) leaks from ears (i.e., CSF otorrhea) or nose (i.e., CSF rhinorrhea)

- Check CSF; if clear, check for glucose (present in CSF) and if blood, check for halo; potential for infection; if leakage of CSF, keep ears/nose clean, do not blow nose/sneeze, DO NOT PACK, do not perform nasal suctioning

Brain Injury (seemingly minor injury can cause serious brain damage)

Concussion

- Temporary loss of neurological function without apparent structural damage, generally involves brief decrease in loss of consciousness (LOC), can produce bizarre behavior (frontal lobe) or temporary amnesia (temporal lobe), can produce postconcussion syndrome (headache, dizzy, lethargy, irritability, anxiety, personality/behavioral changes, memory attention)

- Emergency department discharge instructions—Observe for difficulty awakening, difficulty speaking, confusion, severe headache, vomiting, one-sided weakness

Contusion

- Brain is bruised, possible surface hemorrhage

- Unconscious for period of time

- Manifestations depend on extent of injury and cerebral edema if widespread, poor outcome (brain damage/death) if residual headache, vertigo, impaired mental function, seizures persist

Diffuse Axonal Injury

- No lucid interval, immediate coma, abnormal posturing, global cerebral edema

Laceration

- Intracranial hemorrhage—Manifestations depend on location and speed; if rapid, may be fatal

- Epidural injury involves middle meningeal artery, temporal and basilar fractures, decrease LOC—lucid interval—then decreasing LOC with rapid deterioration, extreme emergency *(continued on pg. 61)*

Head Trauma

Overview

Head injury includes injury to the scalp, skull, or brain. The major risk in head injury is damage to the brain from bleeding, swelling, and increasing intracranial pressure (ICP) with the potential for disability or death.

Two million head injuries occur each year in the United States and approximately 75,000 to 100,000 patients die of the injury. Seventy thousand to 90,000 injuries are severe enough to cause permanent brain dysfunction. The majority of deaths are immediate from direct trauma, massive hemorrhage, and shock. Deaths may occur within a few hours from progressive bleeding or within a couple of weeks from multisystem failure.

The major causes of head injury are motor vehicle accidents (50%), falls (21%), assaults (12%), and sports injuries (10%). Firearms-related head injuries are increasing. Two thirds of head injuries are in individuals younger than 30 years old with males outnumbering females 3:1. The second highest incidence is among the elderly.

Pathophysiology

Mechanisms of trauma include deformation, acceleration-deceleration (associated with coup-countercoup injuries), and rotational (associated with diffuse injury). The injuries may be insignificant or they may lead to poor outcomes. Factors predictive of poor outcomes include intracranial hematoma, increasing age, abnormal motor signs, impaired or absent eye movements or pupil reflexes, early sustained hypotension, hypoxemia/hypercapnia, and ICP >20 mmHg. Scalp injuries (i.e., abrasions, contusions, lacerations, and hematomas) often bleed profusely, but most are benign and only significant if associated with meningeal tears.

Skull fractures occur with or without brain injury. The major complications of skull fractures are intracranial infections, bleeding and hematomas, meningeal tears, brain tissue damage, and increased ICP. The location of a fracture may be significant (e.g., a basilar fracture generally crosses the paranasal sinuses in the frontal bone or the middle ear in the temporal bone, causing meningeal tears that result in cerebrospinal fluid [CSF] fistulas, increasing the risk of infection. Also blood may collect around the eyes or ears).

Injury to the brain can result in alteration of brain cell function or structural damage. *Concussion* involves a brief period of loss of consciousness (LOC) due to temporary altered function of brain cells. It may cause altered behavior or temporary amnesia (i.e., *postconcussion syndrome* with headache, dizziness, irritability, alteration in memory, attention span, and personality) that can last for months. It may also be the beginning of a more serious and progressive problem (e.g., intracranial bleeding).

Contusion, or bruising of brain tissue, results in a longer period of unconsciousness. It often involves a coup-countercoup injury. Its significance depends on the extent of the injury and the amount of cerebral edema.

Diffuse axonal injury results in axonal swelling and disconnection that takes 12 to 24 hours to develop. It results in global cerebral edema, decreased LOC, increased ICP, and decerebrate or decorticate posturing.

Secondary complications may occur with major primary head trauma. Hemorrhaging and hematomas (epidural, subdural, and intracerebral) may develop at various rates, creating an expanding space-occupying mass causing increasing ICP. Temporary seizures may occur due to early inflammation. Later, seizures result from scarring. CSF fistulas that occur may be a factor in intracranial infections. Damage to the posterior pituitary can result in increased production of antidiuretic hormone (ADH) (i.e., syndrome of inappropriate ADH [SIADH]) or decreased production, which results in diabetes insipidus (DI).

Manifestations

Indications of serious head trauma include signs of increasing ICP, such as altered LOC, hemiplegia on the contralateral side, dilated pupil on the ipsilateral side, and alterations in ventilation and vital signs. CSF rhinorrhea or otorrhea may be evident. (CSF tests positive for glucose or will show a "halo" sign when blood is present). Blood behind the ear drum (i.e., hemotympanum) or ecchymosis around the eyes ("raccoon eyes") or over the mastoid (Battle's sign) are indicative of basilar fractures. Seizure activity and indications of infection may be evident. Changes in the volume or tonicity of the urine or serum sodium levels indicate SIADH and DI.

Treatment

Treatment is directed at preserving brain homeostasis and preventing secondary complications. Cardiorespiratory function is stabilized to maintain cerebral blood flow. Hemorrhaging and increasing ICP are aggressively treated and often require surgery. Antibiotics and anticonvulsants may be used prophylactically or acutely.

Spinal Cord Injury

Overview

Spinal cord injuries (SCI) result from vertebral injuries commonly involving cervical vertebrae 5, 6, and 7, thoracic vertebra 12, and lumbar vertebra 1. Partial to complete disruption of the neurons or nerve tracts can occur, resulting in loss of motor, sensory, and reflex activity and bowel and bladder control. Complications include spinal shock, autonomic dysreflexia, and respiratory failure.

Types of Head Injury (Continued)

- Subdural more frequently venous bleed

- Acute subdural hematomas are associated with major head injury, develop over 24 to 48 hours, and are signs of a rapidly developing mass and increasing intracranial pressure (ICP)

- Subacute subdural hematoma is less severe; manifestations appear within 48 hours to 2 weeks

- Chronic subdural hematoma is from a seemingly minor head injury, sometimes forgotten, in the elderly due to atrophy; may present like stroke; may occur 3 weeks to months after injury; clot absorbs fluid and expands slowly

- Intracerebral hemorrhage or hematoma is common when force has been over a small area (e.g., gunshot or stab wound)

Complications
- Cerebral edema/increased ICP (swelling peaks at 48 to 72 hours), impaired LOC, impaired ventilation, diabetes insipidus, syndrome of inappropriate secretion of ADH (SIADH) (impaired fluid balance), CSF fistulas, infections, and seizures

Spinal Cord Injury Syndromes

Syndrome	Area/Cause of Injury	Characteristics
Central cord syndrome	Injury or edema in central cord area, usually cervical	Motor deficits (>upper extremities) Sensory loss varies (>upper extremities) Bowel/bladder function is variable
Anterior cord syndrome	Injuries caused by the following: Hyperflexion Fractures/dislocations Disc herniation Injury to anterior spinal artery	Pain, temperature, motor loss below the level of lesion Light touch, vibration, position sensations intact
Brown-Séquard's syndrome (lateral cord syndrome)	Transection or lesion of one half of the spinal cord Usually penetrating injury or acute ruptured disc	Ipsilateral paresis or paralysis Ipsilateral loss and touch, pressure, and vibration sensations Contralateral loss of pain and temperature sensations

Approximately 10,000 to 20,000 serious SCIs occur each year in the United States. Males between the ages of 15 to 30 who experience motor vehicle accidents (55%), sports injuries (18%), and penetrating injuries (e.g., stab and gunshot wounds) (15%) are at greatest risk. A high correlation exists between SCI and drug and alcohol abuse. Falls in the elderly account for 21% of SCIs.

Pathophysiology

Acceleration, deceleration, or deformation forces compress, pull, or shear tissue or fracture bones. Structures may become displaced and slide into each other. The spinal cord's tough dura is rarely lacerated or transected except in penetrating injuries. After an injury, however, hemorrhages, edema, and metabolic products cause ischemia, which in turn causes necrotic destruction of the spinal cord. After 48 hours, necrosis is complete and the function of any nerves that arise in or pass through the area is lost. Edema extends the level of injury for up to a week, then the exact extent can be determined.

High cervical or thoracic injuries initially cause spinal shock lasting 7 to 10 days and are characterized by decreased reflexes and flaccid paralysis below the level of injury, loss of bowel and bladder function, and loss of sympathetic stimulation (hypotension, bradycardia, loss of sweating). Spasticity, reflex emptying of the bladder, and hyperreflexia indicate the end of spinal shock. Autonomic hyperreflexia, most likely with lesions at T6 or above, is associated with massive, uncompensated cardiovascular response to stimulation. The resulting hypertension and cardiac stimulation may cause cerebral vascular accident or death.

The degree of injury may be complete or partial. Complete cervical injuries lead to quadriplegia and complete thoracic and lumber injuries lead to paraplegia. Three syndromes, related to which nerve tracts are damaged, are associated with incomplete lesions: central (cervical) cord syndrome, anterior cord syndrome, and Brown-Séquard's syndrome (lateral cord syndrome) (see p. 61).

Manifestations

Manifestations are related to the level and degree of injury. Loss of voluntary motor and sensory function, spasticity, and hyperreflexia occur below the level of injury. Cervical injury above C4 results in loss of respiratory muscle function/ventilation. With injuries below C4, diaphragmatic breathing/hypoventilaton occurs and loss of abdominal muscle function decreases cough. Injuries above T5 decrease influence of sympathetic stimulation of the cardiovascular system, causing bradycardia and hypotension. The bladder becomes distended as a result of urinary retention/bladder atony during spinal shock then empties reflexively. With cord injury above T5, the primary gastrointestinal problem is hypomotility with distention and ileus. Gallstones, constipation, and fecal impaction may be problems. Immobility and spasticity lead to contractures and decubitus. Deep vein thrombosis and pulmonary emboli are common.

Treatment

Decompression and surgical fixation may be necessary. Corticosteroids may be used to decrease inflammation. Respiratory, nutrition, skin, and elimination status need to be addressed. Prompt treatment of autonomic hyperreflexia involves removing the stimulus, elevating the head of the bed, and using antihypertensive medications.

17 Cerebrovascular Accident

Stroke Syndromes Related to Cerebral Artery Involved

Cerebral Artery	Manifestations
Middle Cerebral Artery (MCA)	
Most common occlusion	Contralateral; hemiparesis or hemiplegia; arm affected more than the leg
Supplies 80% of cerebral hemispheres	Contralateral sensory impairment (same area as hemiparesis/hemiplegia)
Infarction effects most of hemisphere	Unilateral neglect (if nondominant hemisphere)
	Aphasia (if dominant hemisphere)
	Homonymous hemianopsia (defect of contralateral visual field of both eyes)
Internal Carotid Artery (ICA)	
Manifestations are almost identical to those of strokes of the MCA; however, with MCA strokes, edema is usually extensive, thus deficits are profound	Contralateral hemiparesis or hemiplegia
	Contralateral sensory losses
	Aphasia (if dominant hemisphere)
Vertebrobasilar Artery	
Manifestations reflect its perfusion of the cerebellum and brainstem	Clumsiness, ataxia
	Dysarthria, dysphagia
	Nystagmus and dizziness
	Bilateral sensory and motor deficits
	Facial numbness and weakness

Adapted from Phipps, W., Sands, J., & Marek, J. (1999). *Medical surgical nursing* (6th ed.). St. Louis, MO: C. V. Mosby Co.

Overview

Cerebrovascular accident (CVA), also called *stroke* or *brain attack*, is a focal neurological disorder that develops suddenly because of a pathological process involving the blood vessels to the brain. A CVA may result in disruption of motor, sensory, cognitive, and emotional function that can range from minor to severe disability and death.

The two major types of stroke are ischemic stroke (75%), which results from vessel occlusion due to atherosclerosis, thrombosis, or embolism, and hemorrhagic stroke (15%), which results from bleeding into the brain tissue (intracerebral) or into the subarachnoid space.

CVA remains the third leading cause of death and is the major cause of disability in the United States despite a general decline. What has probably contributed to the decline is an increased awareness of risk factors, improved prophylactic measures, and surveillance of those at risk.

Risk of CVA increases with increasing number of risk factors. The incidence of ischemic CVA, the most common type, increases with age until age 75; however, the incidence of subarachnoid hemorrhage is higher in young adults. The overall incidence in men is higher than women though the incidence in women increases after menopause. CVAs tend to run in families. The incidence of CVA among African Americans is twice that of Caucasians with greater morbidity and mortality. The high incidence among African Americans may be due to their high incidence of hypertension, which is the most important modifiable risk factor for all types. Smoking increases the risk two to five times but risk declines to normal 4 to 5 years after smoking cessation. Obesity, high dietary saturated fat, sedentary lifestyle, excessive alcohol consumption, diabetes, dyslipidemia, atherosclerosis, and recent myocardial infarction are all risk factors. CVA itself is a risk factor for additional CVAs. Atrial fibrillation and valvular disorders, hypercoagulability states such as oral contraception (especially in women who smoke), sickle cell disease, and polycythemia are risk factors for embolic stroke.

Risk factors for hemorrhagic CVAs include hypertension; smoking; sickle cell disease; coagulopathies; iatrogenic anticoagulation; aneurysms; arteriovenous malformations; and alcohol, cocaine, and amphetamine abuse.

Pathophysiology

Ischemic CVAs usually result from blockage of a major artery by a thrombus forming on an atherosclerotic plaque, which is known as an *atherothrombotic stroke*. Rupture of a plaque that has been developing for years leads to clot formation. Dehydration, shock, hypotension, and vasospasm can increase the risk of thrombogenesis.

Thrombotic strokes are usually subdivided into *transient ischemic attack* (TIA), *stroke-in-evolution*, and *completed stroke*. TIAs probably represent microemboli from atherosclerotic plaque in extracerebral arteries causing intermittent occlusion of vessels and temporary neurological deficits. TIAs may be prodromal (i.e., serve as a warning of an impending stroke). Symptoms of thrombotic strokes typically progress slowly over hours to days and, at this stage, are *strokes-in-evolution*. A completed stroke is a stroke that has reached its' maximum destruction. The extent of the neurological damage may depend on collateral circulation. Thrombi can also develop in smaller arteries and are called *lacunar strokes*, in which the prognosis for recovery is usually good.

Ischemic strokes also develop from emboli originating in the heart (resulting from atrial fibrillation, myocardial infarction with aneurysm, valvular disease, or congestive heart failure) and can move into and block cerebral arteries, causing a *cardioembolic stroke*. Cardioembolic strokes generally have a rapid occurrence without prodromal symptoms.

These obstructive processes lead to ischemia and infarction. An area of central necrosis is surrounded by an area of diminished perfusion, the ischemic penumbra. The extent of damage depends on the rapidity of development, size of the lesion, and amount of collateral circulation. Spontaneous or therapeutic reperfusion can limit the size of the infarction.

Hemorrhagic strokes result from bleeding into the brain parenchyma or the subarachnoid space and can last from minutes to days. Intracerebral hemorrhage is most common in people with hypertension and atherosclerosis because the degenerative changes from these processes weaken the vessel wall and the pressure causes rupture. In individuals less than 40 years old, aneurysms and arteriovenous malformations are responsible for the vessel rupture. The bleeding is usually arterial, occurs with activity, and is without prodromal symptoms.

Subarachnoid hemorrhages usually result from aneurysms or malformations of vessels in the circle of Willis that either suddenly rupture or slowly leak. There may be prodromal symptoms because of the pressure the aneurysm puts on surrounding structures.

Manifestations

The specific nature of the neurological deficit resulting from a CVA reflects the specific region of the brain perfused by the involved vessel and the amount of collateral circulation (see p. 65 for areas of brain related to behaviors). Manifestations include motor deficits, communication deficits, affective changes, intellectual deficits, and altered spatial-perceptual function. Typically, signs and symptoms peak within 72 hours as the edema in the area increases. After resolution of the edema, usually within 2 weeks, the signs and symptoms decrease. Typical manifestations are briefly discussed here.

Motor deficits on the contralateral side of the body occur if the CVA affects the motor cortex or pyramidal tracts and may involve voluntary movement, integration, tone, and reflexes. Contralateral weakness (i.e., hemiparesis) or loss of mobility (i.e., hemiplegia), ataxia (i.e., staggering gait), dysarthria (i.e., difficulty forming words), and dysphagia (i.e., difficulty swallowing) may occur. Initial hyporeflexia progresses to hyperreflexia.

In most cases, communication deficits occur with a lesion in the left hemisphere, which is dominant for language. CVAs affecting Broca's motor speech area result in an inability to form words, verbally or in writing, that are understandable (expressive aphasia). CVAs of Wernicke's area impair the ability to comprehend the spoken or written language (receptive aphasia). Massive strokes may affect both expressive and receptive language (global aphasia).

A CVA of the right brain most often results in deficits of spatial-perceptual orientation. With lesions of the parietal area, the individual may have disturbances in visual-spatial relationships. He or she may deny sensory input from one side of his or her body. With lesions of the optic pathways, he or she may experience homonymous hemianopsia, which is blindness in corresponding halves of the visual fields of both eyes on the same side as any motor loss. Sensory losses may involve any modality or the inability to interpret visual, tactile, or

Neurologic Deficits of Stroke: Manifestations

Neurologic Deficit	Manifestation
Visual Field Deficits	
Homonymous hemianopsia (loss of half of the visual field)	• Unaware of persons or objects on side of visual loss • Neglect on one side of the body • Difficulty judging distances
Loss of peripheral vision	• Difficulty seeing at night • Unaware of objects or the borders of objects
Diplopia	• Double vision
Motor Deficits	
Hemiparesis	• Weakness of the face, arm, and leg on the same side (due to a lesion in the opposite hemisphere)
Hemiplegia	• Paralysis of the face, arm, and leg on the same side (due to a lesion in the opposite hemisphere)
Ataxia	• Staggering, unsteady gait • Unable to keep feet together; needs a broad base to stand
Dysarthria	• Difficulty forming words
Dysphagia	• Difficulty swallowing
Sensory Deficits	
Paresthesia (occurs on the side opposite of the lesion)	• Numbness and tingling of body parts • Difficulty with proprioception
Verbal Deficits	
Expressive aphasia	• Unable to form words that are understandable; may be able to speak in single-word responses
Receptive aphasia	• Unable to comprehend the spoken word; can speak but may not make sense
Global aphasia	• Combination of both receptive and expressive aphasia
Cognitive Deficits	
	• Short- and long-term memory loss • Decreased attention span • Impaired ability to concentrate • Poor abstract reasoning

Reproduced with permission from Smeltzer, S. C., & Bare, B. G. (1999). *Brunner and Suddarth's textbook of medical-surgical nursing* (9th ed.). Philadelphia, PA: Lippincott, Williams & Wilkins.

auditory stimuli. This is known as agnosia. Paresthesias (i.e., numbness, tingling, burning) may occur on the side opposite the lesion.

Damage to the frontal lobe may result in cognitive impairment, such as diminished learning capacity, memory attention span, or other intellectual functions may occur. The individual may be unable to control his or her emotions.

A computerized tomography scan is the primary diagnostic test used in diagnosis of CVA. It can indicate the location and size of the CVA and differentiate between an infarction and a hemorrhage. Other diagnostic tests used are magnetic resonance imaging, positron emission tomography scan, and digital subtraction angiography.

Treatment

Measures to prevent stroke include prevention of thrombosis with daily use of platelet aggregation inhibitors and surgical procedures (e.g., endarterectomy and angioplasty to clear vessels).

Acute care includes control of arterial blood pressure and intracranial pressure. Thrombolytic, anticoagulant, and antiplatelet drugs may be used in ischemic strokes. Surgical decompression may be needed in hemorrhagic stroke, and antifibrinolytic drugs may be needed to prevent rebleeding. Aneurysms and arteriovenous malformations may be surgically repaired.

Five Stages of Parkinson's Disease

Stages in the development of parkinsonian symptoms

- Stage 1—Unilateral involvement; blank faces; affected arm in semiflexed position with tremor; patient leans to unaffected side
- Stage 2—Bilateral involvement with early postural changes; show, shuffling gait with decreased excursion of the legs
- Stage 3—Pronounced gait disturbances; moderate generalized disability; postural instability with a tendency to fall

Last stages in the development of parkinsonian symptoms

- Stage 4—Significant disability; limited ambulation with assistance
- Stage 5—Complete invalidism; patient confined to bed or chair; cannot stand or walk even with assistance

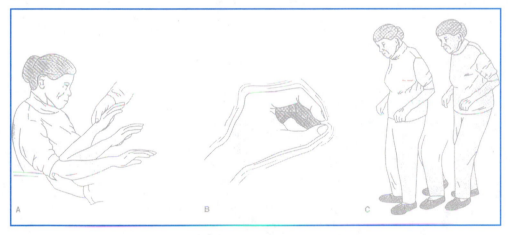

Parkinson's disease is manifested by (A) "cogwheeling" that accompanies passive extremity movement; (B) "pill-rolling" tremor; and (C) postural instability, forward stoop, and shuffling gait (reprinted with permission from Smeltzer, S. C., & Bare, B. G. (1999). *Brunner and Suddarth's textbook of medical-surgical nursing* (9th ed.). Philadelphia, PA: Lippincott, Williams & Wilkins).

Parkinson's Disease

Overview

Parkinson's disease is a commonly occurring degenerative disorder of the basal ganglia involving the dopaminergic (i.e., dopamine-secreting) substantia nigra pathway. *Parkinsonism* is a term applied to the resulting movement disorder (i.e., poverty of movement, stiffness, tremors, and altered posture).

Parkinson's disease is an idiopathic, primary disease. Secondary parkinsonism is caused by disorders other than Parkinson's disease and includes trauma, infection (e.g., postencephalitic parkinsonism), neoplasm, and toxins (e.g., some drugs such as reserpine, methyldopa, haloperidol, and phenothiazine).

Parkinson's disease is one of the most prevalent of the primary central nervous system problems and a major cause of disability in individuals over the age of 65. An estimated 500,000 individuals in the United States are affected. Men and women are affected equally. African Americans are rarely affected.

Pathophysiology

The pathology of Parkinson's disease is associated with the loss of dopamine-producing cells in the substantia nigra in the midbrain, causing depletion of dopamine in the basal ganglia. It is thought that aging may predispose to this damage. A significant reduction in dopamine receptors in the basal ganglia has also been found. Dopamine is an inhibitory neurotransmitter that is necessary for the normal functioning of the extrapyramidal motor system, which regulates subconscious automatic motor activities such as posture control. The depletion of dopaminergic activity leaves a relative excess of cholinergic activity. Acetylcholine is an excitatory neurotransmitter. It is postulated that an imbalance between inhibitory dopaminergic activity and excitatory cholinergic activity causes the movement problems seen in Parkinson's disease.

Manifestations

The classic manifestations of Parkinson's disease are tremors, rigidity, akinesia, and postural abnormalities. These manifestations may develop alone or in combination but all four are usually present as the disease progresses. The onset of the disease is insidious with a gradual progression and long course. It is usually 15 to 20 years before it produces invalidism. Cognitive-affective symptoms may also be a part of the disease.

Initially, only a mild tremor, slight limp, and decreased arm swing may be evident. The tremor is usually the first manifestation. Initially, tremors are asymmetrical and later become symmetrical. They involve the arm more than the leg. The hand tremor is described as "pin rolling." Tremors occur at rest, disappear with movement, and are aggravated with stress.

The first symptom of rigidity may be painful muscle cramps in the toes or hands. The rigidity has a jerky quality to it and is often called *cogwheel rigidity*. It causes sore, achy, tired muscles and slow movement.

Akinesia (i.e., poverty of movement) may be the most crippling of all manifestations. All striated muscles are affected—trunk, ocular, facial (including muscles of chewing, swallowing, blinking, expression, speaking), and swinging of the arms. Akinetic movements include hypokinesia (i.e., absence of movement seen early in the disease) and bradykinesia (i.e., slowness of movement characterized by difficulty initiating, continuing, and synchronizing movements). The facial expression will look blank and speech will be slow and monotonous.

The individual with Parkinson's disease will have a flexed, leaning forward posture. His or her equilibrium will be off and he or she will have a shuffling gait (short, accelerating steps) in an attempt to remain upright.

Because of the connection of the basal ganglia to the hypothalamus, there may also be autonomic and neuroendocrine manifestations. Autonomic and neuroendocrine manifestations include inappropriate diaphoresis, orthostatic hypotension, gastric retention, constipation, urinary retention, and seborrhea (i.e., oily skin).

Fifty percent of individuals with Parkinson's disease have endogenous depression. In the early stages of the disease the mental status is preserved, but 30% of those affected develop dementia later.

Treatment

There is no cure for Parkinson's disease so therapy is directed toward controlling symptoms. Pharmacology therapy attempts to correct the imbalance of neuroreceptors by either enhancing the supply of dopamine with dopaminergic drugs or decreasing the supply of acetylcholine with anticholinergic drugs.

Multiple Sclerosis

Overview

Multiple sclerosis (MS) is a chronic, progressive disease diffusely affecting neurons of the central nervous system (CNS). It is an acquired, primary demyelinating disorder. Without myelin, nerve impulses slow down.

MS is the most prevalent CNS demyelinating disorder and a leading cause of neurologic disability in the young adult. The onset of MS is usually between the ages of 20 to 50 years. It is a relatively common disorder with approximately 250,000 to 350,000 individuals in the United States diagnosed with the disease. It is more prevalent in temperate climates than it is in the tropics. The ratio of males to females is 1:2. It occurs in all races but is more prevalent in Caucasians. Fifteen percent of affected individuals have a relative with the disease.

Pathophysiology

MS is an acquired disease and its cause is unknown. Most theories suggest that MS is related to infectious (viral), immunologic, and genetic factors. The susceptibility to MS appears to be inherited. MS is characterized by chronic inflammation, demyelination, and scarring scattered diffusely in the CNS. The primary pathological mechanism is an immune mediated inflammatory process that damages myelin-producing cells and causes the demyelinization, which may be triggered by a virus. The role of immune factors in the etiology is controversial. Suggested possible precipitating factors include infection, physical injury, stress, excessive fatigue, pregnancy, and poor state of health.

The onset of the disease is often insidious and gradual. Early in the disease the myelin sheath is damaged but the nerve fiber is preserved and can transmit impulses. The individual may complain of some weakness. The myelin can regenerate, symptoms disappear, and a remission occurs. As the disease continues, however, the myelin sheath is destroyed. The myelin is replaced by diffuse lesions and sclerotic plaques in multiple regions of the brain. Eventually, the neurons are destroyed. Without myelin, nerve impulses slow down and with nerve destruction they are totally blocked. Because of the scattered nature of the lesions, the loss of function varies.

Manifestations

The course and type of manifestations of MS vary among individuals. A classification scheme has been developed that identifies the various courses that the disease may take. Usually, individuals with MS initially have a predominant syndrome or grouping of manifestation depending on the area involved. Fifty percent of the individuals develop multiple manifestations after so many years.

Common manifestations include motor, sensory, cerebellar, and emotional problems. Motor symptoms include weakness or paralysis of the limbs, trunk, or head; diplopia; scanning speech; and spasticity of muscles. Sensory symptoms include numbness, tingling, and other paresthesias; patchy blindness; blurred vision; color vision defect; defective pupillary reflex; vertigo; tinnitus; and decreased hearing. Cerebellar symptoms include nystagmus, ataxia, dysarthria (i.e., difficulty pronouncing words), and dysphagia (i.e., difficulty swallowing).

Bowel problems result in constipation. The individual may develop a spastic bladder (frequency, urgency, dribbling, incontinence) or a flaccid bladder (retention) depending on the location of the lesion. Sexual dysfunction (e.g., erectile problems, decreased libido, painful intercourse) may occur though MS has no apparent effects on pregnancy.

Intellectual function is generally preserved though there may be some problems with memory, attention, and word finding. Emotional stability may be affected. Mood alterations are common with depression occurring more than euphoria.

Treatment

Drug therapy is aimed at treating the disease process and providing symptomatic relief. Adrenocorticotropic hormone (ACTH), glucocorticoids, and immunosuppressive drugs are used in treating acute episodes. Muscle relaxants are used for reducing spasticity. Physical and speech therapy may also be helpful.

1. What is the role of myelin that surrounds the axon of the neuron?

(A) Protection from injury

(B) Nourish the cell body

(C) Provide energy

(D) Speed transmission of impulse

2. Where do motor fibers originating in the precentral gyrus cross to the other side of the body?

(A) At the level of the spinal segment from which they emerge from the spinal cord

(B) At the level of the medulla

(C) One or two segments above the level from which they emerge

(D) One or two segments below the level from which they emerge

3. From what area of the brain do the cell bodies of the third cranial nerve originate?

(A) Medulla

(B) Cerebellum

(C) Midbrain

(D) Frontal lobe

4. Which of the following statements regarding the autonomic nervous system is correct?

(A) Acetylcholine is the neurotransmitter of the sympathetic nervous system.

(B) Beta 1 receptors are found in the myocardium.

(C) Stimulation of alpha 1 receptors causes vasodilation of the arterioles.

(D) Pupil dilation is a result of parasympathetic stimulation.

5. Which of the following is the earliest compensatory mechanism for increasing intracranial pressure?

(A) Increased systemic blood pressure due to systemic arterial vasoconstriction

(B) Displacement of cerebrospinal fluid (CSF) into the spinal column

(C) Vasodilation of intracranial arteries

(D) Herniation of brain tissue

6. The nurse is caring for a patient who sustained a head injury in a motor vehicle accident. In her assessment of the patient, the nurse should keep in mind that one of the earliest signs of increased intracranial pressure in a supratentorial lesion is what?

(A) Pupillary changes

(B) Changes in the level of consciousness

(C) Respiratory pattern alterations

(D) Widened pulse pressure and tachycardia

7. Which of the following changes in vital signs occurs in the late decompensation stage of increased intracranial pressure?

(A) Rapid respirations

(B) Slow pulse

(C) Widening pulse pressure

(D) Rapid pulse

8. What does a loss of consciousness during a seizure indicate?

(A) An infection is causing the seizure

(B) That the locus of seizure activity is in the frontal lobe

(C) That the seizure activity involves both hemispheres of the brain

(D) The individual has status epilepticus

9. The individual with bacterial meningitis may present with which of the following manifestations?

(A) Decreased body temperature

(B) Decreased blood pressure

(C) Edema of the eyelids

(D) Stiff neck

10. Clinical manifestations of bacterial meningitis include which of the following?

(A) Fever, swollen tongue, and diminished level of consciousness

(B) Photophobia, elevated blood pressure, and skin rash

(C) Fever, stiff neck, and diminished level of consciousness

(D) Diminished level of consciousness, nausea, and low body temperature (hypothermia)

11. Which of the following is included among the complications of meningitis?

(A) Septic shock, hearing loss, and hydrocephalus

(B) Chronic pain, cardiac dysrhythmias, and seizures

(C) Visual loss, paralysis, and arthritis

(D) Seizures, hydrocephalus, and arthritis

12. In what way do subdural hematomas differ from epidural hematomas?

(A) Subdural hematomas result from arterial damage, thus bleeding forcefully and occurring rapidly.

(B) Subdural hematomas exhibit a classic picture of momentary loss of consciousness, lucid interval, and rapid deterioration.

(C) Subdural hematomas should be suspected if the individual has a fracture that crosses the middle meningeal artery.

(D) Subdural hematomas may develop weeks to months following a head injury.

13. The patient who sustained a head injury now has clear fluid dripping from his nose that tests positive for glucose. The nurse suspects that the patient has which of the following complications of head injury?

(A) Meningitis

(B) Syndrome of inappropriate secretion of antidiuretic hormone

(C) CSF fistula

(D) Damage to the hypothalamus

14. Which of the following statements regarding spinal shock following a spinal cord injury is correct?

(A) It results in a massive, uncompensated cardiovascular response to stimulation.

(B) It results in decreased reflexes and flaccid paralysis.

(C) It may cause death or stroke.

(D) It may occur approximately 7 to 10 days after the injury.

15. Respiratory muscle function is disrupted with spinal cord injuries above which level of the spinal cord?

(A) C4

(B) C13

(C) T1

(D) T5

16. Which of the following is a risk factor for embolic stroke?

(A) Atherosclerosis

(B) Atrial fibrillation

(C) Hypertension

(D) Smoking

17. A stroke that involves the left hemisphere may have which of the following consequences?

(A) Paralysis on the right side and loss of hearing

(B) Loss of sweating and communication problems

(C) Paralysis on the left side and loss of gag reflex

(D) Paralysis on the right and communication problems

18. A cerebrovascular accident causing damage to which area of the brain would result in cognitive impairment?

(A) Temporal lobe

(B) Parietal lobe

(C) Frontal lobe

(D) Occipital lobe

19. Which of the following pathophysiological mechanisms explains the movement disorder seen in Parkinson's disease?

(A) Deficit of dopamine

(B) Excess of dopamine

(C) Deficit of acetylcholine

(D) Excess of acetylcholine

20. Which of the following is correct regarding characteristics of multiple sclerosis?

(A) It occurs most commonly in the elderly.

(B) It results from a deficit of myelin.

(C) It always has a rapidly deteriorating course.

(D) It results in motor rigidity.

1. The correct answer is D.

The myelin sheath insulates the axon and is interrupted periodically at the nodes of Ranvier, which enables the impulse to "jump" more quickly.

2. The correct answer is B.

Motor fibers cross at the level of the medulla, thus the left hemisphere controls all the activities on the right side of the body and vice versa.

3. The correct answer is C.

The midbrain is at the level of the tentorial notch, thus third cranial nerve function/pupillary function is compromised with herniation through the tentorial notch with increased intracranial pressure.

4. The correct answer is B.

Beta 1 receptors on the heart are stimulated by the sympathetic nervous system, resulting in increased impulse formation, conduction, and myocardial contraction. Acetylcholine is the neurotransmitter of the parasympathetic nervous system. Stimulation of alpha 1 receptors causes vasoconstriction. Pupillary dilation is a result of sympathetic stimulation.

5. The correct answer is B.

Movement of CSF is easiest to accomplish, thus it is the earliest compensatory mechanism mobilized. According to the Monro-Kellie hypothesis, when one of the components of the cranium (i.e., brain tissue, blood, and CSF) expand another component must contract in order to maintain the normal level of intracranial pressure. The other mechanisms mentioned occur at stages when the earlier mechanisms are exceeded

6. The correct answer is B.

The cerebral cortex and the reticular activating system are involved in consciousness, and these areas are the first to be affected by increased intracranial pressure. The other functions are regulated in the brainstem at a lower level and, thus, are not affected until later.

7. The correct answer is B.

As the severity of the increased cranial pressure increases, the perfusion to the vital center in the brain stem diminishes, functions of the cardiovascular and the respiratory system slow down, and regulation of blood pressure is disrupted. The pulse rate slows, the respiratory rate slows, and the pulse pressure narrows as the systolic blood pressure falls.

8. The correct answer is C.

A pathological process must involve both cerebral hemispheres for a loss of consciousness to occur.

9. The correct answer is D.

Irritation of the meninges due to inflammation causes stiff neck or nuchal rigidity.

10. The correct answer is C.

The infection causes the fever, meningeal irritation causes the stiff neck, and increased intracranial pressure can alter the level of consciousness. Photophobia, petechial skin rash, and nausea are other manifestations; however, the tongue does not swell, the body temperature does not become hypothermic, and the blood pressure is unaffected.

11. The correct answer is A.

The organisms can enter the blood stream and cause septicemia; damage to the eighth cranial nerve can cause hearing loss; and scarring can block the ventricles, leading to hydrocephalus. Irritation of brain tissue and scarring can cause seizures. Other cranial nerves can be damaged, leading to visual impairment. Damage to motor pathways can cause paralysis. Cardiac dysrhythmias, chronic pain, and arthritis are not complications of meningitis.

12. The correct answer is D.

Subdural hematomas are a result of venous bleeding. The breakdown products of the clot absorb fluid slowly, becoming an expanding mass so it may take weeks to develop. Epidural hemorrhaging occurs more rapidly because it results from arterial tears most often involving the middle meningeal artery.

13. The correct answer is C.

CSF normally contains glucose. An individual with fractures involving the sinuses may develop dural tears that allow CSF to leak, thus increasing the risk of infection.

14. The correct answer is B.

For 7 to 10 days following the spinal cord injury, edema in the area of injury suppresses function of the spinal nerves, resulting in decreased reflexes and paralysis. The other choices apply to autonomic hyperreflexia, a condition that may begin following the period of spinal shock when the peripheral autonomic nerves have recovered.

15. The correct answer is A.

The nerves that innervated the muscles for respiratory ventilation emerge from the spinal cord at this level. There is no C13. Nerves innervating respiratory muscles emerge above the thoracic area.

16. The correct answer is B.

Stasis of blood in the heart due to atrial "quivering" with atrial fibrillation causes mural clots to form that, if released, travel through the arterial system to the brain and obstruct blood vessels. The other factors mentioned cause stroke through ischemia and vasoconstriction.

17. The correct answer is D.

The left brain is involved with language. Motor tracts cross to the contralateral side in the medulla, thus motor loss would be on the side opposite the cerebrovascular accident.

18. The correct answer is C.

The frontal lobe is responsible for cognitive functions. The other answers do not apply.

19. The correct answer is A.

Dopamine is an inhibitory neurotransmitter. Acetylcholine is an excitatory neurohormone both necessary for the proper functioning of the extrapyramidal motor system. A deficit in the production of dopamine in Parkinson's disease leads to imbalance and the motor problems that are seen.

20. The correct answer is B.

A deficit of myelin explains the motor weakness that occurs.

PART V

Endocrine System

Suzanne MacAvoy, EdD, APRN-C

Pamela J. Dudac, MS, MSN, APRN-C

19 Anatomy and Physiology of the Endocrine System

Definitions

- Endocrine glands—Ductless glands that secrete hormone directly into the circulation (e.g., adrenal, thyroid).
- Exocrine glands—Secrete hormone to epithelial surface either directly or through a duct (e.g., sweat, salivary).

Common Abbreviations

TRH—Thyroid-releasing hormone
TSH—Thyroid-stimulating hormone
CRH—Corticotropin-releasing hormone
ACTH—Adrenocorticotropic hormone

T_4—Thyroxine
T_3—Triiodothyronine
PTH—Parathyroid hormone

Relationship Between Hypothalamic, Pituitary, and Selected Endocrine Glands and Hormones

TRH from hypothalamus
CRH from hypothalamus

TSH from anterior pituitary
ACTH from pituitary

T_3 and T_4 from thyroid
Cortisol and aldosterone from adrenal cortex

Effects of Aging

- Increased amount of connective tissue
- Structural changes (nodules)
- Variable changes in hormone secretion
- Decreased sensitivity of target organs
- Decreased receptor binding

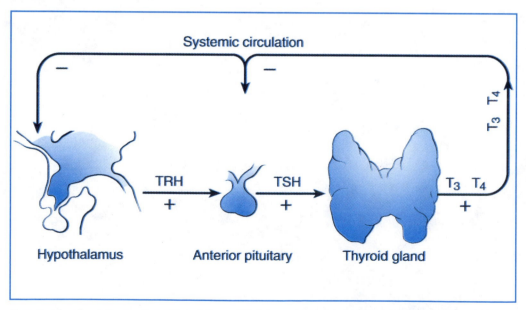

Negative feedback loop—Secretion of T_3 and T_4 into systemic circulation inhibits the release of TSH and TRH.

Hormones are secreted in any of three patterns—diurnal, pulsatile, or cyclic—or in patterns that are dependent upon the levels of circulating substrates (e.g., electrolytes, minerals). Generally, hormones are metabolized in the liver and excreted by the kidneys. Hormone release can be regulated by chemical factors, endocrine or hormonal factors, and/or neural factors. Feedback systems function to keep hormone levels within physiologic ranges. The complexity of the feedback systems of the endocrine glands contributes to the difficulty of diagnosing endocrine disorders.

Negative feedback is the most common feedback system in hormonal regulation. For example, reduced levels of circulating thyroid hormone stimulate the release of thyroid-stimulating hormone (TSH) from the anterior pituitary, which in turn causes the thyroid gland to secrete additional thyroxine. Conversely, if circulating levels of thyroxine are too high, the anterior pituitary decreases production of TSH, thereby reducing the level of thyroid hormone in the blood. *Positive feedback* is less common and occurs when the release of hormone from the target organ stimulates the endocrine gland to secrete additional hormone.

Hormones that are lipid soluble diffuse through the walls of the capillaries. Thyroid hormones and adrenal hormones are among the lipid-soluble hormones. For the most part, they are bound to proteins for transport in the blood. Conditions that affect the amount of protein available to act as a carrier can affect the concentration of hormone available for bodily functions. Lipid soluble hormones are metabolized more slowly than water-soluble hormones. Metabolism can also take place through degradation of the hormone by the target cell after being bound to the receptors. In some instances, metabolism increases hormonal activity, as in the case of the metabolism of the thyroid hormone T_4 to T_3, which is a more biologically active form. Hormones that are water-soluble (e.g., epinephrine) generally circulate in free or unbound form and enter capillaries through pores in their walls.

Target cells are cells with specific receptors appropriate for, or responsive to, a particular hormone and are the only cells that will be affected by that particular hormone. Some receptors, which are proteins, are located on the cell membrane; others are intracellular. The receptors for lipid soluble hormones are intracellular. The sensitivity of a target cell is related to the number of receptors it contains. If concentrations of a hormone are low, the target cells will increase their number of receptors. This is known as *up regulation*. Likewise, if concentrations are high, target cells will decrease their number of receptors, which is known as *down regulation*. This process allows the cells to adjust their sensitivity to the concentration of circulating hormone, thereby facilitating homeostasis. Another process known as *permissiveness* increases the number of receptors in target cells for other hormones (e.g., thy-

roid hormone increases the number of receptors on adipose tissue [the target cells] for epinephrine). The physiological effect of this is that greater amounts of fatty acids are released for cellular metabolism than would occur in the absence of thyroid hormone.

Plasma concentrations of hormones depend upon the rate of synthesis and release of the hormone as well as its rate of metabolism and excretion. If the end-organ fails to respond to the hormone and the hormone levels are normal or elevated, this indicates end-organ resistance, which can be to both endogenous and exogenous hormone. Ectopic hormone production is usually caused by a malignant tumor (e.g., some lung tumors produce antidiuretic hormone [ADH]). Medical treatment can also result in endocrine disorders (e.g., cushingoid syndrome when glucocorticoids are used to treat autoimmune disorders; hypothyroidism following thyroidectomy). These disorders are termed *iatrogenic*.

Affinity is the degree of "adhesion" between the hormone and the receptor. The amount of hormone required to elicit a response is dependent upon the degree of affinity (i.e., the higher the affinity, the less hormone needed to elicit a response). *Cross specificity* or *cross sensitivity* may occur between hormones if their structures are similar. For example, some hypothalamic hormones may affect the secretion of more than one hormone from the anterior pituitary. Which hormone takes precedence at a given time is to some degree dependent on the concentration of the hormone in the body, as are the types of clinical manifestations seen in patients. For example, thyroid-releasing hormone (TRH) stimulates both TSH and prolactin, so effects of both of these hormones may be seen in patients (i.e., gynecomastia as a side effect of thyroid hormone replacement). If hormones are administered exogenously, the effects seen may not reflect the actions of the hormones at physiologic levels. Certain medications can also act as agonists or antagonists of hormones, thereby increasing or decreasing their effects.

The hypothalamic-pituitary axis (HPA) is an important dimension of the physiology of the endocrine system. It produces various releasing/inhibitory hormones and tropic hormones that affect the function of various glands and body processes. Releasing/inhibitory hormones are produced and secreted by the hypothalamus (TRH, corticotropin-releasing hormone [CRH]) and tropic hormones are produced and secreted by the pituitary (TSH, adrenocorticotropic hormone [ACTH]). Tropic hormones, in turn, cause the release of hormones from other glands, which act on target cells in particular organs. There are both neural (posterior pituitary) and vascular (anterior pituitary) connections between the hypothalamus and the pituitary.

Endocrine pathology can result from hyposecretion, hypersecretion, or altered responsiveness of the target cells. These can occur because of altered function anywhere along the HPA or in the target gland itself. Therefore, diagnosis of specific disorders needs to take into account the complex mechanisms among these organs. Primary disease is of the endocrine gland itself, and secondary disease is a consequence of abnormalities of the pituitary or other ectopic sources. For example, hypothyroidism could be caused by decreased secretion of thyroid hormone (primary disease) or by decreased concentrations of TSH (secondary disease). Therefore, accurate diagnosis requires determination of levels of tropic as well as target organ hormones. Endocrine disorders may also be referred to as *functional* if caused by nonendocrine disease. Hyporesponsiveness of the target organ is usually a result of receptor deficiency (e.g., insulin resistance with diabetes).

Effects of Aging

It is difficult to establish the precise relationship between normal aging and endocrine function because of the complexities of the endocrine system and the many other factors that play a role in its' function. For example, changes in organ function and metabolism, and excretion; nutrition; medication use; and various acute and chronic diseases can all influence endocrine function, particularly in the elderly. This helps explain how drug toxicity occurs with relative ease in the elderly, as well as those with renal and liver disease. It also explains the need for control of polypharmacy, careful dosing, and conscientious monitoring of drug regimens in the elderly.

20 Thyroid

Thyroid Gland

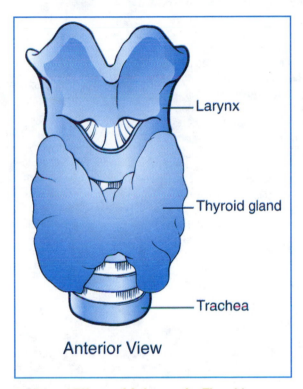

Larynx

Thyroid gland

Trachea

Anterior View

Additional Effects of Aging on the Thyroid
- Decrease in serum T_3
- Decrease in calcitonin
- Decrease in production and clearance of T_3 and T_4

Pathophysiology

The thyroid gland contains follicular and nonfollicular cells. The thyroid gland produces thyroxine (T_4) and triiodothyronine (T_3), which control metabolism, and calcitonin, which lowers serum calcium levels by opposing bone resorption (inhibition of osteoclastic activity). The follicular cells synthesize and secrete some of the thyroid hormones, and the nonfollicular cells (C cells) secrete various polypeptides including calcitonin, which is also called *thyrocalcitonin*. The metabolic effects of calcitonin excess and deficiency are not well understood and continue to be studied. The follicular cells also contain a gelatinous substance called *thyroglobulin*. If iodine, which is necessary for the formation of T_4 and T_3, is deficient, inadequate amounts of T_4 and T_3 are produced. If the thyroid does

20: THYROID 79

not produce enough hormone to inhibit thyroid-stimulating hormone (TSH), the thyroid will produce additional thyroglobulin, which is not affected by iodine, in an effort to increase circulating levels of thyroid hormone. This results in hypertrophy of the thyroid gland known as *goiter*. An enlarged thyroid gland can occur with either hypothyroidism or hyperthyroidism although it is not necessarily indicative of thyroid dysfunction. If the thyroid is enlarged but not associated with identifiable clinical manifestations, it is referred to as a *nontoxic goiter*. Thyroid nodules may result from malignancy (usually solitary) or may be benign (often multiple).

TSH is synthesized and stored in the anterior pituitary. Once released, it binds to receptors located on cell membranes of the thyroid gland. This causes a release of stored thyroid hormones, increases iodine uptake and oxidation, increases thyroid hormone syntheses, and increases the synthesis and secretion of prostaglandins by the thyroid. Thyroid hormone is regulated through a negative feedback loop involving the hypothalamus, anterior pituitary, and thyroid gland. Thyrotropin-releasing hormone (TRH) is synthesized and stored in the hypothalamus. It is released and travels to the anterior pituitary through vascular channels where it stimulates the release of TSH. Thyroid hormones, thus produced, have a negative feedback effect and inhibit TRH and TSH, which in turn decreases thyroid hormone synthesis and secretion. Normally, the thyroid gland produces 90% of T_4 and 10% of T_3. T_4 is converted to T_3 in body tissues; it is T_3 that has the greatest metabolic effect. Ninety percent of these hormones are bound to protein for transport to body tissue. T_4 and T_3 have a diurnal variation that peaks in the late evening. Their secretion is influenced by gender, pregnancy, nutrition, and levels of selected hormones or chemicals. TRH is increased with exposure to cold, stress, and decreased levels of T_4.

In addition to TSH, the thyroid gland is also stimulated to produce thyroid hormone by low iodide levels and by drugs that interfere with uptake of iodide. Because there is a high concentration gradient of iodine between the thyroid gland and the blood, iodide is moved into the follicular cells of the gland via active transport. There it is oxidized to iodine. A glucoprotein, thyroglobulin, is also necessary for the formation of the T_3 and T_4.

The thyroid hormones regulate protein, fat, and carbohydrate metabolism; metabolic rate; and, therefore, the production of body heat. Because of its influence on cellular function, thyroid hormones play a role in the function of other body systems (e.g., cardiac, respiratory, gastrointestinal, musculoskeletal, humoral, and neurological). They also influence growth and development and the effectiveness of growth hormone. In the United States iodine is added to salt and flour so iodine deficiency is less common here than in some other countries.

Effects of Aging

Atrophy and fibrosis with nodule formation and an increase in inflammatory infiltrates are normal changes in the thyroid gland due to aging. Because of the multiple factors that can affect endocrine function in the elderly, it is difficult to determine how much of an effect the changes in the gland itself have on the physiological function of the thyroid. However, research seems to indicate that there is a decrease in T_4 secretion and turnover, a decline in serum T_3 levels, an increase in hypothyroidism, variation in TSH secretion, and decreased responsiveness of plasma TSH concentrations to exogenous TRH administration, particularly in men.

Hypothyroidism

In *primary hypothyroidism*, decreased thyroid hormone levels cause an increase in TSH levels, resulting in hypertrophy of the thyroid or goiter. *Secondary hypothyroidism* is most commonly caused by failure of the pituitary to produce sufficient TSH. Hypothyroidism is caused by a deficiency in thyroid hormone and may be classified as congenital or acquired as well as primary or secondary. The most common cause of acquired, primary hypothyroidism is Hashimoto's thyroiditis or autoimmune thyroiditis, in which antibodies destroy thyroid tissue. Infiltration of lymphocytes contributes to enlargement of the gland and often nodules. Cellular destruction caused by inflammation can initially release large amounts of T_4 and T_3. Ultimately, however, hormone production is decreased, causing increased secretion of TSH by the anterior pituitary in an effort to increase the amount of circulating thyroid hormone. As the disease progresses, the thyroid gland atrophies and becomes fibrotic and hypothyroidism results. Anemia is often associated with hypothyroidism due to a decrease in erythropoiesis.

Hyperthyroidism

Thyrotoxicosis is a broad term that may be assigned to any condition resulting in excess thyroid hormone regardless of cause. Iatrogenic thyrotoxicosis can be caused by ingestion of excessive thyroid hormone or iodine preparations. Hyperthyroidism is a form of thyrotoxicosis in which excess hormones are secreted by the thyroid gland. It can be caused by increased synthesis and secretion of T_4 and T_3; follicular cell destruction, which causes a release of stored T_4 and T_3; or thyroid cancer. Stimulation of thyrotropin receptors by TSH or stimulation of thyrotropin receptor antibodies (TRAb) can also result in elevated T_4 and T_3 levels. Stimulation of thyrotropin receptors by TRAb is the mechanism underlying Graves' disease, the most common cause of hyperthyroidism. Graves' disease is an autoimmune process in which the negative feedback mechanism is ineffective in lowering circulating levels of thyroid hormone. It is often triggered by stress or viral infections. It is reported that thyroid autoantibodies are found in more than 95% of subjects with Graves' disease. Immunoglobulins bind to TSH receptors, ultimately causing thyroid hypertrophy. This condition is more common in women and increases with puberty, pregnancy, and menopause. Ocular manifestations are associated with sympathetic nervous system hyperactivity and infiltrative changes involving the orbital contents with associated enlargement of orbital muscles. Arrhythmias are commonly associated with hyperthyroidism. There is also increased cardiovascular and metabolic sensitivity to catecholamines. This is most likely due to an increase in the number and reactivity of beta and alpha adrenergic receptors.

Enlargement of the thyroid from an increased number of follicular cells is normal during puberty, pregnancy, or with some infectious disorders and is a compensatory mechanism. If the gland does not revert to its normal size when the need for excess thyroid hormone subsides, hyperthyroidism may result and is often referred to as *toxic multinodular goiter*. Thyrotoxic crisis is rare but can be fatal if not treated within 48 hours. It occurs most commonly in undiagnosed persons, following thyroid surgery, or in those under extreme physical or emotional stress.

Management

The goal of management is to produce an euthyroid state. Once treatment is begun, the goiter usually regresses. Primary *hypothyroidism* is ordinarily treated with oral medications. If the deficiency is caused by a nonthyroid disorder, that condition needs to be managed. Thyroid replacement doses in the elderly should be lower than those in other adults, ordinarily starting at no more than one half of the normal adult dose with adjustments being made as indicated. It is thought that peripheral metabolism of thyroid hormone decreases with age. Signs of thyroid disease are less easy to detect in the elderly. Extreme care must be taken in treating those with angina or myocardial infarction. Early detection and treatment of congenital hypothyroidism is essential for normal central nervous system development and to prevent mental retardation. With *hyperthyroidism*, treatment consists of the use of antithyroid medications and perhaps B adrenergic antagonists to reduce cardiovascular insult. Although the size of the goiter may decrease with treatment, exophthalmos ordinarily does not. Long-term treatment (18 months) is necessary and frequent monitoring is important. Relapse after treatment may occur. Radioactive iodine is the treatment of choice for most adults and is often used for ablation. Treatment commonly results in hypothyroidism, which then requires life long management. Surgical removal increases the risk of secondary hypoparathyroidism and is less commonly used. *Thyroid storm* is a life-threatening form of thyrotoxicosis and must be treated promptly and aggressively.

21 Parathyroid

Primary Diagnostic Tests for Parathyroid Conditions
Parathyroid hormone (PTH), Ca, PO_4, HCO_3, Mg, Cl, pH, UA for Ca, x-ray/bone density, cAMP (cyclic adenosine monophosphate levels), 1 to 25 vitamin D levels

Causes of Hyperparathyroidism
- Chronic renal failure
- Familial tendency
- Dietary deficiencies in vitamin D and calcium
- Malabsorption of vitamin D and calcium
- Certain drugs (e.g., phenytoin, laxatives, phenobarbital)

Physical Examination Signs
- Chvostek's sign—Ipsilateral contraction of facial muscles elicited by tapping facial nerve anterior to the ear.
- Trousseau's sign—Carpal spasm related to ischemia of nerves in upper arm during inflation of blood pressure cuff (wait 3 to 5 minutes) above systolic pressure.

Parathyroid Glands

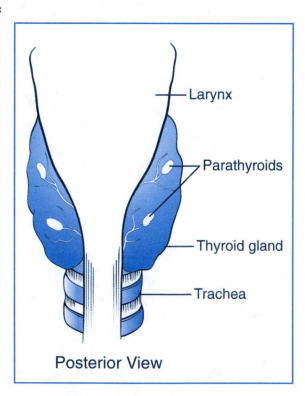

Larynx

Parathyroids

Thyroid gland

Trachea

Posterior View

Pathophysiology

The parathyroid glands are located behind the upper and lower poles of the thyroid. There are commonly four, although the range can be from two to six. The parathyroid glands produce parathyroid hormone (PTH), which maintains calcium homeostasis. PTH is primarily regulated by the serum level of ionized calcium. If serum calcium is low, PTH is released. If it is high, PTH is suppressed. PTH is not part of the hypothalamic-pituitary feedback mechanism, so marked increases or decreases can have severe consequences. Magnesium and phosphate levels also influence PTH secretion (e.g., hyperphosphatemia leads to hypocalcemia, which in turn influences PTH secretion). The relationship among these three minerals is complex. Calcitonin, produced by the thyroid, also plays a role in controlling serum calcium levels by increasing bone formation by osteoblasts and decreasing bone breakdown by osteoclasts. Its effect is to decrease serum calcium levels and conserve bone matrix.

PTH is the most important hormone in the regulation of serum calcium levels. It is secreted in response to lowered serum calcium levels and acts directly on bone (the body's primary reservoir of calcium) and on the kidneys. PTH causes bone resorption (i.e., breakdown), thereby increasing serum calcium levels. If PTH release is chronically stimulated, it results in bone remodeling. PTH also acts in the proximal and distal tubules of the kidneys to increase reabsorption of calcium and decrease reabsorption of phosphorus. In addition, it influences tubular reabsorption of bicarbonate and stimulates the synthesis of biologically active vitamin D. Vitamin D facilitates calcium and phosphorus transport through the intestinal wall.

Effects of Aging

With aging, the level of parathyroid hormone increases. In addition, intestinal adaptation to variations in calcium intake is reduced, leading to a decrease in intestinal absorption. There may also be a defective renal response to decreased calcium intake and decreased levels of circulating vitamin D. Dietary intake of calcium also tends to decrease with aging. All of these factors may contribute to changes in calcium metabolism apparent in the elderly, although there is insufficient evidence to explain the changes more fully.

Hyperparathyroidism

Hyperparathyroidism is a consequence of increased secretion of PTH and is classified as either *primary* or *secondary*. In primary hyperparathyroidism, the normal feedback mechanism fails to inhibit PTH secretion in response to elevated serum levels of ionized calcium. Primary hyperparathyroidism is usually due to adenoma but can also be due to cancer or hyperplasia. Decreased synthesis of vitamin D and renal phosphate retention promote hyperplasia of the parathyroid gland and, therefore, increased secretion and synthesis of parathyroid hormone. Secondary hyperparathyroidism is caused by an increase in PTH secondary to a chronic disease or condition that causes hypocalcemia. For example, in chronic renal failure, hypocalcemia stimulates PTH secretion as well as renal and gastrointestinal calcium absorption, which ultimately leads to hyperparathyroidism (as the parathyroid responds to increased demand for hormone) and hypercalcemia. Bone turnover is accelerated in hyperparathyroidism. Hypercalcemia affects many body systems because of the role it plays in cellular/tissue function throughout the body. For example, bone resorption puts one at risk for fractures; hypercalcemia can produce renal calculi and cause metabolic acidosis because it alters renal tubular function. Chronic hypercalcemia is also associated with insulin resistance. Extreme levels of hypercalcemia are rarely of parathyroid origin; rather, they are associated with ectopic sources from elsewhere in the body (e.g., metastatic tumors). Mild hyperparathyroidism may be asymptomatic and discovered through routine blood chemistries. It predisposes one to fractures and renal stones.

Hypoparathyroidism

Hypoparathyroidism is the result of decreased secretion of PTH that can be because of decreased tissue responsiveness, autoimmune destruction, or, more commonly, damage to the parathyroid glands during surgery. It can also be a consequence of hypomagnesemia associated with a variety of chronic illnesses or drugs. Lack of circulating PTH depresses serum calcium levels, increases phosphate levels, and impairs calcium resorption from bone. The most serious consequence of hypocalcemia is lowering of the threshold for neuromuscular excitation. Therefore, neuromuscular irritability, spasm, hyperreflexia, and convulsions may occur. Phosphate retention also impairs vitamin D conversion to its active form, which further exacerbates depression of serum calcium levels. In primary hypoparathyroidism, calcium levels are decreased and phosphate levels are increased, while PTH levels are usually normal.

Management

The goal of management in hyperparathyroidism is to reduce hypercalcemia through the use of hydration, diuretics, and other drugs that decrease resorption of bone. Definitive treatment is surgical excision of hyperplastic glands. In hypoparathyroidism, vitamin D and calcium replacements (1 to 3 gm) are prescribed. Drugs to decrease phosphate absorption from the gastrointestinal tract are used if phosphate levels are significantly elevated.

22 Adrenal Physiology

Additional Actions/Effects of Glucocorticoids

Gluconeogenesis
Increased appetite
Increased fat deposition
Decreased growth hormone
Melanocyte stimulation

Increased circulating red blood cells
Mood changes
Increased uric acid secretion
Decreased serum calcium levels
Decreased secretion/synthesis of adrenocorticotropic hormone (ACTH)

Additional Stimuli to Adrenal Medullary Secretion

Hypoglycemia
Hypercapnia
Hemorrhage
Nicotine
Histamine

Hypoxia
Acidosis
Glucagon
Pilocarpine
Angiotensin II

Common Diagnostic Tests

Radioimmunoassay (RIA)
Dexamethasone suppression test
Complete blood count
Serum and urinary electrolytes/hormones

Urine catecholamines
CT scan
Blood chemistry
Enzyme-linked immunosorbent assays (ELISAs)

Signs and Symptoms of Hypercorticalism

Weight gain
Truncal obesity
Glucose intolerance
Polyuria
Pathologic fractures
Kyphosis
Capillary fragility
Hyperpigmentation
Poor wound healing
Increased susceptibility to infection
Altered mental status
Hirsutism

"Moonface"
Glycogenesis
Gluconeogenesis
Overt diabetes mellitus
Weakness
Renal stones
Ecchymosis
Vasoconstriction
Fungal infections
Emotional lability
Psychosis
Acne

"Buffalo hump"
Sodium and water retention
Insulin resistance
Protein/muscle wasting
Osteoporosis
Thinning of skin
Purple striae
Hypertension
Decreased immune response
Euphoria
Menstrual irregularities

The adrenal glands are composed of two parts: the outer part called the *cortex* and the inner part called the *medulla*. The cortex comprises 80% of the gland and secretes several steroid hormones: the mineralocorticoids (e.g., aldosterone), androgens, and glucocorticoids (e.g., cortisol). The medulla makes up the remaining volume (20%) and secretes epinephrine, norepinephrine, and dopamine and is enervated by the parasympathetic and sympathetic nervous systems. The hormones of the adrenal cortex are synthesized from cholesterol. Most corticosteroids (steroids) are produced in response to stimulation of the cortex by adrenocorticotropic hormone (ACTH) from the anterior pituitary, which in turn is stimulated by corticotropin-releasing hormone (CRH) in the hypothalamus. The secretion of ACTH is regulated by negative feedback (i.e., high levels of cortisol or exogenous glucocorticoids suppress CRH and ACTH). Secretion peaks 3 to 5 hours after sleep begins and declines throughout the day (i.e., diurnal rhythm). ACTH secretion and consequently cortisol levels are also increased due to stress. In addition, the adrenals produce small amounts of androgens that are converted in peripheral tissues to estrogen and testosterone.

The *glucocorticoids* (e.g., cortisol) have metabolic, anti-inflammatory, and growth suppressing effects as well as others. They increase blood glucose levels by promoting gluconeogenesis in the liver, decreasing cellular uptake of glucose, and stimulating protein catabolism and inhibiting protein synthesis. In addition they promote lipogenesis and increase blood cholesterol. They inhibit immune and inflammatory responses by suppressing the mediators of these responses and by depressing the action of lymphocytes and macrophages. The glucocorticoids produce a variety of additional effects because of the presence of receptors on extra-adrenal tissues. These are listed on p. 84. In addition, they potentiate the effects of catecholamines, thyroid hormone, and growth hormone on adipose tissue. Cortisol is necessary for maintenance of life and protection from stress.

Mineralocorticoids are those steroids that maintain normal salt and water balance by promoting sodium retention and potassium loss. *Aldosterone* is the most potent of these, and its primary role is to conserve sodium (Na) and increase the excretion of potassium (K) and hydrogen ions. Its synthesis and secretion are regulated primarily by the renin-angiotensin system (as opposed to ACTH control) in response to decreases in blood volume, renal circulation, and potassium levels. High levels of aldosterone may also result in alkalosis and hypokalemia.

The adrenal glands produce small amounts of *androgens*. Under normal circumstances, these play a minor role in the development and maintenance of secondary sex characteristics. The amount of estrogen converted peripherally from the androgens (i.e., androstenedione) is minimal and is physiologically unimportant; however, it becomes the major source of endogenous estrogen in postmenopausal women. Weak androgens are converted in peripheral tissues to stronger ones such as testosterone and thus have some androgenic effect. Certain conditions (e.g., obesity, aging), however, increase peripheral conversion, leading to more obvious effects (e.g., hirsutism).

The *catecholamines* (e.g., epinephrine [adrenaline] and norepinephrine) are the main products secreted by the adrenal medulla. Epinephrine comprises approximately 75% to 85% of catecholamines secreted by the adrenal medulla. Epinephrine is significantly more potent than norepinephrine in producing direct metabolic effects. The catecholamines are synthesized from the amino acid phenylalanine. Their secretion is increased by ACTH and the glucocorticoids and is effected by a variety of other stimuli (see p. 84). Catecholamines bind to receptors throughout the body, accounting for the widespread effects of their secretion in response to stressors and in the well-known "fight or flight" response.

Effects of Aging

Metabolic clearance of cortisol decreases because of declines in liver and kidney function. There is also a decrease in the amount of cortisol used by the body as a function of the decrease in lean body mass associated with aging. Diurnal variations and feedback mechanisms remain intact. Adrenal androgens decrease to 50% to 75% of young adult levels.

Adrenal Dysfunction

Hyperfunction of the adrenals can result in *Cushing's syndrome or disease* (i.e., too much cortisol), virilization/feminization (e.g., androgens and estrogen), and hyperaldosteronism (e.g., aldosterone). *Hypofunction* leads to *Addison's disease*.

Cushing's Syndrome/Disease

Cushing's syndrome is due to excess circulating cortisol from adrenal cortical disease or exogenous steroid administration, while Cushing's disease is caused by excessive secretion of ACTH by the anterior pituitary. Cushing's disease is more common in adults and in females. Cushing's syndrome is more common in adults between the ages of 30 to 50 and elderly adults, particularly men. Adrenal tumors are more common in children.

Hypercortisolism is usually caused by Cushing's disease (75% to 80%) but may also result from ACTH or cortisol-secreting tumors. Most persons with Cushing's disease have a pituitary microadenoma and a loss of normal feedback mechanisms to control CRH and ACTH secretion. A variety of ectopic tumors can produce CRH and ACTH that are not effected by the normal feedback mechanisms. Cortisol from cortisol-secreting tumors suppresses CRH and ACTH, leading to atrophy of normal adrenal cortical tissue. With these conditions diurnal activity is lost as is the body's ability to increase ACTH and cortisol production under stress.

Hypocorticalism, or adrenal insufficiency, involves either inadequate stimulation of the adrenal glands by CRH and ACTH (i.e., secondary hypocorticalism) or inability of the adrenals to produce and secrete adrenocortical hormone (i.e., primary hypocorticalism), also known as *Addison's disease*. Idiopathic or organ specific autoimmune causation is most common. More than 90% of adrenal tissue must be destroyed before manifestations become evident. Addison's disease is often associated with other autoimmune disorders, and a genetic predisposition is suggested in come cases. Secondary hypocorticalism is due to low levels of ACTH from a variety of disorders or exogenous administration of glucocorticoids. Abrupt withdrawal of these medications can be life threatening. Manifestations involve a number of body systems; hypoglycemia, hyperkalemia, hypotension, and possibly hyperpigmentation will be most evident. Acute adrenal insufficiency is an emergency.

Management

Treatment is essential. It is directly related to the cause and can include drugs, radiation, and/or surgery.

Hyperaldosteronism

Hyperaldosteronism can be caused by either a *primary* adrenal disorder (i.e., adrenal tumor) or extra-adrenal stimulation, a *secondary* adrenal disorder (i.e., extra-adrenal stimulation [e.g., excessive angiotensin II]). Pathophysiologic alterations are manifestations of fluid and electrolyte changes, which include Na and H_2O retention, hypokalemia, hypokalemic alkalosis, and hypertension.

Hypersecretion of Androgens

Hypersecretion of adrenal androgens can be caused by a tumor, Cushing's syndrome, or other pathology. Manifestations (e.g., feminization, virilization, early sexual development, and bone aging) depend upon age, gender, and which hormone is secreted.

Management

The goal of management of these disorders is to normalize hormone levels. This is accomplished by surgery or drugs, depending upon the particular disease and its cause. Sometimes dietary modification is indicated.

Adrenal Medulla Disorders

The adrenal medulla secretes two important catecholamines—epinephrine and norepinephrine. These hormones bind to receptors in the sympathetic nervous system to prolong and enhance the effects of sympathetic stimulation. *Hypofunction* of the adrenal medulla does not produce any known physiologic problems. *Hyperfunction*, however, can be life threatening. *Pheochromocytoma* (an uncommon disorder) is caused by an adrenal medullary tumor that primarily produces norepinephrine. Manifestations are those associated with sustained catecholamine release (i.e., persistent hypertension, tachycardia, headaches, diaphoresis, hypermetabolism, glucose intolerance, palpitations, etc.).

Management

The usual management is surgical excision with medications being used to stabilize the patient preoperatively, as well as to normalize hormone levels if needed postoperatively.

23 Diabetes Mellitus

Comparison of Type I and Type II Diabetes Mellitus

I. Type 1 (Juvenile Diabetes Mellitus [DM]; Ketosis Prone)
  A. Etiology
    1. Genetic susceptibility (HLA-DR3)
    2. Environmental exposure to virus/infection leading to immune destruction of beta cells
    3. Family history of autoimmune disease
    4. Islet cells antibodies
    5. Insulin antibodies
    6. Absence of C peptide
    7. Ten percent of DM, <20 years old and of European ancestry
  B. Manifestations
    1. Symptomatic
      a. Onset is usually sudden and severe
      b. Early stage—Polyuria, polydipsia, polyphagia; weight loss; normal or increased appetite; blurred vision; fatigue/weakness; nausea/vomiting; vaginal itch, infection; skin rashes; ketones in blood/urine
      c. Advanced disease (long-term complications)—Loss of appetite, bloating; dehydration; diabetic ketoacidosis (DKA); neurogenic/microvascular paresthesias, visual impairment, constipation, nocturnal diarrhea, nocturia, neurogenic bladder, impotence, nephropathy, foot deformity, silent myocardial infarction (MI), cold extremities
    2. Physical Examination
      a. Early—Thin, decreased weight; ill appearance; orthostatic hypotension
      b. Advanced disease—Skin ulcers, "shin spots," hair loss; poor eyes: retinopathy, cataracts, glaucoma; cardiovascular: cool, pale extremities, diminished peripheral pulses, decreased capillary refill, pretibial edema; neurological: sensory loss, absent reflexes, deficits of extraocular movement
II. Type II (Adult Onset; Ketosis Resistant)
  A. Etiology
    1. Strong genetic link-familial pattern
    2. Insulin resistance, decreased insulin receptors in target cells
    3. Postreceptor defect impairing glucose uptake into cells
    4. Insulin resistance>, hyperinsulinemia> diminished insulin production
    5. Relationship to obesity, unknown genetic link, or increased demand
    6. Eighty percent to 90% of DM, >40 years old, overweight, sedentary, family history
  B. Manifestations
    1. Symptomatic
      a. Onset is usually insidious
      b. Early stage—Polyuria, polydipsia, polyphagia; blurred vision; fatigue; sores that heal slowly; recurrent infections (vaginal *Monilia*, urinary tract infections [UTIs], furuncles, poor dentition); and spontaneous abortion
      c. Advanced disease (long-term complications)—Similar to Type 1 but macrovascular problems are more prominent; dyslipidemia, atherosclerosis; hypertension; arterial insufficiency; coronary artery disease; and hyperosmolar hyperglycemic nonketotic coma

(continued on p. 89)

Overview

Diabetes mellitus (DM) is a group of heterogeneous disorders characterized by abnormalities in glucose homeostasis, resulting in chronic hyperglycemia. Hyperglycemia is caused by a decrease in the secretion or activity of insulin. The insulin alteration results in disordered metabolism of carbohydrates, fats, and proteins, which may lead to acute, life-threatening complications or chronic complications including vascular and neurological deficits.

DM affects 16 million Americans (6%) with one third undiagnosed. The number is expected to double in the next decade. African Americans, Hispanics, and Native Americans are particularly vulnerable to the disease and its complications. It is the seventh leading cause of death in the United States and is a significant contributing factor to deaths from other causes. Life expectancy is reduced by about 15 years and the quality of life is impacted. It is the leading cause of end-stage renal disease, blindness, and nontraumatic lower extremity amputations. Approximately 80% of diabetics have cardiovascular complications. The economic cost is estimated to be $102 billion per year.

The American Diabetes Association identifies four types of DM: Type I (absolute insulin deficiency, ketosis prone), Type II (insulin resistant, nonketosis prone), gestational (glucose intolerance first recognized during pregnancy, usually the third trimester), and "other specific types" (due to less common secondary conditions such as pancreatic disorders, drug related).

Pathophysiology

Type I DM accounts for approximately 10% of the cases with a higher incidence among Caucasians, a 10% to 13% incidence among first degree relatives, a peak incidence at age 12, and more cases reported during autumn and winter.

Two distinct types of Type I have been identified: immune mediated Type I (more common in Caucasians) and nonimmune/idiopathic Type I (more common in African and Asian Americans). In immune mediated Type I DM, genetic and environmental factors have been implicated in cell mediated pancreatic beta cell destruction with autoantibodies found in 85% to 90% of individuals. Studies indicate that there is a long preclinical period when autoantibodies are detectable before the abrupt onset of clinical manifestations when 80% to 90% of the beta cells are destroyed, resulting in an insulin deficit. C peptide, which is formed in the process of converting proinsulin to insulin, can be measured in the blood and used as an indicator of the level of functioning beta cells. Type I DM is associated with HLA-DR3 and HLA-DR4 antigens, suggesting a genetic susceptibility to environmental factors, such as drugs and chemicals, viruses, and nutritional factors in the etiology. Nonimmune Type I DM has no identified etiology.

Carbohydrate, fat, and protein metabolism are affected by the lack of insulin and relative excess of glucagon. As a result, insulin mediated glucose uptake by hepatic and skeletal muscle cells is disrupted, thus glucose accumulates in the blood and spills into the urine when the renal threshold is exceeded. Breakdown of fats and protein leads to weight loss and also to high circulating levels of ketones and metabolic acidosis. The metabolic disruption may also cause cardiovascular and neurological problems.

Type II DM accounts for 90% of the cases with the highest percentage among African Americans, Hispanics, and Native Americans. It mainly affects individuals over age 40 and those who are obese. The etiology of Type II DM is unknown. Genetic factors interact with environmental factors to affect both insulin action and secretion. Abdominal obesity and high intake of calories and fats are the strongest risk factors and are associated with insulin resistance. It appears that there are two genetic loci involved: one for obesity and one for insulin resistance. The mechanism for insulin resistance is related to defects in insulin receptors, glucose transport mechanisms, and enzymes involved in postreceptor activities in skeletal muscle and hepatic and adipose tissue (see p. 87). The sequence of progression of the disorder begins with the inability of the skeletal muscle cells to take up glucose, especially after meals, resulting in mainly postprandial hyperglycemia. The pancreas may secrete more insulin to counteract the hyperglycemia, causing hyperinsulinemia. The hyperglycemia appears to have a toxic affect on the pancreatic beta cells, which then results in a decrease secretion of insulin as the disease progresses.

Abnormal secretion of glucagon has also been demonstrated. Insulin no longer suppresses hepatic gluconeogenesis and glycogenolysis, thus, in addition to postprandial hyperglycemia, fasting blood glucose, HgbA1c, triglycerides, and possibly ketones rise later in the disease.

Manifestations

DM is diagnosed based on random and fasting blood glucose levels and symptoms. Four clinical stages of glucose tolerance have been identified and are delineated on p. 89: normoglycemic, impaired glucose tolerance, impaired fasting glucose, and diabetes. Patients may be diagnosed while asymptomatic, with early symptoms, with chronic complications established, or at the time of an acute life-threatening complication.

The hypertonicity of the blood that results from the hyperglycemia causes some of the symptoms such as polyuria, polydipsia, temporary blurred vision, and dehydration and later acute complications such as hypovolemia, shock, and hyperglycemic hypertonic nonketotic syndrome (HHNKS). Hyperglycemia and ketogenesis can be aggravated by counterregulatory hormones such as catecholamines, cortisol, growth

2. Physical Examination
    a. Early—Usually obese; hypertension
    b. Advanced disease—Similar to Type I

Criteria for Diagnosis of Diabetes

Diabetes Mellitus

- A fasting plasma glucose (FPG) >126 mg/dl on more than one occasion, a random PG of >200 with symptoms, or a PG value in the 2 hour sample (2hPG) of the standard oral glucose tolerance test (OGTT) of >200 mg/dl PG

Impaired Fasting Plasma Glucose (IPFG)

- A fasting plasma glucose of 110 to 125 mg/dl

Impaired Glucose Tolerance (IGT)

- A 2hPG on standard OGTT of 140 to 199 mg/dl

Normoglycemia

- FPG <110 mg/dl, random PG <140 mg/dl, or 2hPG on standard OGTT <140 mg/dl

Note: Individuals with IGT and IFPG are at increased risk for progressing to diabetes mellitus.

Normal Actions of Insulin

- Facilitates glucose transport into cells (except neurons and hepatic cells)
- Facilitates glycogenesis (i.e., the synthesis of glycogen from glucose for storage in liver and skeletal muscles)
- Facilitates lipogenesis (i.e., the storage of excessive glucose as lipid in adipose tissue)
- Inhibits glycogenolysis (i.e., the breakdown of glycogen stores that is facilitated by glucagon and epinephrine)
- Inhibits gluconeogenesis (i.e., the formation of glucose from breakdown of protein and lipids that is facilitated by cortisol and glucagon)

Hyperglycemic Hypertonic Nonketotic Syndrome (HHNK) versus Diabetic Ketoacidosis (DKA)

HHNK

- Severe hyperglycemia
- Severe osmotic diuresis
- Severe hypovolemia (tachycardia, hypotension, shock)
- Severe dehydration (dry mucous membranes, poor turgor)
- Oliguria/anuria
- Neurological abnormalities (altered sensorium, somnolence, coma, seizures, paresis, aphasia)
- Lactic acidosis
- Minimal or absent ketosis

DKA

- Hyperglycemia (polyuria, polydipsia, blurred vision)
- Dehydration/hypovolemia (weakness, tachycardia, hypotension)
- Ketoacidosis (acetone breath, Kussmaul's breathing [deep/rapid], nausea, vomiting, abdominal pain)
- Headache

hormone, and glucagon (which may be released in situations of stress/infection/trauma), resulting in another acute complication, diabetic ketoacidosis (DKA). While DKA is more prevalent in Type I DM because of the absolute insulin deficit and relative excess glucagon, HHNKS is more prevalent in Type II DM because of the profound hyperglycemia that can result (see above).

In addition to the acute problems, chronic problems (i.e., neuropathies, macrovascular, and microvascular problems) can result and are commonly present for years prior to diagnosis. Neuropathies are the most common chronic complications of DM and are relevant in both types of DM. They are thought to result from a combination of metabolic, genetic, and environmental factors and result in problems with motor (e.g., Charcot's joints, foot drop), sensory (e.g., painful paresthesias, silent MI), and autonomic dysfunction (e.g., orthostatic hypotension, gastroparesis, diabetic diarrhea, bladder atony, impotence). Macrovascular problems result from premature atherosclerosis. Hyperglycemia, dyslipidemias (high triglycerides [TGs], oxidized low density lipoproteins [LDLs], and low high density lipoproteins [HDLs]), and glycation end products damage vascular endothelium, stimulate smooth muscle proliferation, and increase lipid deposits in plaque. Macrovascular problems lead to hypertension, coronary artery disease (most common cause of death in Type II diabetics, also common in Type I), stroke, and peripheral vascular disease.

Microvascular disorders result from a thickening of the basement membrane of the capillaries, resulting in ischemia and hypoxia of tissues. Two areas often affected are the eyes and kidneys. Retinopathy develops more readily in Type II DM and can lead to retinal detachment and progressive loss of vision. Diabetic nephropathy develops in 30% of Type I diabetics and 5% to 10% in Type II diabetics. The exact mechanism that results in glomerulosclerosis is unknown. Proteinuria is a reliable sign of renal damage.

The neurological and vascular problems contribute to increased risk of infection throughout the body (e.g., skin, bladder, gingiva). Neurological deficits prevent awareness of skin breaks; vascular deficits prevent delivery of defensive cells and oxygen; diminished protein synthesis reduces healing; and elevated glucose provides source of nutrition for pathogens, and white blood cells are abnormal in DM.

Treatment

The main goals of diabetic treatment focus on normalization of blood sugar and prevention of acute and chronic complications. Controlling hypertension and dyslipidemias are essential aspects of a treatment plan. Dietary measures, exercise, and weight management are part of all treatment regimens. Endogenous insulin is required to sustain life in Type I diabetics. Type II diabetics may be managed with diet and exercise alone, oral hypoglycemic agents (OHAs), and/or insulin. OHAs may act by diminishing intestinal absorption of glucose, increasing insulin sensitivity, decreasing insulin resistance, or increasing pancreatic insulin. Areas of research include genetic engineering, stem cell research, and beta cell/islet cells transplantation.

1. The sensitivity of a target cell to a circulating hormone is a result of what?

(A) The number of receptors for that hormone

(B) The amount of hormone in the blood

(C) The amount of bound hormone in the blood

(D) The percentage of body fat

2. Which of the following is an example of an iatrogenic endocrine disorder?

(A) Graves' disease

(B) Cushingoid syndrome from exogenous glucocorticoids

(C) Ectopic hormone production by a malignant tumor

(D) Addison's disease

3. If thyroxine levels are too high, the anterior pituitary produces less TSH. What is this an example of?

(A) Positive feedback

(B) Negative feedback

(C) Facilitated diffusion

(D) Pituitary dysfunction

4. Aging affects endocrine physiology. With aging, there may be:

(A) Increased sensitivity of target organs

(B) Increased receptor binding

(C) Glandular structural changes

(D) Decreased amount of connective tissue

5. Increases in parathyroid hormone levels result in which of the following?

(A) Bone catabolism

(B) Bone deposition

(C) Renal excretion of calcium

(D) Renal reabsorption of phosphorus

6. Hyperparathyroidism puts one at risk for what?

(A) Hypothyroidism

(B) Hypertension

(C) Fractures

(D) Gingivitis

7. Which hormone from the parathyroid gland controls calcium homeostasis?

(A) Parathyroid hormone

(B) Calcitonin

(C) Thyroid hormone

(D) Parathyroid-releasing hormone

8. What is the most common cause of hyperparathyroidism?

(A) Graves' disease

(B) Adenoma of the parathyroid

(C) Hashimoto's disease

(D) Surgical excision of the parathyroids

9. What measure has been taken in the United States to help prevent dietary deficiencies that lead to thyroid dysfunction?

(A) Adding vitamin B to flour

(B) Adding calcium to orange juice

(C) Adding iodine to salt

(D) Adding vitamin D to milk

10. Because of the thyroid's role in metabolic function, which of the following manifestations would you expect in someone with hyperthyroidism?

(A) Lethargy

(B) Decreased appetite

(C) Weight gain

(D) Heat intolerance

11. The thyroid gland produces all of the following except:

(A) T_3

(B) T_4

(C) Calcitonin

(D) TSH

12. All of the following are normal changes in the thyroid gland with aging except:

(A) Atrophy

(B) An increased risk of malignant changes

(C) Fibrosis

(D) An increase in inflammatory infiltrates

13. When does cortisol secretion peak?

(A) In the morning

(B) In the late afternoon

(C) In the evening

(D) During the night

14. Your patient is on long-term glucocorticoid treatments. All of the following are important for her to learn. Which is the most important?

(A) Do not stop taking the drug abruptly

(B) Take the medication with food

(C) Monitor cuts for healing

(D) Contact her primary care provider if she has signs of infection

15. Which of the following is the correct sequence of events in glucocorticoid (cortisol) production?

(A) ACTH-CRH-cortisol

(B) CRH-cortisol-ACTH

(C) CRH-ACTH-cortisol

(D) Cortisol-CRH-ACTH

16. What is an uncommon but potentially life-threatening disorder of the adrenal medulla?

(A) Addison's disease

(B) Pheochromocytoma

(C) Cushing's disease

(D) Hyperaldosteronism

17. Which of the following insulin functions is lost in diabetes mellitus?

(A) Insulin facilitated breakdown of protein

(B) Insulin facilitated uptake of glucose by the hepatic and skeletal muscle cells

(C) Insulin facilitated breakdown of adipose tissue

(D) Insulin facilitated excretion of glucose by the kidneys

18. Which of the following characteristics more commonly applies to Type I diabetes, differentiating it from Type II?

(A) Stronger genetic component

(B) More common in obese individuals

(C) Greater tendency for ketosis

(D) More common in older individuals

19. Which of the following individuals would be diagnosed with diabetes mellitus?

(A) Individual 1 with a fasting plasma glucose of 126 mg/dl

(B) Individual 2 with a random plasma glucose above 200 and symptoms of diabetes

(C) Individual 3 with a random plasma glucose less than 140 mg/dl

(D) Individual 4 with a fasting plasma glucose between 110 mg/dl and 125 mg/dl

20. Which of the following is a complication of diabetes related to autonomic neurological dysfunction?

(A) Orthostatic hypotension

(B) Coronary artery disease

(C) Painful paresthesias of the lower extremities

(D) Renal failure/nephropathy

1. **The correct answer is A.**

Receptors are necessary for hormones to produce their effects on the target tissue. Choices B, C, and D all play a role in the action and effects of hormones but not sensitivity of the target cell.

2. **The correct answer is B.**

Iatrogenic disorders are those caused by medical care. The other choices are all diseases.

3. **The correct answer is B.**

Negative feedback is a process by which a substance secreted centrally (TSH) is reversed or decreased based upon feedback received from the periphery (thyroxine levels). Choices A, C, and D represent different processes/problems.

4. **The correct answer is C.**

This is the only change associated with aging among the options given.

5. **The correct answer is A.**

The main function of the parathyroid hormone is to maintain serum calcium levels by releasing stored calcium from the bone. Choices B, C, and D are related to bone metabolism in some way but not directly related to increases in parathyroid hormone.

6. **The correct answer is C.**

Hyperparathyroidism causes the release of calcium from bone into the blood, resulting in demineralization that puts one at risk for fractures. The other choices are not related to hyperparathyroidism.

7. **The correct answer is A.**

The other choices regulate other processes.

8. **The correct answer is B.**

This is the most common cause. Choices A and C are related to the thyroid. Choice D results in hypoparathyroidism.

9. **The correct answer is C.**

Iodine is necessary for the formation of thyroxine. The other nutritional additives do not relate to the thyroid.

10. **The correct answer is D.**

Heat intolerance is one of many manifestations of a hypermetabolic state. The others can be anticipated with hypothyroidism.

11. **The correct answer is D.**

TSH is produced by the anterior pituitary.

12. **The correct answer is B.**

Malignant changes are more likely in a younger population.

13. **The correct answer is D.**

Diurnal variation is an important consideration in understanding the pathophysiology of certain diseases and administration of selected medications. Choices A, B, and C are incorrect.

14. **The correct answer is A.**

Abrupt cessation of exogenous glucocorticoids can cause adrenal insufficiency due to iatrogenic adrenal atrophy that can be reversed by tapering the dose before discontinuing the drug. The other options are important but have less immediate life-threatening consequences.

15. **The correct answer is C.**

Corticotropin-releasing hormone from the hypothalamus stimulates adrenocorticotropic hormone from the pituitary which stimulates cortisol secretion from the adrenal cortex. The other options are not in the correct sequence.

16. **The correct answer is B.**

This is the best choice because it is most immediately life threatening. The others are chronic diseases and can usually be managed effectively. Choices A, C, and D are chronic problems not likely to be immediately life threatening if managed correctly.

17. **The correct answer is B.**

In diabetes, the relative or total lack of insulin prevents uptake of glucose by hepatic and skeletal muscle cells, thus leading to hyperglycemia (i.e., the accumulation of glucose in the blood). Without glucose for energy production, fats may be broken down, creating ketone bodies leading to acidosis. Insulin facilitates the synthesis, not breakdown, of protein, thus leading to problems of skin breakdown and poor tissue healing. Insulin facilitates the storage of fats in adipose tissue, not the breakdown. It is lack of insulin that leads to the breakdown of adipose tissue leading to serum lipid problems.

18. The correct answer is C.

Because of the absolute lack of insulin in Type I diabetes, glucose can't enter hepatic and skeletal muscle cells; therefore, fats are broken down for energy, leading to the creation of ketone bodies causing ketosis/metabolic acidosis. The other answers apply to Type II diabetes.

19. The correct answer is B.

A random plasma glucose of 200 mg/dl or above with symptoms of diabetes meets the criteria for a diagnosis of diabetes. Other criteria for the diagnosis of diabetes are a fasting plasma glucose of 126 mg/dl or above on two occasions or a plasma glucose value equal to or above 200 mg/dl in the 2 hour sample on a glucose tolerance test. A random plasma glucose of 140 mg/dl or less is normoglycemic. A fasting plasma glucose of 110 mg/dl to 125 mg/dl is considered impaired fasting plasma glucose (IPFG), represents an increased risk for diabetes and a need for lifestyle changes to prevent the onset of diabetes.

20. The correct answer is A.

Disruption of function of the sympathetic nerves in the lower extremities may lead to orthostatic hypotension. Other manifestations of autonomic dysfunction include gastroparesis, diabetic diarrhea, bladder atony, and impotence. Coronary artery disease is related to the macrovascular problems. Painful paresthesias are related to dysfunction of sensory nerves. Renal failure is due to microvascular problems.

PART VI

Respiratory System

Bernadette R. Madara, EdD, APRN-CS

24 Anatomy and Physiology of the Respiratory System

Laboratory Tests

Test	*Rationale*
Arterial blood gases	Evaluates acid-base balance
	Respiratory acidosis: Caused by respiratory depression or pulmonary disease—retention of carbon dioxide decreases pH below 7.35
	Kidneys compensate by increasing the production and retention of bicarbonate
	Respiratory alkalosis: Caused by hyperventilation—carbon dioxide rapidly exhaled, leading to a pH increase above 7.45
	Kidneys compensate by excreting bicarbonate
	Metabolic acidosis: Caused by increased production or retention of hydrogen ions as in shock, ketoacidosis, renal failure; pH decreases, bicarbonate decreases
	Lungs compensate by increasing ventilation rate
	Metabolic alkalosis: Caused by loss of hydrogen ions or ingestion of bicarbonate as in prolonged vomiting or bicarbonate overdose; pH increases, bicarbonate increases
	Lungs compensate by slow ventilation in order to retain carbon dioxide
Bronchoscopy	Allows for visualization of the larynx, trachea, and bronchi
	Local or general anesthesia or conscious sedation may be used
	Biopsies are collected to test for infection or cancer
	Aspirated foreign objects, such as peanuts, are removed
	Requires nothing by mouth (NPO) status until gag reflex returns
Pulmonary function tests	Measures the amount of air inhaled and exhaled during a normal breath (tidal volume: about 500 mL) and after maximum inspiration and/or expiration
	Abnormal readings signal pulmonary disease
	Effectiveness of bronchodilators is evaluated by comparing results before and after their use
Ventilation/perfusion scan (V/Q scan)	Perfusion of the pulmonary vessels is determined by injecting radiotagged albumin IV
	Pulmonary blood flow distributes the albumin
	Ventilation scan detects areas of poor ventilation
	Radiotagged gas is inhaled and lungs are scanned for gas distribution
	If all lung areas are ventilated and perfused equally, a pulmonary emboli is ruled out
	If the lungs are equally ventilated but not perfused, a pulmonary emboli is suspected

The functions of the respiratory system are to provide oxygen to cells during inhalation; to remove carbon dioxide, which is a by-product of cell metabolism, during exhalation; and to help regulate serum pH. Oxygen is needed to produce adenosine triphosphate (ATP), which is a nucleic acid that in turn powers cellular activity. Cellular activity produces carbon dioxide that must be removed in order to prevent a build-up of carbonic acid (carbon dioxide + water = carbonic acid) in the blood stream, which would lower blood pH to life-threatening levels. Although the term *respiration* is frequently used to denote respiratory activity, *ventilation* and *respiration* are more precise descriptors. *Ventilation* means the movement of air and thus denotes inhalation and exhalation, while *respiration* denotes the exchange of oxygen and carbon dioxide between cells, the alveoli, and the environment.

Functional Anatomy

The pulmonary system consists of the airways (nasal passages, mouth, nasopharynx, larynx, trachea), lungs (two lobes on the left, three on the right), diaphragm, and pulmonary blood vessels. Turbinates are tissue protrusions in each nostril that create air turbulence. Large pollutants, such as dust, are trapped by nasal hairs, while the tiny capillaries of the nares warm and humidify the air. Stimulation of nasal irritant receptors by triggers such as pollen activates the sneeze reflex and clears the nares. Insensible water loss of approximately one pint per day occurs as we provide humidity to the air we breathe. The frontal, maxillary, and ethmoid sinuses are air-filled spaces that provide resonance to the voice. The larynx contains the vocal cords. Aspiration is prevented by the epiglottis, a tissue flap that closes over the tracheal opening during swallowing.

The trachea branches into the right and left bronchus and then further divides 16 times finally ending in terminal bronchioles. Mucous and cilia, which line the airway, trap and remove inspired foreign particles by an escalator motion. When the mucous reaches the pharynx, it is either swallowed or expectorated. If tracheal or large airway irritant sensors are triggered, the cough reflex is activated and the lower airways are cleared. The ability to clean and humidify the airway and prevent an environment in which bacteria can flourish is impaired by anything that damages the mucociliary system, such as dehydration, smoking, dry air, or by mouth breathing or a tracheostomy, which bypasses the nares.

There is a double-layered membrane that lines the inside of the thoracic cavity (i.e., parietal pleura) and the outside of the lungs (i.e., visceral pleura) so that the lungs slide up and down easily during inhalation and exhalation. A thin layer of serous fluid lubricates the pleura and reduces friction associated with ventilation. Accumulation of excess pleural fluid is called *pleural effusion* and results in lung tissue compression and inadequate ventilation.

Ventilation

The medulla oblongata in the lower brainstem contains "pacemaker" cells that stimulate autonomic ventilation. The phrenic nerve, which innervates the diaphragm and internal intercostal muscles, transmits neural impulses that trigger inhalation. Stimulation of the apneustic center in the pons triggers gasping ventilation when the higher respiratory center is damaged by trauma.

Chemoreceptors located in the carotid and aortic bodies, the brainstem, stretch and irritant receptors in the airways, and motion receptors in the joints and muscles also help regulate the rate and depth of ventilation. If we require additional oxygen, such as occurs during exercise, the ventilatory rate and volume increases. Although ventilation is mainly an involuntary process controlled by the brainstem, the rate and depth of breathing can be consciously altered up to a point.

When peripheral chemoreceptors in the carotid and aortic bodies sense a rise in the level of arterial carbon dioxide or a decrease in arterial oxygen or serum pH, the respiratory center is stimulated to increase the ventilatory rate and depth. When the central chemoreceptors located near the respiratory center sense a drop in cerebrospinal fluid pH, which closely mirrors serum pH, the respiratory center is again stimulated, resulting in a deeper and faster rate of ventilation in order to blow off carbon dioxide and lower carbonic acid production.

The diaphragm and external intercostal muscles contract during inhalation, causing an enlarged chest wall and decreased pressure in the lungs enabling air to enter. Approximately 500 cc of air is inhaled and exhaled with a normal, relaxed breath. Accessory muscles are used during dyspnea to assist in ventilation and include the sternocleidomastoid and scalenus muscles in the neck and possibly facial muscles.

Airway diameter plays an important role in successful ventilation. Bronchodilation occurs because of sympathetic nerve stimulation in an attempt to increase the body's oxygen supply during times of stress. Irritant receptors in the pharynx, trachea, and bronchus, when stimulated by cold air, secretions, or pollutants such as pollen, dust, and tobacco smoke, cause bronchoconstriction and/or coughing and sneezing. If bronchoconstriction continues, the ventilatory effort increases, resulting in dyspnea.

Oxygen and Carbon Dioxide

Adults have approximately 300 million alveoli, each of which contains macrophages on the inner surface to fight bacteria, chemicals, and other irritants. A fluid called *surfactant* coats the inner surface of each alveoli and allows it to remain partially opened during exhalation.

The pulmonary artery, which receives deoxygenated blood from the right ventricle, divides into arterioles and finally pulmonary capillaries, which are composed of capillary endothelium and a basement membrane.

These pulmonary capillaries surround the alveoli. Each surfactant-coated alveolar wall consists of epithelial cells and a basement membrane. A very thin layer of interstitial fluid separates the pulmonary capillary basement membrane from the alveolar basement membrane. Oxygen and carbon dioxide diffuse across this alveolocapillary respiratory membrane. A thick or damaged respiratory membrane will impair this diffusion process.

Hemoglobin, a protein contained in red blood cells (RBCs), is responsible for transporting 99% of dissolved oxygen to the cells, with 1% transported in plasma. Oxygen and hemoglobin combine in the lungs to form oxyhemoglobin. At the cellular level the oxygen is released in a process called *hemoglobin desaturation*. Acidosis, hypercapnia, high altitude, heart failure, and anemia cause the oxygen/hemoglobin bond to weaken, thereby easily releasing oxygen to the cells. In contrast, alkalosis or a subnormal body temperature make the oxygen/hemoglobin bond stronger.

An enzyme in RBCs called *carbonic anhydrase* causes 60% of the carbon dioxide produced by cell metabolism to rapidly combine with water and create carbonic acid. The carbonic acid, in turn, rapidly ionizes in the RBCs to form bicarbonate and hydrogen ions. Hemoglobin acts as a buffer by combining with the hydrogen ions while the bicarbonate diffuses into the plasma. Some carbon dioxide (30%) also forms a weak bond with hemoglobin (carbaminohemoglobin), which transports it to the alveoli. The remaining 10% of carbon dioxide produced is dissolved in the plasma.

25 Asthma

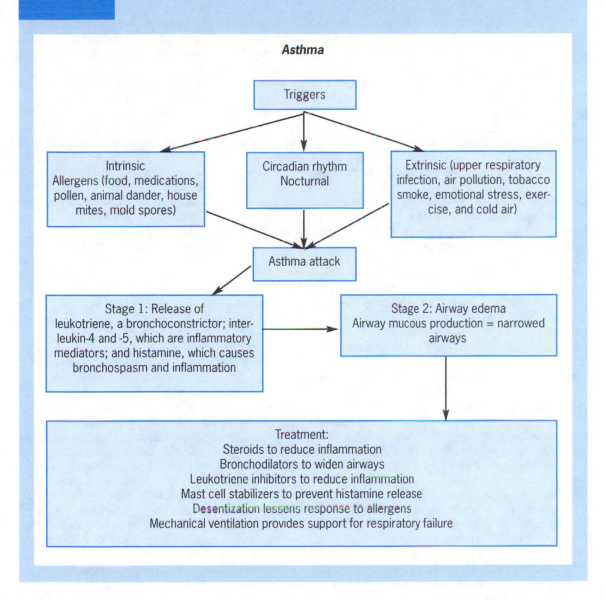

Asthma

Triggers

Intrinsic
Allergens (food, medications, pollen, animal dander, house mites, mold spores)

Circadian rhythm
Nocturnal

Extrinsic (upper respiratory infection, air pollution, tobacco smoke, emotional stress, exercise, and cold air)

Asthma attack

Stage 1: Release of leukotriene, a bronchoconstrictor; interleukin-4 and -5, which are inflammatory mediators; and histamine, which causes bronchospasm and inflammation

Stage 2: Airway edema
Airway mucous production = narrowed airways

Treatment:
Steroids to reduce inflammation
Bronchodilators to widen airways
Leukotriene inhibitors to reduce inflammation
Mast cell stabilizers to prevent histamine release
Desentization lessens response to allergens
Mechanical ventilation provides support for respiratory failure

Overview

Chronic airflow limitation (CAL) consists of three common respiratory diseases: asthma, chronic bronchitis, and emphysema. Asthma is the only one of the three disease entities that produces intermittent, reversible airway obstruction. Asthma, which is characterized by acute airway inflammation, bronchoconstriction, bronchospasm, edema of the bronchioles, and increased production of mucous, is the most common chronic illness in children. Of the 15 million people in the United States, approximately 5% of adults and 8% of children are diagnosed with asthma. Characteristic signs and symptoms of asthma are chest tightness, cough, tachypnea, wheezing, anxiety, and dyspnea caused by airway narrowing. Unless treated promptly, asthma can lead to ineffective gas exchange and death. Status asthmaticus is a severe, prolonged asthma attack that does not respond to usual treatment and is life threatening. Approximately 5,000 people die each year from asthma.

Wearing a face mask, which warms the air and retains airway humidity, is helpful in preventing exercise-induced asthma. Asthma caused by allergens can be managed by removing as much of the offending allergen as possible from the person's environment. Air filters, absence of tobacco smoke, hard wood floors rather than carpets, and dusting daily are some of the measures used to control dust mites and other allergens. Desensitization treatments are also useful in controlling extrinsic asthma.

Pathophysiology

Asthma may be classified according to cause (e.g., extrinsic [allergic], intrinsic [idiopathic], nocturnal, exercise induced, occupational, drug induced) or more precisely by severity (e.g., mild intermittent, mild persistent, moderate persistent, and severe persistent). Extrinsic asthma is a result of increased IgE synthesis and hypersensitivity of the airways, resulting in mast cell destruction and release of inflammatory mediators. When stimulated by allergens such as house mites, food additives, pollen, animal dander, drugs (e.g., aspirin [ASA], nonsteroidal anti-inflammatory drugs [NSAIDs], nonselective beta blockers), or mold spores, mast cells in the bronchial tissue release leukotrienes, which cause bronchoconstriction; histamine, which causes increased vascular permeability; and prostaglandins, which cause increased mucous production. The onset of extrinsic asthma generally occurs in childhood or adolescence and is more common in males than females.

In contrast to extrinsic asthma, intrinsic asthma commonly occurs after age 35. Triggers for intrinsic asthma are an upper respiratory infection, air pollution, tobacco smoke, emotional stress, exercise, and exposure to cold air. Exercise-induced asthma is fairly common, affecting approximately 70% of the people who have asthma. In this type of asthma, the attack usually begins 5 to 10 minutes after the activity begins. Hypotheses related to exercise-induced asthma focus on increased airway cooling and drying of the mucosa.

Occupational asthma is caused by a reaction to substances, such as fumes from plastic, formaldehyde, or cedar dust. Each exposure to the offending substance produces increasingly severe asthma attacks. Time away from work, such as during the weekend, results in clearing of symptoms.

A common cause of drug-induced asthma is ASA and it may be fatal. ASA intolerance usually develops in patients who have nasal polyps, sinusitis, and asthma. Delayed reactions may occur 12 hours after the ingestion of ASA or may occur shortly after taking the drug. There appears to be a cross-sensitivity to NSAIDs in the person with ASA-induced asthma. Both ASA and NSAIDs prevent the conversion of arachidonic acid to prostaglandins, thereby stimulating leukotriene release, which is a powerful bronchoconstrictor. Food additives, such as yellow dye no. 5 used in pharmaceutical, hair, and food products; monosodium glutamate (MSG); and hops, commonly found in beer, have also been indicated in asthma attacks.

Nocturnal asthma, which generally occurs between 3 am and 7 am, is thought to be related to circadian rhythms. At night natural cortisol and epinephrine levels decrease and plasma histamine levels increase. Epinephrine is a naturally occurring bronchodilator, thus a decrease in epinephrine release produces bronchoconstriction. Nocturnal airway diameter in asthmatics can decrease by as much as 50%. This narrowing coupled with airway cooling and drying, impaired mucociliary clearance, increased vagal tone, and gastroesophageal reflex disease (GERD) causing microaspiration are thought to be contributing factors for nocturnal asthma. The role of late-phase response to allergens, which may occur 6 to 12 hours after exposure, is also under investigation.

Regardless of classification, asthma attacks are the body's response to bronchial inflammation. Stage one of an acute asthma attack, generally signaled by coughing, is primarily bronchospastic in nature and reaches a peak within 15 to 30 minutes of the beginning of the attack. Chemical inflammatory mediators responsible for stage one include leukotrienes, interleukin-4 and -5, and histamine.

Stage two of an asthma attack peaks within 2 to 6 hours of onset and is a result of airway edema and mucous production. The mucous produced during stage two is generally thick and contains bronchial casts. Air trapping during expiration with resulting alveolar hyperinflation is common. Bronchospasm, smooth muscle contraction, inflammation, and increased mucous production combine to produce a narrowed airway.

Pulmonary function tests, arterial blood gas analysis, complete blood count (CBC), challenge testing, and allergy testing are mainstays of asthma diagnosis. Pulmonary function testing in a person with asthma reveals a decreased peak expiratory flow rate, indicating trapped air. Arterial blood gas analysis reveals a decreased carbon dioxide level and respiratory alkalosis related to tachypnea. As respiratory exhaustion takes place, there is an increase in the arterial carbon dioxide level and a decrease in the oxygen level. Eosinophilia, as reflected in a CBC, indicates the body's response to an allergen. Allergy testing is used to pinpoint the offending allergen(s).

Management

Inhaled steroids, nebulizer treatments, inhaled bronchodilators, and leukotriene modifiers are some of the pharmaceutical agents used to control and/or prevent asthma attacks. Beta agonists are useful in preventing exercised-induced asthma, as is cromolyn sodium, which is a mast cell stabilizer. Ipratropium bromide, an inhaled anticholinergic, is used to relax bronchial smooth muscle. During status asthmaticus, intravenous (IV) steroids, IV bronchodilators, and mechanical ventilation may be necessary.

Prevention of nocturnal asthma is vital because the majority of asthma-related fatalities occur during the early morning hours. The treatment for nocturnal asthma includes longer-acting beta agonists and histamine blockers to control GERD. Left untreated, long-term asthma may result in bronchial tissue damage and scarring, which in turn leads to increased hyperreactivity of the airways.

26 Acute Respiratory Distress Syndrome and Pulmonary Emboli

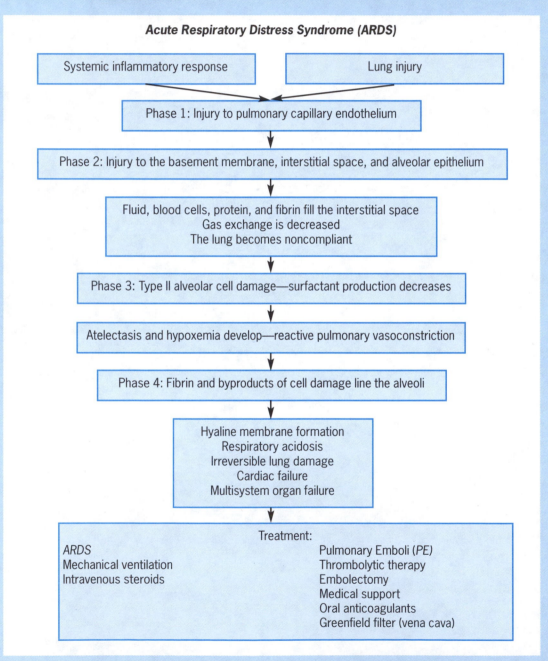

Acute Respiratory Distress Syndrome (ARDS)

Systemic inflammatory response — Lung injury

Phase 1: Injury to pulmonary capillary endothelium

Phase 2: Injury to the basement membrane, interstitial space, and alveolar epithelium

Fluid, blood cells, protein, and fibrin fill the interstitial space
Gas exchange is decreased
The lung becomes noncompliant

Phase 3: Type II alveolar cell damage—surfactant production decreases

Atelectasis and hypoxemia develop—reactive pulmonary vasoconstriction

Phase 4: Fibrin and byproducts of cell damage line the alveoli

Hyaline membrane formation
Respiratory acidosis
Irreversible lung damage
Cardiac failure
Multisystem organ failure

Treatment:

ARDS
Mechanical ventilation
Intravenous steroids

Pulmonary Emboli (*PE*)
Thrombolytic therapy
Embolectomy
Medical support
Oral anticoagulants
Greenfield filter (vena cava)

Acute Respiratory Distress Syndrome

Overview

Acute respiratory distress syndrome (ARDS), which is also known as *shock lung, wet lung, Vietnam lung,* and *adult hyaline membrane disease*, was first identified in 1967 as a cause of pulmonary edema resulting from alveolocapillary membrane injury. This noncardiogenic type of pulmonary edema affects approximately 150,000 patients per year and has a mortality rate of around 60%. Patients who survive ARDS may have permanent lung damage. Risk factors for developing this noncardiogenic pulmonary edema include aspiration of gastric contents, all types of shock, oxygen toxicity, fat embolism, major trauma, smoke inhalation, multiple blood transfusions, viral pneumonia, and burns. Prevention of ARDS relies on avoidance of the occurrences that cause the syndrome.

Pathophysiology

ARDS develops rapidly, often within 90 minutes of a systemic inflammatory response and within 24 to 48 hours of an initial lung injury. There are four phases of the ARDS process during which there is progressive respiratory distress caused by atelectasis resulting from reduced surfactant production, reactive pulmonary vasoconstriction caused by hypoxemia, and cardiac failure caused by an increase in right ventricular afterload. The pulmonary capillary endothelium is injured during phase 1. Phase 2 follows with injury to the basement membrane, interstitial space, and alveolar epithelium. The damaged capillaries and alveolar walls become permeable during phase 2, allowing fluid, blood cells, protein, and fibrin to fill the space around the alveoli, decreasing gas exchange, creating a noncompliant lung, and increasing the work of breathing. The protein-rich fluid filling the alveoli causes damage to type II alveolar cells that produce surfactant in phase 3, ultimately leading to atelectasis and hypoxemia. Fibrin and by-products of cell damage line the inside of the alveoli in phase 4, leading to hyaline membrane formation, respiratory acidosis, irreversible lung damage, and possibly multisystem organ failure.

Assessment of a patient who has ARDS reveals tachypnea, dyspnea, crackles related to pulmonary edema, hypoxemia not relieved by oxygen therapy, respiratory acidosis, restlessness, anxiety, and right-sided heart failure. Stress ulcers frequently occur. Clinical and x-ray examinations cannot differentiate between pulmonary edema that has a cardiogenic cause and one that has a noncardiogenic cause. Pulmonary capillary wedge pressure (PCWP) reflecting left ventricular filling pressure enables a definitive diagnosis to be made. The PCWP is elevated in pulmonary edema caused by congestive heart failure, but it is normal (6 to 12 mmHg) in pulmonary edema caused by ARDS since the edema is created by damage to the alveolar-capillary membrane, not a deficient heart muscle.

Management

The treatment goals for a patient with ARDS include supplying oxygen to vital organs by supporting the respiratory system with mechanical ventilation until the process has reversed itself and the prevention of bronchopulmonary dysplasia. Although the lowest concentrations of oxygen, tidal volume, and airway pressure are used in order to accomplish these goals, high concentrations of oxygen may be necessary to maintain the PO_2 around 90%. Intravenous (IV) steroid therapy is used to halt the progression of late-stage fibrin deposits, enabling the lungs to function at an optimal level.

Pulmonary Emboli

Overview

Any bolus of bloodborne material such as air from an IV line, fat from a long bone fracture or trauma, amniotic fluid that enters the circulation during childbirth, tumor tissue, or a thrombus that blocks a pulmonary artery is termed a *pulmonary embolism* (PE), the third most common cardiovascular disease process in the United States. Approximately 64% of autopsies reveal a PE regardless of the cause of death. PE causes a sudden obstruction of blood flow to lung tissue and may cause death, especially within the first 1 to 2 hours after the initial insult. The most common sources of blood clots include the right ventricle, as a consequence of atrial fibrillation, and deep vein thrombosis (DVT) arising in the pelvis or calf. DVT is the most common cause of PE, accounting for approximately 5 million cases in the United States each year, of which 600,00 are severe. Annually, PEs cause approximately 300,000 deaths and 250,000 hospitalizations.

Prevention of PE lies in removing or reducing risk factors that create clots. Low dose subcutaneous (SQ) heparin every 12 hours helps to reduce the likelihood of DVT after surgery or during periods of immobility. Activities that discourage venous stasis, such as encouraging movement and using sequential compression devices (Venodyne boots) in postoperative or bed ridden patents, avoiding oral contraceptives in women who smoke, using anticoagulant medication for patients with atrial fibrillation, and using an inferior vena cava filter (Greenfield filter) to stop clots from traveling to the heart, are some of the measures employed to reduce the risk of PE.

Pathophysiology

As clots pass through the right atrium to the right ventricle of the heart they are broken into smaller units that can subsequently block peripheral branches of the pulmonary artery. This blockage results in decreased perfusion and ventilation ability. Respiratory distress may be slight if only a few small capillaries are blocked or major if larger vessels are blocked. If one or more large clots block a large pulmonary vessel, the right ventricle pumps harder in a futile attempt to bypass the

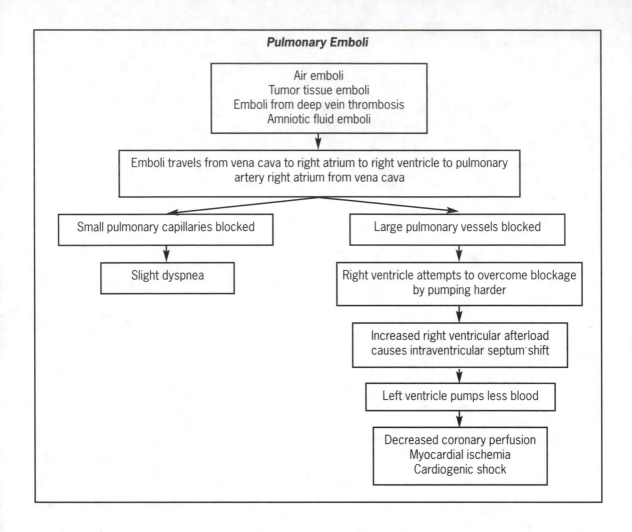

Pulmonary Emboli

Air emboli
Tumor tissue emboli
Emboli from deep vein thrombosis
Amniotic fluid emboli

↓

Emboli travels from vena cava to right atrium to right ventricle to pulmonary artery right atrium from vena cava

Small pulmonary capillaries blocked

↓

Slight dyspnea

Large pulmonary vessels blocked

↓

Right ventricle attempts to overcome blockage by pumping harder

↓

Increased right ventricular afterload causes intraventricular septum shift

↓

Left ventricle pumps less blood

↓

Decreased coronary perfusion
Myocardial ischemia
Cardiogenic shock

blockage. As blood builds up in the right ventricle (right ventricular afterload) the intraventricular septum shifts to the left, making the left ventricle smaller. As a result the left ventricle is able to pump far less blood to the circulation, leading to decreased coronary perfusion, myocardial ischemia, and cardiogenic shock.

Assessment of a patient who has a small PE may reveal no signs or symptoms of hypoxia. Large PEs cause abrupt onset of signs and symptoms of respiratory distress such as dyspnea, pain on inspiration, chest pain, anxiety, cough, tachypnea, and crackles. Massive clots cause cyanosis, syncope, and sudden death.

In contrast to emboli caused by clots, fat emboli occur as fat droplets and enter the circulation after orthopedic surgery, bone fracture, or surgery on an obese patient. As the pulmonary fat emboli is hydrolyzed free fatty acids are released, resulting in increased capillary permeability. Sections of alveolar collapse occur, resulting in dyspnea and rapid heart and ventilatory rates. Confusion, delirium, and petechiae on the chest and arms are also signs of a fat emboli.

Most diagnostic tests are not conclusive and only suggest a diagnosis of PE. Blood gas analysis will reveal a PO_2 of less than 80 mmHg, chest x-ray that may show pulmonary infiltration, and a lung scan (ventilation/perfusion [V/Q] scan) may demonstrate ventilation but lack of perfusion. A definitive test for PE is the pulmonary angiogram. During this test a contrast medium is injected into the pulmonary arteries and the vessels are visualized.

Management

Treatment for a PE includes thrombolytic therapy directly into the pulmonary artery to dissolve clots if the patient has immediate access to medical care or possible surgical embolectomy and medical support of cardiac and respiratory functions. IV heparin administered as a continuous infusion for approximately 5 days then oral anticoagulant therapy for several months is utilized if a diagnosis of PE has been made and the patient survives. Treatment for a fat emboli includes respiratory support via oxygen and/or mechanical ventilation and systemic steroids to reduce the inflammatory response.

27 Chronic Bronchitis and Emphysema

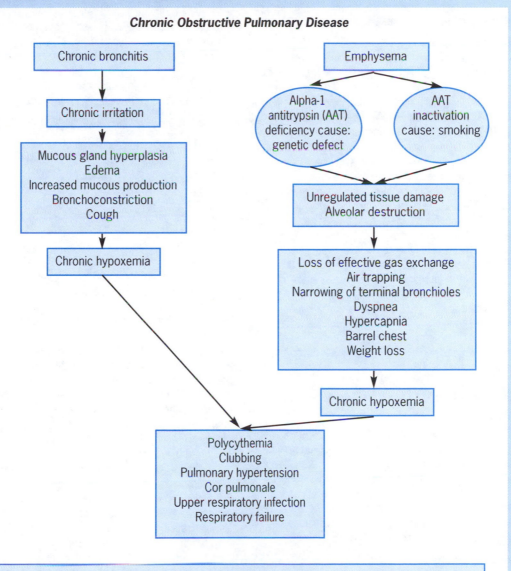

Chronic Obstructive Pulmonary Disease

Chronic bronchitis
↓
Chronic irritation
↓
Mucous gland hyperplasia
Edema
Increased mucous production
Bronchoconstriction
Cough
↓
Chronic hypoxemia

Emphysema

Alpha-1 antitrypsin (AAT) deficiency cause: genetic defect

AAT inactivation cause: smoking

↓
Unregulated tissue damage
Alveolar destruction
↓
Loss of effective gas exchange
Air trapping
Narrowing of terminal bronchioles
Dyspnea
Hypercapnia
Barrel chest
Weight loss
↓
Chronic hypoxemia
↓
Polycythemia
Clubbing
Pulmonary hypertension
Cor pulmonale
Upper respiratory infection
Respiratory failure

Treatment:

Smoking cessation
Antibiotics for infection
Percussion and postural drainage
Bronchodilators
Inhaled or systemic steroids

Replacement of ATT enzyme if deficiency exists
Surgical removal of lung segments
Low flow oxygen for maintenance
Lung transplant
Mechanical ventilation during respiratory failure

Chronic Bronchitis

Overview

Approximately one out of four adults in the United States has chronic bronchitis, which is defined as inflammation of the bronchi, a productive cough, and increased mucous production for at least 3 months of the year for 2 consecutive years. Current or former smokers are at greatest risk for developing this disease, as are people exposed to inhaled irritants such as second-hand cigarette smoke and air pollution.

Pathophysiology

As a defense against airborne irritants, the upper and midairways set up an inflammatory response that results in mucous gland hyperplasia, edema, increased thick mucous production, bronchoconstriction, and cough. Airway resistance affects both inspiration and expiration, resulting in hypoventilation, hypoxemia, cyanosis, hypercapnia, increased red blood cell production (i.e., polycythemia), clubbing of the fingers, and eventually shortness of breath even at rest.

Chronic hypoxemia causes reflexive pulmonary vascular narrowing called *pulmonary hypertension*. As the right ventricle hypertrophies in an attempt to overcome increased pulmonary artery resistance, cor pulmonale (i.e., right-sided heart failure) develops.

Patients with chronic bronchitis are, for unknown reasons, unable to increase their ventilatory effort in order to effectively overcome airway resistance and eventually develop cyanosis ("blue bloaters"). Impaired pulmonary defenses, including cilia damage and decreased phagocytic activity, result in frequent respiratory infections and, in some cases, respiratory failure requiring mechanical ventilation.

Emphysema

Overview

Emphysema, which affects 2.5 million Americans, is an anatomical term that denotes loss of lung elasticity as a result of the breakdown of connective tissue support of the lower airways, abnormal dilatation of air spaces distal to the terminal bronchioles, and abnormal enlargement and eventual destruction of the alveoli. Risk factors for developing emphysema include chronic bronchitis, smoking, and air pollution.

Pathophysiology

Approximately 2% of emphysema cases are caused by a genetic deficiency of the alpha-1 antitrypsin (AAT) enzyme. Lung tissue normally undergoes a process of remodeling during periods of growth and repair related to lung infections and inflammation. Proteolytic enzymes, such as trypsin, involved in this process are normally inactivated by AAT so that tissue damage is controlled. A deficiency of AAT results in early onset (before age 40) of unregulated tissue damage mainly in the lower lobes. Smoking, which causes an inflammation of lung tissue, also results in the release of proteolytic enzymes and the inactivation of AAT, resulting in upper lobe structural changes.

Two major patterns of emphysema are centrilobular (centriacinar) and panlobular (panacinar). Centrilobular emphysema is associated with both smoking and chronic bronchitis, primarily affecting the respiratory bronchioles, while panlobular emphysema is associated with AAT deficiency and senile emphysema, which affects the terminal and respiratory bronchioles and alveoli. Senile emphysema is a normally occurring degenerative change and does not usually cause symptoms.

Alveoli destruction causes a loss of surface and pulmonary capillary bed area, which reduces effective gas exchange, decreases surfactant production, and produces large, ineffective air spaces called *bullae* or *blebs*. The loss of elastic recoil of lung tissue results in air trapping during expiration, and hyperinflation of the alveoli causes a narrowing of the terminal bronchioles. Inspiration is not affected, and cough is not a usual symptom. Assessment will reveal diminished breath sounds and a rapid, shallow respiratory pattern ("pink puffers").

A person with emphysema initially presents with dyspnea upon exertion. In later stages of the disease weight loss is marked due to severe dyspnea and tachypnea even at rest. The work of breathing is so difficult that most calories taken in are expended in maintaining respiration and normal pH blood gas levels. Hypercapnia (i.e., elevated carbon dioxide level) because of CO_2 trapping is evident, as is the use of accessory muscles, leading to the development of a barrel chest as the lungs maintain a hyperinflated state. Normally, the diaphragm does 65% of the work of respiration and the accessory muscles do 35% of the work. In emphysema, lost lung elasticity and hyperinflation of the airways causes the accessory muscles to work more and the diaphragm to work less.

Pursed-lip breathing, either instinctive or learned, and assuming a tripod position ease the work of breathing. Pursed-lip breathing increases the resistance to the expiratory phase of respiration and produces airway backpressure, which helps to prevent alveolar and airway collapse. The tripod position is assumed when the person sits up and leans forward, thus supporting the ribcage and allowing for fuller chest expansion.

A patient with chronic obstructive pulmonary disease (COPD) will have an abnormal pulmonary function test, most notably a reduction of the forced expiratory volume, forced vital capacity, increased residual volume, and increased airway resistance. Decreased elastic recoil results in an increased residual volume and an increased total lung capacity. Arterial blood gases may reflect hypercapnia, hypoxemia, and respiratory acidosis, especially in patients with airway obstruction due to chronic bronchitis. Pulse oximetry of less than 95% is generally considered normal in patients with chronic hypoxemia. Because of tachypnea, some patients will have mild respiratory alkalosis. Chest x-rays will show increased anterior-posterior (A-P) diameter, low flat diaphragm, and possibly bullae and blebs.

COPD produces an increased hemoglobin and hematocrit count as the body attempts to overcome hypoxemia by supplying more red blood cells (RBCs) to carry oxygen. If infection is present, the white blood cell (WBC) count will be increased with a shift to the left, indicating release of immature WBCs. Long-term, severe COPD may eventually result in cor pulmonale, which can be diagnosed by a noninvasive Doppler echocardiogram.

Management

Prevention of chronic bronchitis and emphysema focuses on smoking avoidance or cessation, yearly flu vaccines and a Pneumococcal vaccine to prevent pneumonia, and support of clean air legislation. Antibiotic therapy for bacterial respiratory infections, mucolytics, increased fluid intake to thin secretions, bronchodilators, inhaled or systemic steroids, oxygen, and mechanical ventilation during periods of respiratory failure are treatment options.

Percussion and postural drainage may be required to assist in mobilizing thick secretions and prevent mucous plug formation. Pulmonary rehabilitation programs are aimed at increasing respiratory function through participation in regular exercise programs. Education and psychosocial support are achieved through the use of support groups. To prevent weight loss, small frequent feedings and vitamins are encouraged.

Continuous, low flow (1 to 2 L/min) oxygen therapy has been shown to reduce mortality in persons with severe COPD and PO_2 levels below 55 mmHg. Episodes of hypoxemia during sleep are common because of shallow breathing. Oxygen therapy is titrated to maintain PO_2 around 60 mmHg. In COPD the drive to breath is controlled by the amount of oxygen in the blood, not by the amount of carbon dioxide. Flooding the person with oxygen will, therefore, decrease the respiratory drive.

If emphysema is caused by an ATT deficiency, enzyme replacement is a treatment option; however, this treatment is expensive and it's efficacy is uncertain. Screening should be done for people with a family history of this genetic defect.

The most recent advance in treatment for severe emphysema is surgical lung volume reduction, which removes bullous lung segments. This procedure seems to restore support to the distal airways, improving expiration. Lung transplantation has also been utilized for patients with severe COPD and has a 75% 2-year survival rate.

28 Lung Cancer

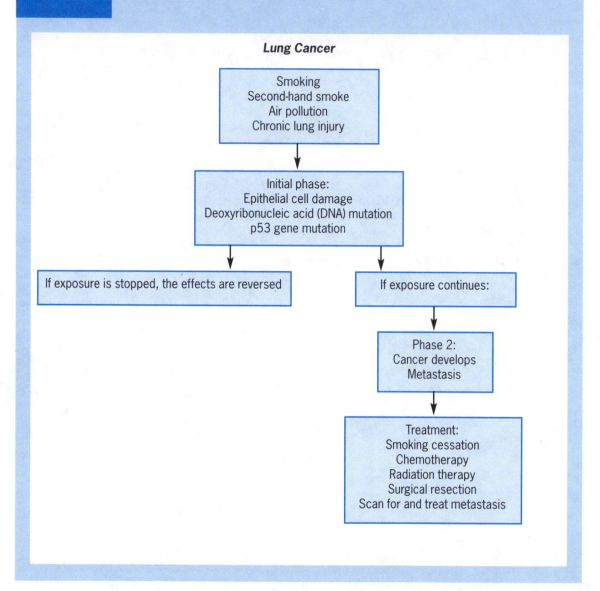

Lung Cancer

Smoking
Second-hand smoke
Air pollution
Chronic lung injury

↓

Initial phase:
Epithelial cell damage
Deoxyribonucleic acid (DNA) mutation
p53 gene mutation

If exposure is stopped, the effects are reversed

If exposure continues:

↓

Phase 2:
Cancer develops
Metastasis

↓

Treatment:
Smoking cessation
Chemotherapy
Radiation therapy
Surgical resection
Scan for and treat metastasis

Overview

Lung cancer is a neoplasm that arises out of lung tissue or develops as a result of cancer metastasis from another site, most notably breast cancer. It is currently the leading cause of cancer deaths among both men (32%) and women (25%) with more African Americans than Caucasians developing the disease. Mortality rates for lung cancer approach 90% with a 5-year sur-vival rate after diagnosis approaching only 15%. Each year approximately 180,000 new cases of lung cancer are diagnosed and the vast majority of these cases (80% to 90%) are directly linked to smoking. Cigarette smoke contains 4,000 chemicals, 43 of which are known carcinogens including tar, which paralyzes cilia. Other causes of lung cancer include second-hand smoke inhalation, which causes between 500 and

5,000 deaths per year; inhaled carcinogens such as asbestos; and chronic lung disease such as chronic obstructive pulmonary disease (COPD) in which mucociliary action is diminished, resulting in poor removal of airborne carcinogens.

There is a direct correlation between the age a person began smoking, how much and how long he or she smoked, and the likelihood of developing lung cancer. People who began smoking in their teenage years, inhale deeply, and smoke at least one-half pack per day have the highest risk of developing the disease. Someone who stops smoking experiences a gradual decline in lung cancer risk. Recently, attention has focused on the risk of developing lung cancer for those exposed to second-hand smoke such as someone living with a smoker and restaurant/bar workers. Research has indicated that second-hand smoke may contain more carcinogens than inhaled smoke. It takes between 10 and 30 years after exposure to the carcinogens in cigarettes for lung cancers to develop. This accounts for the incidence of lung cancers in people who develop the disease years after they stop smoking. Smokers who are also exposed to other environmental carcinogens, such as air pollution, are at a very high risk for developing lung cancer.

Pathophysiology

Bronchogenic cancers arise from epithelial cells of the respiratory tract and are aggressive. The first phase of lung cancer development involves irreversible cell deoxyribonucleic acid (DNA) mutation of oncogenes and tumor suppressor genes because of exposure to carcinogenic substances. One of the genes that is mutated is the p53 gene, a tumor suppressor gene responsible for controlling cell replication. Over time exposure to carcinogenic environmental agents alters the growth and reproduction of the affected cells. If exposure to the carcinogens is stopped, the effects are reversible. If the exposure to carcinogens continues, cancer develops.

Lung cancer is classified as squamous cell, adenocarcinoma, large cell, and small cell. Small cell cancers generally occur in the central part of the lungs and are also called *oat cell cancers*. They tend to be more aggressive than large cell cancers, invade local tissue, and metastasize readily by way of the lymphatic system. Small cell cancers make up approximately 25% of all lung cancers, are the most strongly associated with smoking, and have a poor prognosis. These tumors grow aggressively, metastasize readily, and have paraneoplastic characteristics, meaning that the tumors can produce indirect effects such as the secretion of inappropriate antidiuretic hormone or hyperparathyroidism, producing hypercalcemia. Other paraneoplastic syndromes associated with lung cancer include Cushing's syndrome, myasthenia-like syndrome, peripheral neuropathy, endocarditis, and anemia.

Nonsmall cell cancers account for 75% of all lung cancers. Included in this group are adenocarcinomas, squamous cell carcinomas, and large cell carcinomas. Squamous cell cancer, which arises from epithelial cells, is generally located in the hila (i.e., the areas where the bronchus splits into the right and left bronchi), tends to be slow growing, is strongly associated with smoking and air pollution, and may take 4 years to become large enough to cause symptoms. Ninety percent of squamous cell cancers occur in men, cause bronchial obstruction, and account for approximately 30% to 40% of lung cancers. Half of the patients diagnosed with squamous cell lung cancer will survive 5 years.

Adenocarcinomas arise primarily at sites of previous pulmonary damage such as fibrotic areas and are the most common lung tumors in nonsmokers and women. This cancer arises from the bronchial glandular epithelium including the alveoli and terminal bronchioles. Although this type of lung cancer is slow growing, it also has a tendency to metastasize. The 5-year survival rate for adenocarcinoma is poor.

Large cell undifferentiated cancers carry a poor prognosis because of early metastasis. Metastasis to the brain, bone, liver, central nervous system (CNS), and adrenal glands is common with this type of lung cancer, and it tends to invade surrounding structures such as the heart, major blood vessels, esophagus, and trachea.

The patient will be asymptomatic early in the course of lung cancer. Later signs and symptoms include a chronic cough similar to "smoker's cough" as irritant receptors are stimulated, wheezing as airway obstruction increases, fatigue, and aching joints. Upper respiratory infections may develop because airway defense mechanisms are hampered. Hemoptysis is a late sign. Superior vena cava syndrome (SVCA) may occur as the tumor compresses that vessel and impairs blood return to the right atrium. Signs of SCVA include headache, upper extremity edema, and facial flushing.

By the time most lung tumors are detectable by x-ray, they are already 1 cm large and the likelihood of metastasis is great. Fiberoptic bronchoscopy, which enables bronchial washings and the recovery of bronchial cells, can detect lung cancer early in the disease process; however, the prognosis is generally poor because of the tendency of lung cancer to metastasize.

Management

The most efficient method to prevent lung cancer is to eliminate cigarette smoking and exposure to occupational carcinogens. Smoking has been a common activity since ancient times when it was thought to have medicinal properties. Today smoking is recognized as the primary cause of chronic bronchitis, emphysema, and lung cancer and is associated with the development of pancreatic and bladder cancer. Although cigarette smoking is slightly declining in the United States due to aggressive marketing techniques, its use is increasing in underdeveloped countries. Because the nicotine in cigarettes is a highly addictive psychoactive substance most people find it difficult to stop smoking. The use of nicotine patches, which replace inhaled nicotine with a gradually declining amount of transdermally absorbed nicotine, has enabled some people to stop smoking without suffering from nicotine withdrawal. Smoking cessation support groups, psychotherapy, and hypnosis have also been successful. As with any addiction the key to the success of any smoking cessa-tion program lies with the commitment the person has to give up the addiction.

Treatment for large cell cancers includes pneu-monectomy, which is removal of the entire lung, or lobectomy, which is removal of the affected lung seg-ment if distant metastasis has not occurred. Chemo-therapy and radiation therapy are also treatment options if local lymph node involvement is detected. Because of their bronchial location small cell cancers are treated with palliative measures such as chemother-apy and radiation therapy but not surgery.

Pneumonia and Atelectasis

29

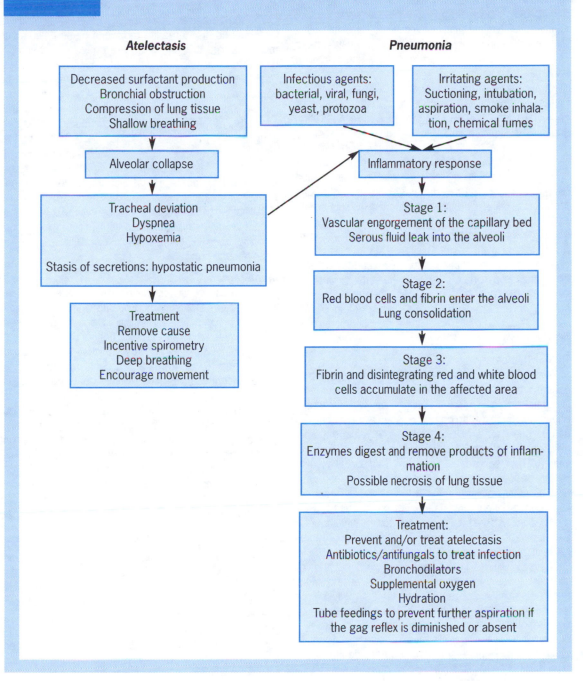

Atelectasis

Decreased surfactant production
Bronchial obstruction
Compression of lung tissue
Shallow breathing

↓

Alveolar collapse

↓

Tracheal deviation
Dyspnea
Hypoxemia

Stasis of secretions: hypostatic pneumonia

↓

Treatment
Remove cause
Incentive spirometry
Deep breathing
Encourage movement

Pneumonia

Infectious agents:
bacterial, viral, fungi,
yeast, protozoa

Irritating agents:
Suctioning, intubation,
aspiration, smoke inhala-
tion, chemical fumes

↓

Inflammatory response

↓

Stage 1:
Vascular engorgement of the capillary bed
Serous fluid leak into the alveoli

↓

Stage 2:
Red blood cells and fibrin enter the alveoli
Lung consolidation

↓

Stage 3:
Fibrin and disintegrating red and white blood
cells accumulate in the affected area

↓

Stage 4:
Enzymes digest and remove products of inflam-
mation
Possible necrosis of lung tissue

↓

Treatment:
Prevent and/or treat atelectasis
Antibiotics/antifungals to treat infection
Bronchodilators
Supplemental oxygen
Hydration
Tube feedings to prevent further aspiration if
the gag reflex is diminished or absent

Pneumonia

Overview

Pneumonia, the sixth leading cause of death in the United States and the leading cause of death from infection, is an inflammatory process that may be caused by numerous infectious agents such as bacteria, viruses, fungi, yeast, or protozoa. *Streptococcus pneumoniae* is a bacteria responsible for up to 75% of all cases of pneumonia. In contrast to bacterial pneumonia, viral pneumonia is usually mild and heals without intervention; however, it can lead to a more virulent bacterial pneumonia.

Irritating agents/events, such as suctioning, intubation, aspiration of gastric juice, inhalation of smoke or chemical fumes, can also lead to pneumonia. Aspiration pneumonia may occur because the gag reflex is impaired as the result of a brain attack or because a nasogastric tube prevents the lower esophageal sphincter from closing, allowing gastric juice or tube feeding formula to enter the lungs. Gastric secretions and tube feeding formulas are irritating to lung tissue and set up an inflammatory response when aspirated.

Other common causes of pneumonia are stasis of respiratory secretions and thickened secretions. Stasis of secretions in immobile patients can lead to pneumonia because bacteria can grow in the static secretions. When respiratory secretions become thick, as in a patient with fluid volume deficit, ciliary action cannot remove the bacteria-laden mucous and pneumonia may result.

Pathophysiology

Pneumonia may be classified by the agent that causes it or by its location in the lung. Lobar pneumonia is confined to a single lobe of the lung, while bronchopneumonia, the most common type, is described as patchy pneumonia in several lobes. Atypical pneumonia, usually caused by viruses (e.g., type A or B influenza) or some bacteria (e.g., *Legionella*) is also patchy but does not involve the alveoli. Pneumonia may also be classified according to where it was acquired. Nosocomial pneumonia is pneumonia acquired while the patient is hospitalized, and community-acquired pneumonia is pneumonia acquired outside of a hospital/health care setting.

When the cough/gag reflex, mucociliary system, or immune system is compromised, bacteria and other pneumonia-causing agents enter the normally sterile lung fields. Bacteria can enter the lungs by inhalation or via the blood stream. The inflammatory process is responsible for the four stages of pneumonia. The first stage is the *24-hour congestion stage,* during which time there is vascular engorgement of the capillary bed and serous fluid leaks into the alveoli. During this time the patient may complain of fever, chills, aching chest, malaise, dyspnea, and watery phlegm and the white blood cells (WBCs) will begin to rise. Auscultation will reveal fine crackles over the affected area.

The second stage is also called the *red hepatization stage* as red blood cells and fibrin enter the alveoli, creating a red, firm lung appearance. Lung sounds in the consolidated area will be absent. The patient may complain of dyspnea (a subjective symptom) and tachypnea.

The third stage is called the *gray hepatization stage* as fibrin and disintegrating red/white blood cells accumulate in the affected area. The cough may become blood-tinged or purulent. If the pneumonia has not been treated with antibiotics, the resolution stage begins in approximately 8 to 10 days. This is the "clean-up" stage during which time enzymes digest and remove the products of inflammation. The exudate is either coughed up or removed by WBCs. Necrosis of lung tissue may occur.

Diagnostic tests for pneumonia include a chest x-ray, which will show areas of consolidation; culture and sensitivity of collected sputum; complete blood count (CBC); arterial blood gases to determine oxygenation needs, including intubation and ventilation support; and possibly a bronchoscopy to collect samples and/or remove secretions.

Management

Careful and consistent handwashing will help to prevent nosocomial infections. Patients who are in a high risk group for community-acquired pneumonia benefit from influenza and pneumococcus vaccines. Postoperative patients should be turned every 2 hours, encouraged to deep breath and cough, and taught to use an incentive spirometry. All three acts will assist in preventing atelectasis, a frequent cause of pneumonia in this population. The elderly and immunocompromised patients are most at risk for developing pneumonia.

Once pneumonia develops treatment focuses on eradicating the infection and/or correcting the underlying cause of the inflammation. Bacterial and fungal infectious agents are treated with antibiotic therapy. Few antiviral agents are available at this time. Bronchodilators may be prescribed to reduce or prevent bronchospasm.

Supportive measures include careful monitoring of respiratory and oxygenation status, hydration to thin secretions so that they can be expectorated, supplemental oxygen, rest to promote healing, and, in some cases, chest physiotherapy. If aspiration pneumonia occurs, treatment is aimed at eliminating the cause of the aspiration and includes having the patient take nothing by mouth (NPO) until swallowing studies have been completed and evaluated and possibly placing a permanent feeding tube.

Atelectasis

Overview

Atelectasis, or incomplete alveolar expansion or collapse, occurs when the walls of the alveoli stick together, producing impaired gas exchange. Atelectasis is caused by a decrease of surfactant, a lipoprotein that coats the inside of the alveoli and allows them to remain open at the end of expiration; by obstruction of a bronchus; or by compression of lung tissue as a result of a tumor, pleural effusion, or pneumothorax. To prevent atelectasis postoperative patients and those on bed rest should be encouraged to deep breath and cough every 1 to 2 hours. Effective pain management and incisional splinting postoperatively will allow the patient to deep breath and cough.

Pathophysiology

Small areas of atelectasis may produce few, if any, symptoms, while larger areas of involvement will result in inadequate ventilation and hypoxemia, producing signs such as diminished breath sounds, dyspnea, and restlessness. Tracheal deviation to the affected side will occur if the area of alveolar collapse is large. Atelectasis is diagnosed by chest x-ray and if left untreated, it may lead to pneumonia and/or respiratory failure.

Management

Treatment focuses on removing the cause (e.g., utilizing bronchoscopy to remove a mucous plug or antibiotic therapy to combat infection). Incentive spirometry is effective because it encourages the patient to hold, take, and hold a deep breath, increasing the likelihood of keeping the alveoli open.

30 Tuberculosis

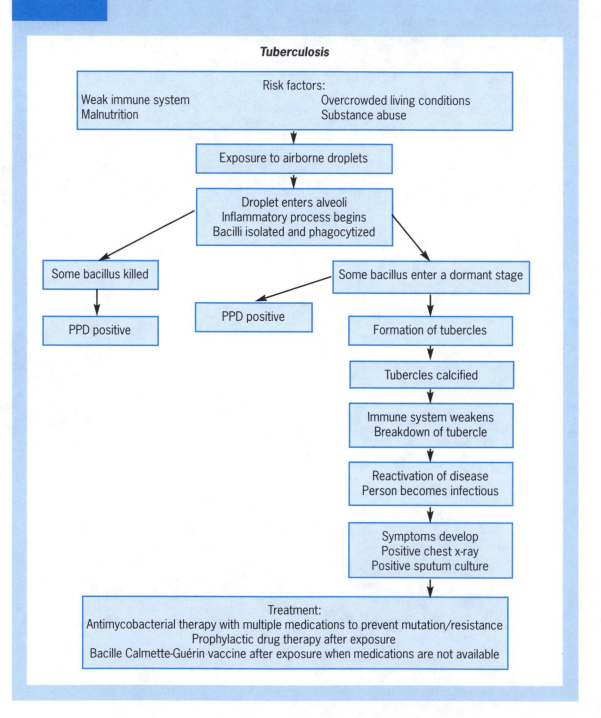

Tuberculosis

Risk factors:

Weak immune system | Overcrowded living conditions
Malnutrition | Substance abuse

↓

Exposure to airborne droplets

↓

Droplet enters alveoli
Inflammatory process begins
Bacilli isolated and phagocytized

Some bacillus killed

↓

PPD positive

Some bacillus enter a dormant stage

PPD positive

↓

Formation of tubercles

↓

Tubercles calcified

↓

Immune system weakens
Breakdown of tubercle

↓

Reactivation of disease
Person becomes infectious

↓

Symptoms develop
Positive chest x-ray
Positive sputum culture

↓

Treatment:
Antimycobacterial therapy with multiple medications to prevent mutation/resistance
Prophylactic drug therapy after exposure
Bacille Calmette-Guérin vaccine after exposure when medications are not available

Overview

Tuberculosis (TB) is a chronic, recurrent infection involving the lung and less commonly other tissues, specifically the meninges, liver, kidney, brain, and bone marrow. The aerobic bacillus responsible for causing the infection is called *Mycobacterium tuberculosis*, and it has been around since ancient times. It is estimated that one third of the world's population has been infected with this bacillus, and it remains a major health problem in developing countries. Approximately 20 million people worldwide have TB, and it is responsible for 3,000 deaths annually. In the United States men are infected more than women and the incidence is highest among Asians and Pacific Islanders followed by African Americans, Hispanics, Native Americans, and Caucasians. The incidence of TB is rising in the United States because of the emergence of drug-resistant strains.

TB is often classified as an opportunistic infection because it is likely to develop in someone with a weakened immune system. People at high risk for contracting TB are those with AIDS, malnutrition, diabetes, and/or alcoholism. Poverty, overcrowding, homelessness, and drug abuse also place people at risk for the disease.

TB may be classified as primary (i.e., disease occurs 2 years after infection), reactivation (i.e., disease occurs later than 2 years after infection), pulmonary (i.e., disease occurs in the lungs), or extrapulmonary/miliary (i.e., disease occurs in other tissues).

Transmission of TB occurs via airborne droplets when a person with active disease, approximately 5% to 15% of those infected, talks, sings, coughs, or sneezes. High concentrations of the bacilli in the air, such as in small, closed, nonventilated areas, and numerous exposures to the bacilli increase the risk for transmission of the infection.

The incidence of TB can be reduced by education aimed at stopping the transmission of the disease and screening measures to identify persons who have been exposed to the bacillus so that additional further testing and medical treatment can begin.

Pathophysiology

The droplet nuclei that harbor the bacilli are so small that when they are inhaled they travel directly to the alveoli. Once the bacilli enter the alveoli, usually settling in an upper lobe, an inflammatory response begins. The bacilli are isolated and phagocytized but not all are destroyed. Some enter a dormant state and can reactivate. From 1 to 3 weeks after the initial infection, tubercles (granulomatous lesions or Ghon's focus) begin to form. These tubercles are comprised of fused, elongated macrophages that have engulfed the bacilli and are surrounded by lymphocytes. In time the central section of the tubercle becomes necrotic and forms a yellow, "cheesy" mass called a *caseous necrosis*. As the immune response continues, scar tissue forms around the tubercle and it eventually calcifies. The breakdown of a tubercle releases the bacilli and signals an active disease process. If the primary TB progresses, it can erode the bronchus. If the infection spreads to the bloodstream, it can be disseminated to other body areas. Partial immunity develops from infection and offers protection against reinfection.

Secondary, or reactivation, TB occurs if the sealed-off primary lesion breaks apart and can lead to pleural effusion, empyema, and spread of the disease to others. This is most likely to happen if the person's immune system weakens due to events such as malnutrition, use of systemic steroids, chemotherapy, or AIDS.

A person initially infected with TB may be asymptomatic, have nonspecific symptoms, or may show signs of pneumonia. Common signs and symptoms of active disease include a low grade fever, weight loss, weakness, anorexia, night sweats, and malaise. Hemoptysis, chest pain, and cough indicate advanced necrosis.

The tuberculin skin test will convert to positive during the granuloma formation stage of the disease. People exposed to the bacilli will develop a cellular response within 3 to 10 weeks after exposure, and injecting a small amount of purified protein derivative (PPD) of tuberculin will activate a local inflammatory response, yielding a positive test result. A positive PPD indicates that the person has been infected and developed a cellular response to the bacillus, not that he or she currently has active disease and is infectious. Intradermal PPD is also called a *Mantoux test*, while multiple-puncture test is termed a *tine test*. The tine test is less accurate than the Mantoux test.

Active TB is diagnosed by a positive chest x-ray and positive culture. Eighty-five percent of patients with TB will have an abnormal chest x-ray involving the apical and posterior segments of the upper lobes, especially in the right lung. Early morning sputum cultures, generally three consecutive specimens, will be examined for the acid-fast bacillus. A culture positive for *Mycobacterium tuberculosis* is definitive for the disease. Ten days is required for the slow-growing bacillus to produce positive culture results.

Management

Treatment for TB requires an average of 9 months of antimycobacterial therapy. The slow growing bacilli have a high rate of mutation and develop resistance when exposed to monotherapy, so multiple medications are required to treat this disease. Primary drugs used include medications by mouth (PO) such as isoniazid, rifampin, ethambutol, pyrazinamide, and parenteral streptomycin. Because TB is a public health risk, antituberculin medications are provided free of charge by the United States Public Health Service. Sputum cultures and chest x-rays are used to evaluate the effectiveness of the treatment regime.

In cases in which a person is suspected of having a subclinical case of TB, a year-long treatment with isoniazid is recommended in order to prevent active disease. Persons who are HIV positive and have a positive PPD or persons who are close contacts of a person with newly diagnosed TB and who have a positive PPD fall into this category.

The bacille Calmette-Guérin (BCG) vaccine is administered when prophylactic isoniazid therapy cannot be used. This vaccine is widely used in developing countries and in the United States it is recommended for infants, children, and health care workers with a negative PPD who are repeatedly exposed to ineffectively treated or untreated persons with TB. After the vaccine is administered, subsequent PPD tests will be positive.

1. What mainly controls the ventilatory rate?

(A) Medulla oblongata

(B) Serum bicarbonate level

(C) Pons' apneustic center

(D) Sympathetic nervous system

2. Which of the following statements about carbon dioxide is true?

(A) Ninety-nine percent of the carbon dioxide produced by cellular metabolism combines with hemoglobin.

(B) Carbon dioxide combines with water to form carbonic anhydrase.

(C) Serum carbon dioxide levels drive the rate and depth of ventilation in individuals who do not have chronic obstructive pulmonary disease.

(D) A high serum carbon dioxide level results in respiratory alkalosis.

3. Medications that may cause asthma in hypersensitive individuals include:

(A) Cardiac glycosides

(B) Beta blockers

(C) Carbonic anhydrase inhibitors

(D) Serotonin reuptake inhibitors

4. What is a cause of nocturnal asthma?

(A) Increased cortisol levels

(B) Decreased vagal tone

(C) Decreased epinephrine levels

(D) Increased plasma histamine levels

5. Which of the following acid-base imbalances occurs in ARDS?

(A) Respiratory acidosis

(B) Respiratory alkalosis

(C) Metabolic acidosis

(D) Metabolic alkalosis

6. Which of the following statements concerning ARDS is true?

(A) One of the causes of ARDS is congestive heart failure.

(B) Pulmonary capillary wedge pressure is elevated in ARDS.

(C) Surfactant production is reduced in ARDS.

(D) ARDS has a low mortality rate.

7. When assessing a client who has fat emboli, the nurse is likely to note which of the following?

(A) Petechiae on the chest

(B) Bradycardia

(C) Bradypnea

(D) Pedal edema

8. What is the major cause of chronic bronchitis?

(A) A deficiency of AAT

(B) Smoking

(C) Aging

(D) Asthma

9. Lung changes that occur in emphysema include:

(A) Increased elastic recoil

(B) Increased pulmonary capillary permeability

(C) Increased surfactant production

(D) Narrowing of the terminal bronchioles

10. Which of the following statements about lung cancer is true?

(A) Metastasis is rare.

(B) When someone stops smoking their risk of developing lung cancer declines rapidly.

(C) Second-hand smoke is more likely to cause lung cancer than inhaled smoke.

(D) The 5-year survival rate for adenocarcinoma is high.

11. Signs of superior vena cava syndrome related to lung cancer include:

(A) Headache

(B) Pallor

(C) Wheezing

(D) Pedal edema

12. Which of the following statements regarding pneumonia is true?

(A) It is the third leading cause of death in the United States.

(B) It is most often caused by a bacteria.

(C) It generally produces mild symptoms if the cause is bacterial.

(D) It generally resolves within 3 to 4 days.

13. Auscultation of lung sounds in a patient with atelectasis will reveal what?

(A) Rhonchi

(B) Rales

(C) Wheezing

(D) Diminished breath sounds

14. Which of the following statements concerning TB is true?

(A) A PPD indicates active infection.

(B) bacille Calmette-Guérin vaccine is used prophylactically.

(C) The dormant stage generally lasts a few months.

(D) Developing resistance to antimycobacterial therapy is rare.

15. What is a classic sign of active pulmonary TB?

(A) High fever

(B) Absence of cough

(C) Night sweats

(D) Wheezing

PART VI ANSWERS

1. **The correct answer is A.**

The medulla oblongata contains "pacemaker" cells that control the rate and depth of respiration.

2. **The correct answer is C.**

Chemoreceptors in the carotid and aortic bodies react to high serum carbon dioxide levels and trigger ventilation in healthy individuals.

3. **The correct answer is B.**

Nonselective beta blockers block sympathetic nervous system stimulation and cause bronchoconstriction.

4. **The correct answer is C.**

Epinephrine is a natural bronchodilator. In the early morning hours epinephrine levels decrease by as much as 50%.

5. **The correct answer is A.**

Alveoli damage results in a decreased ability to exchange carbon dioxide for oxygen. Carbon dioxide + water = carbonic acid.

6. **The correct answer is C.**

Type II alveolar cells are damaged as part of the ARDS cascade, leading to a decrease in surfactant production and alveolar collapse.

7. **The correct answer is A.**

Petechiae on the arms and chest are a classic sign of a fat emboli.

8. **The correct answer is B.**

Smoking and/or inhalation of second-hand smoke are the major causes of chronic bronchitis.

9. **The correct answer is D.**

Loss of elastic recoil and alveolar hyperinflation results in narrowing of the terminal bronchioles.

10. **The correct answer is C.**

Second-hand smoke contains more carcinogens than inhaled smoke.

11. **The correct answer is A.**

Impaired blood return to the right atrium because of vessel compression by a tumor results in a headache as cerebral blood vessels become engorged.

12. **The correct answer is B.**

Streptococcus pneumonia is responsible for causing 75% of all pneumonia cases.

13. **The correct answer is D.**

Areas of alveolar collapse will result in absent breath sounds.

14. **The correct answer is B.**

After exposure to TB, the bacille Calmette-Guérin vaccine may be used as a prophylactic measure if antimycobacterial medications are not available.

15. **The correct answer is C.**

Night sweats are a classic sign of active pulmonary TB.

PART VII

Cardiovascular System

Pamela J. Dudac, MS, MSN, APRN-C

Anatomy and Physiology of the Cardiovascular System: Part I

Phases of the Cardiac Cycle

Diastole

Phase 1—Isovolumetric Relaxation
At the beginning of diastole, all valves are closed. The atria are filling. The ventricular muscles begin to relax.. As atrial pressures rise and ventricular pressures fall, the tricuspid and mitral valves open.

Phase 2—Rapid Ventricular Filling
Seventy percent to 80% of the blood flows into the ventricles, increasing ventricular volume and pressure.

Phase 3—Atrial Kick
The atria contract, sending 30% more blood into the ventricles, after which ventricular pressure rises above atrial pressure. The mitral valve closes immediately followed by the tricuspid valve. The closing of the mitral and tricuspid valves causes the first heart sound, the "lub," signifying the beginning of systole. [During diastole, blood in the aorta and pulmonary artery flow out to the body and lungs, diminishing the pressure in these two vessels.]

Systole

Phase 1—Isovolumetric Contraction
At the beginning of systole, all valves are closed and the myocardial muscle tension begins to rise. When the pressure in the ventricles exceeds the pressure in the aorta and pulmonary artery, the aortic and pulmonic valves open.

Phase 2—Rapid Ejection
About 60% to 75% of the blood in the ventricles is ejected into the aorta and pulmonary artery. The pressures in these vessels rise.

Phase 3—Reduced Ventricular Ejection
Blood flow from the ventricles diminishes. When the pressure in the ventricles falls below aortic and pulmonic pressure, the aortic and pulmonic valves close, creating the second heart sound, the "dub," signifying the beginning of another diastole.

The role of the heart and blood vessels is to deliver to the body tissues constituents of the blood (e.g., oxygen, nutrients, defensive cells, etc.) needed for their function and integrity and to remove waste products (e.g., carbon dioxide, nitrogenous wastes, acids, etc.). The heart provides a pumping mechanism and the blood vessels provide the transport system. The arterial system delivers the blood to the tissues and the venous system returns the blood to the heart. The cardiovascular system works in an integrated fashion and has both intrinsic and extrinsic control mechanisms to accomplish its' task.

The anatomy and physiology of the heart is designed so that the right side of the heart receives carbon dioxide-laden, deoxygenated blood from the body via the venous system and delivers it to the lungs for carbon dioxide removal and oxygenation. Oxygenated blood returns to the left side of the heart for delivery out to the body via the arterial system.

The heart is a four chambered muscular organ divided into right and left sides. The two sides of the heart function separately but simultaneously and in a coordinated fashion. The superior and inferior vena cava deliver deoxygenated blood to the right atrium.

The blood then passes through the tricuspid valve into the right ventricle. The blood leaves the right ventricle through the pulmonic valve and is conducted via the pulmonary artery to the lungs. Blood enters the left atria via the pulmonary veins and passes through the mitral valve into the left ventricle. It is then ejected through the aortic valve and out the aorta. The two sides of the heart are separated by the septum.

The heart wall has three layers. The endocardium is the smooth, innermost layer that covers the heart valves and is continuous with the endothelium that lines all the blood vessels. The myocardium is the middle layer, consisting of cardiac muscle. It is the thickest layer, thicker in the left ventricle than the right because of the greater pressures against which the left ventricle must pump. The pericardium is a double walled membranous sac that surrounds the heart. The visceral and parietal pericardia are separated by the pericardial cavity and lubricated by pericardial fluid.

Blood vessels have three layers: the innermost intima composed of smooth endothelium, the middle tunica media composed of elastic and smooth muscle fibers, and the outermost adventitia. The endothelium produces substances that promote relaxation (e.g., prostacyclin and nitric oxide) and others that promote constriction (e.g., endothelial derived constricting factor [EDCF]). Prostacyclin also inhibits platelet aggregation. Another substance, thromboxane, is produced and promotes platelet aggregation. Elastic arteries (e.g., aorta and major branches) and pulmonary arteries have many elastic fibers to withstand the pressure of the blood pumped from the heart. Muscular arteries are medium and small sized arteries, and arterioles precede capillaries. Capillaries are thin, single layers of endothelial cells that allow for exchange of substances between blood and tissues.

Veins are thinner than arteries and have fewer elastic fibers, thus they are more distensible and serve as capitance vessels. The veins in the lower extremities have one way valves.

Stimulation of parasympathetic cholinergic receptors on the heart decreases the rate. Stimulation of sympathetic adrenergic beta 1 receptors increases the heart rate, conductivity, and contractility. Stimulation of beta 2 receptors causes vasodilation of the coronary arteries as well as the arteries of skeletal muscles and lungs. Stimulation of alpha 1 receptors on the peripheral arterioles and veins causes vasoconstriction.

The heart achieves its pumping action by means of the relaxation and contraction of the myocardium and the opening and closing of valves in a cyclic, coordinated fashion. This creates pressure gradients that move the blood forward. Events on the left side of the heart occur at approximately the same time as events on the right. The period of the cardiac cycle during which the ventricles relax and fill is diastole and the period of ventricular contraction is systole (see p. 122). Normally, diastole is longer in duration than systole. It is also the phase during which the coronary arteries are perfused because their ostia are not covered by the aortic valve cusps as they are in systole. With excessive heart rates, ventricular filling and coronary artery perfusion are diminished.

Direction of Blood Flow Through the Heart

Superior vena cava
Inferior vena cava

(No valve)

Right atrium

(Tricuspid valve)

Right ventricle

(Pulmonic valve)

Pulmonary artery

Right and left
pulmonary arteries

Lungs

(No valve)

Right and left*
pulmonary veins

Left atrium

(Mitral valve)

Left ventricle*

(Aortic valve)

Aorta*

Arterial system*

Venous system

Bold is arterial (oxygenated) blood, nonbold is venous (deoxygenated) blood.

Conduction System of the Heart

Sinoatrial node (right atrium)

Intranodal tracts

Anterior tract ——— Bachmann's bundle ——→ Left atrium
Middle tract
Posterior tract

Atrioventricular node

Bundle of His

Right bundle branch   Left bundle branch

Purkinje system   Purkinje system

Distribution of Coronary Arteries

Aorta

Left coronary artery (LCA)

Left anterior descending (LAD)
(anterior interventricular branch) ——→ Anterior wall, left ventricle, and inter-ventricular septum

Left circumflex branch (LCX) ——→ Lateral walls of the left atrium and left ventricle

Posterior descending branch
(posterior interventricular branch) ——→ Posterior walls of both ventricles and interventricular septum

Right coronary artery (RCA)
(main supplier of the right ventricle and inferior wall) ——→ Sinoatrial node
Atrioventricular node

Margin branch ——————→ Lateral wall of the right ventricle

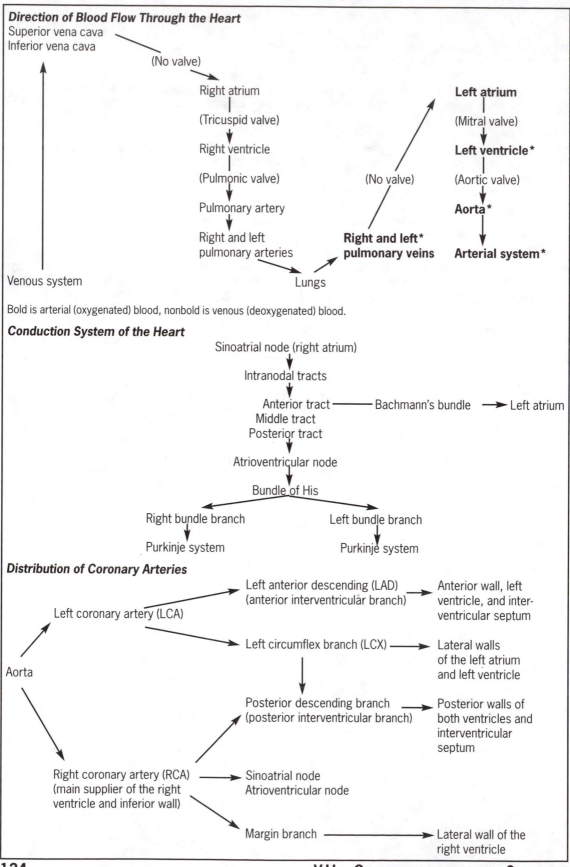

32 Anatomy and Physiology of the Cardiovascular System: Part II

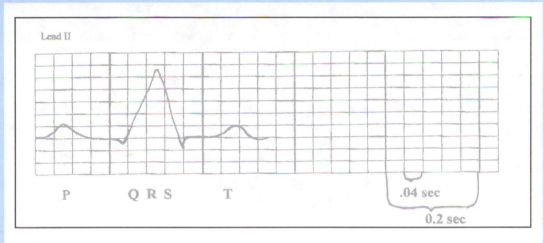

P wave
- Begins with firing of the sinoatrial (SA) node and represents depolarization of the atria
- Duration is 0.06 to 0.12 seconds

QRS wave
- Represents depolarization of the atrioventricular (AV) node through the ventricles
- Duration is 0.04 to 0.12 seconds (The height of the Q wave should be <one third the height of the R wave)

T wave
- Represents repolarization of the ventricle
- Duration is 0.16 seconds

P-R interval
- A measure of time required for the impulse to spread from the SA node through the ventricles
- Duration is 0.12 to 0.20 seconds

QT interval
- Represents the time it takes for depolarization of the ventricles
- Duration varies with the pulse; at a heart rate of 72, it is 0.31 to 0.38 seconds

Regulation and coordination of contractions of the atria and ventricles are essential for effective pumping of the heart. There are both intrinsic and extrinsic mechanisms to accomplish these goals.

Intrinsic mechanisms achieve coordination through precise timing and routing of electrical impulse formation and conduction, which are tied to stimulation of contractility. In the healthy heart, impulses originate in the sinoatrial (SA) node and spread rapidly through the atrial myocardial fibers that respond by contracting. The impulses are also conducted toward the atrioventricular (AV) node where they are delayed slightly before being transmitted to the ventricles. The impulse then spreads through the His-Purkinje system and up through the ventricles, ultimately stimulating ventricular contraction.

Four properties of cardiac tissue enable the initiation and conduction of impulses and myocardial contractility: automaticity, excitability, conductivity, and contractility. Automaticity is the ability of specialized tissue cells in the SA node, parts of the atria, and AV node to spontaneously initiate impulses. Excitability is the ability of the myocardial tissue to be depolarized by a stimulus. Conductivity is the transmission of impulses from one fiber to another, and contractility is the ability of the myocardial fibers to shorten.

Cardiac cells achieve these tasks by initiating and conducting action potential (APs) (i.e., self-propagating waves of depolarization followed by repolarization). The APs are generated by sodium ions (NA+), potassium ions (K+), and calcium ions (CA+) moving in and out of cells through channels in the cell membranes. In a resting myocardial cell, negatively charged ions line up inside the cell membrane while positively charged ions line up outside, creating an electrical charge difference, and the cell is said to be polarized. With stimulation or sometimes spontaneously, channels in the membrane open allowing positive ions to enter and eliminating the charge differences and the cell is then said to be depolarized. Following depolarization, the positively charged ions are extruded and the cell membrane repolarized.

Cardiac excitation normally begins in the SA node where autorhythmic fibers undergo rapid spontaneous depolarization, initiating APs at a rate of 90 to 100 times per minute, prior to any spontaneous depolarization in other regions. APs from the SA node spread to other areas of the conduction system, stimulating them before they are able to generate an AP at their own slower rate. Thus, the SA node becomes the primary pacemaker for the heart. Hormones or neurotransmitters can slow or speed pacing of the heart. Slow conduction in the small size fibers of the AV node allows time for the atria to contract, moving blood forward into the ventricles before they contract.

If, because of disease or damage, the SA node fails to initiate an impulse, the slower AV node fibers can pick up the pacing chores; however, with AV pacing, the pacing rate is 40 to 50 beats per minute. If activity in the nodes is suppressed, the heartbeat may be maintained by autorhythmic fibers in the ventricles (i.e., the AV bundle, a bundle branch, or conduction myofibrils). These fibers fire AVs very slowly, only about 20 to 40 beats per minute, a rate too slow to adequately perfuse the brain. Sometimes a site other than the SA node develops abnormal self-excitability. Such a site is called an *ectopic focus*.

The level of excitability of myocardial cells is determined by the length of time since the previous depolarization. The recovery time is called the *refractory period* and is subdivided into the *absolute refractory period*, which extends through depolarization and most of repolarization when no other AP can be stimulated, and *relative refractory period*, which occurs slightly later when excitability is more likely (i.e., approximately on the second half of the T wave on an electrocardiogram [ECG]). The refractory period is normally longer than the period of contraction, giving the ventricles time to fill before another contraction can occur.

The electrical activity of the heart leads to myocardial muscle fiber contraction by initiating the influx of Ca+ through calcium channels in the cell membranes, raising its' concentration among contractile fibers. Ca+ binds to a regulator protein, troponin, which allows actin and myosin fibers to slide past one another, tension mounts, and fibers shorten. The muscle contraction moves the blood out of the heart. The volume expelled with each contraction is called the *stroke volume* (SV). The portion of the end diastolic volume that is ejected is called the *ejection fraction*.

The electric currents produced by the impulses as they are conducted in the heart can be detected on the body surface by an electrocardiogram tracing. The tracing represents the net electrical activity of the atria and ventricle as they depolarize and repolarize. Conventionally, 12 leads are placed on different areas of the chest wall and limbs to evaluate electrical activity from different perspectives. A lead is a pair of electrodes with a positive and a negative pole that can detect electrical current. The electrical currents drive a stylus that can make a tracing of the impulse. An impulse traveling toward the positive pole will cause an upward deflection in the ECG tracing, and one traveling away from the positive pole will cause a downward deflection. In addition to the direction of the current, the voltage and timing of the electric current can be determined by the vertical and horizontal calibrations of the graphic paper. The deflections or waves on the ECG graph, which have been arbitrarily designated as P, Q, R, S, and T, represent events during the cardiac cycle (see p. 125).

Extrinsic neurohumoral control mechanisms also influence cardiac function. These mechanisms are initiated by changes in the *cardiac output* (CO), which is a function of the SV times the heart rate (CO = SV x R). The stroke volume is influenced by the preload, contractility, and afterload.

Preload refers to the stretch in the wall of the heart at the end of diastole and reflects the end diastolic volume (EDV) or venous return. Venous return is a function of both the blood volume of the body and venous constriction. Stretch determines the amount of tension in the wall and, according to the Frank-Starling law of the heart, within limits, the greater the stretch of the fibers, the greater the force of contraction. The renin-angiotensin-aldosterone system (RAAS), which is activated when decreased CO diminishes renal blood flow, increases the blood volume. Sympathetic nervous system (SNS) stimulation also activates the RAAS and increases secretion of antidiuretic hormone (ADH), contributing to the increased blood volume. SNS stimulation causes venous vasoconstriction. All of these mechanisms increase venous return. Overstretching (e.g., excessive fluid volume), however, can diminish contractility. Contractility is the ability of the myocardial fibers to shorten. It is a function of the amount and quality of the fibers, the physiological environment (e.g., adequate oxygen and calcium), and sympathetic stimulation. Increased contractility improves the SV.

Afterload is the amount of pressure that the ventricles must develop to overcome the opposing pressure in the pulmonary artery or aorta in order to move blood forward. It is most commonly a factor of blood pressure (Bp). SNS stimulates arteriole constriction and increases the Bp and afterload. Increased afterload decreases SV.

The factors that determine CO (i.e., SV [preload, contractility, and afterload] and the heart rate) are all influenced by the nervous system.

Nervous system control of the heart stems from the cardiovascular center in the medulla oblongata, which receives sensory input from receptors in blood vessels. The SNS is the first mechanism to be activated when CO falls. Changes in CO alter pressure in blood vessels, which is sensed by baroreceptors located in the aortic arch, carotid arteries, and other arteries and veins. The baroreceptors have connections to the cardiovascular (CV) center in the brainstem, which then provides output to the heart and blood vessels via the autonomic nervous system. Other influences on the CV center are higher brain centers, such as the limbic system and cerebral cortex; chemoreceptors that monitor chemical changes in blood, such as oxygen changes; and proprioceptors that are stimulated during exercise.

Sympathetic stimulation increases heart rate, conduction, and contractility, all of which increase CO. SNS stimulation of beta receptors in the kidneys increases the production of renin and ultimately the preload. Alpha 2 receptors in the smooth muscle walls of arterioles and veins are also stimulated by norepinephrine. The venous constriction increases the preload. Decreased pressure sensed by baroreceptors also increases ADH secretion, thus also contributing to preload.

The activation of the RAAS and ADH secretion are later compensatory responses to decreased CO than is the SNS.

CO is one of the factors that influences systemic arterial Bp. Bp is a function of the CO times the systemic vascular resistance (SVR) (Bp = CO x SVR). SVR is a factor of the caliber of the arterioles that is influenced by the SNS. Thus, the neuroendocrine mechanisms that influence heart function and CO are the same mechanisms that regulate Bp. Decreased Bp increases firing of the baroreceptor, which activates SNS, thus increasing heart rate, contractility, arteriole and venous constriction, ADH secretion, and renin production all of which serve to increase Bp. With an elevation of Bp, these mechanisms are not initiated and the Bp falls. A substance produced in the atria known as *atrial natriuretic hormone* promotes excretion of fluids, thereby reducing Bp.

33 Dyslipidemias and Atherosclerosis

Classifications of Hyperlipidemia*

Lipoprotein	Desirable	Borderline	High
Cholesterol	<200**	200 to 239	>240
LDL	< 130	130 to 159	>160
TG	<200	200 to 399	>400

HDL <35 is low
**Concentration = (mg/dL)
60% to 70% of total cholesterol is LDL cholesterol

Treatment Goals Based on LDL Levels*

Patient Category	Goal LDL (mg/dL)	Diet RX	Drug Rx
without CAD <2 risk factors	<160	>160	>190
without CAD >2 risk factors	<130	>130	>160
with CAD	<100	>100	>130

Diet Therapy for Hyperlipidemia*

Nutrient	Step 1	Step 2 (for those who don't reach goals with Step 1)
Total Fat	<30%	<30%
Saturated Fats	8% to 10%	<7%
Polyunsaturated Fats	up to 10%	up to 10%
Monounsaturated Fats	up to 15%	up to 15%
Carbohydrates	>55%	>55%
Cholesterol	<130 mg/day	<120 mg/day

*National Cholesterol Education Program Expert Panel

Overview

Dyslipidemias, also called *hyperlipidemias*, are important because of their relationship to atherosclerotic vascular disease, especially coronary artery disease (CAD), cerebrovascular disease, and peripheral vascular disease (PVD). Alterations in the lipid profile are associated with the increased risk of CAD and are classified as to level of risk (see above).

It is estimated that anywhere from 38% to 50% of Americans have dyslipidemia. There is a high incidence of dyslipidemia in diabetics, hypertensives, and African Americans. Familial or inherited forms of hypercholesterolemia are relatively rare.

Atherosclerosis is a chronic disease characterized by thickening and hardening of the arterial wall. Lesions/plaques containing lipids develop and calcify, causing vessel obstruction, platelet aggregation, and abnormal vasoconstriction.

Atherosclerotic heart disease is the leading cause of death in the United States, and atherosclerotic cerebrovascular disease is the leading cause of stroke. Peripheral vascular disease is an important cause of disability.

The risk factors for atherosclerotic vascular disease include dyslipidemia, cigarette smoking, hypertension (HTN), male or postmenopausal female, age >50, diabetes/insulin resistance, increased serum fibrinogen, hyperhomocystinemia, a diet high in saturated fat, obesity, sedentary lifestyle, and family history.

Pathophysiology

The two main lipids in the blood are triglycerides (TGs) and cholesterol. Saturated fats in the diet are the source of serum TGs. Some cholesterol is absorbed from food, but most is synthesized by the liver from breakdown products of saturated fats.

Because lipids are insoluble, they combine with carrier proteins (i.e., apoproteins) as lipoproteins and are carried in the blood. The lipoproteins are classified on the basis of their density, which is determined by the amount of TG, which makes them less dense, and protein, which makes them more dense. The main classes of lipoproteins are chylomicrons, very low density lipoproteins (VLDLs), low density lipoproteins (LDLs), and high density lipoproteins (HDLs).

The least dense lipoproteins are the chylomicrons, which are found in blood and appear only after a fatty meal. Chylomicrons are mostly TGs and some cholesterol. TGs are fats and oils that are absorbed from the diet. Chylomicrons transport dietary TGs, a highly concentrated energy source, to peripheral cells for energy needs (broken down into fatty acids to form adenosine triphosphate [ATP]). If there is no need to use TGs this way, a limited amount is stored in the liver and the rest is stored in adipose. The capacity to store TGs in the adipose tissue is unlimited. Excess dietary carbohydrates, proteins, fats, and oils are all stored in the adipose tissues as TGs. The stored TGs can be broken down by lipolysis if needed by cells.

Some cholesterol is absorbed from the diet, but most is endogenously produced in the liver at night. Increases in dietary cholesterol produce only a slight elevation of blood cholesterol because ingestion reduces endogenous hepatic production. An increase in dietary saturated fats (i.e., TGs), however, produces a substantial increase in blood cholesterol because they serve as a substrate for endogenous cholesterol production.

From its' fat and carbohydrate stores, the liver manufactures VLDL particles, which are mainly TGs and some cholesterol. The VLDL particles transport the TGs to cells to meet their needs. After losing enough TGs, the VLDL particles become LDL particles, which are mainly cholesterol and provide cholesterol for cellular needs. HDL particles, which are mainly apoprotein with some cholesterol, participate in reverse cholesterol transport, bringing cholesterol back to the liver and clearing the blood. HDL is reduced by smoking and is increased by exercise.

Plaque found in the arterial walls of individuals with atherosclerosis contains large amounts of cholesterol. Epidemiological studies have established that the higher the level of serum LDL cholesterol, the higher the risk of atherosclerotic heart disease; conversely, the higher the level of HDL, the lower the risk. Because most serum cholesterol is LDL cholesterol, high total cholesterol levels are also associated with increased risk. The relationship of VLDL and TGs in atherogenesis is less certain. The levels of VLDL and HDL are inversely related, thus individuals with high TGs/VLDL are likely to have low HDLs and for this reason alone are likely to have a higher risk of atherosclerosis. High blood levels of one of the apoproteins, apoprotein A, have been identified as a risk factor.

The initiating event in atherogenesis is *endothelial injury*. Dyslipidemia, HTN, cigarette smoking, diabetes/insulin resistance, hyperhomocystinemia, autoimmune processes, and possibly infection (e.g., chlamydia) have been implicated as causes of injury. The injured cells become more permeable, have increased levels of oxygen radicals, and become inflamed; thus, they recruit leukocytes and macrophages that produce more oxygen radicals, increasing the injury. They also release cytokines and mitogens that stimulate smooth muscle cell proliferation and inhibit the endothelial cells from secreting endogenous vasodilators, such as nitric oxide.

Serum LDLs are oxidized by the oxygen radicals and phagocytized by the macrophages, becoming foam cells that penetrate into the intima. This creates further inflammation and injury, forming a lesion called a *fatty streak*. Fibrous tissue and smooth muscle cells migrate and cover the foam cells, forming a cap. Protrusion into the lumen causes narrowing and diminished blood flow (i.e., ischemia). This lesion is called a *fibrous plaque*. This is a relatively stable plaque and probably represents the stage of chronic angina in CAD.

Necrosis and calcification occur below the cap, and as the plaque progresses, it can ulcerate and rupture. This is called a *complicated plaque*. Platelets can aggregate and adhere to the surface of the plaque. Coagulation may be initiated with thrombus formation that may completely obliterate the lumen, possibly resulting in death of tissue/infarction perfused by the artery. This probably represents unstable angina or infarction of CAD.

The end result of the pathological process is a narrowed artery vulnerable to abnormal constriction and thrombosis. If the process occurs slowly, collateral circulation may bypass the lesion and maintain perfusion.

Manifestations

Dyslipidemias and atherosclerosis are often asymptomatic for a long period of time, often until the degree of arterial obstruction (e.g., 50% to 70% blockage in CAD) is sufficient to compromise blood supply to the target organ. The individual may then complain of symptoms of CAD (i.e., dyspnea, fatigue, chest pain, etc.), of cerebral vascular disease (i.e., transient or permanent neurological deficits), or of arterial insufficiency (i.e., intermittent claudication, hair loss, skin ulcers, etc.). Physical examination may reveal evidence of plaque or findings related to damage to the organs supplied. Evidence of lipid abnormalities or plaque might include xanthomas and xanthelasma, arcus senilis, abdominal bruits, peripheral thrills, bruits, and diminished pulses. Cholesterol screening and lipid profile will identify specific lipid abnormalities. Angiography, ultrasound, or nuclear scanning may be used to specifically locate an atherosclerotic lesion.

Treatment

The goals of treatment for dyslipidemias and atherosclerosis are to normalize lipids, prevent plaque progression, and restore blood supply. Lifestyle adjustments that reduce the risk are critical components of the therapeutic regimen.

Pharmacological interventions include lipid-lowering agents, antiplatelet/anti-inflammatory agents (e.g., aspirin), thrombolytics, angiotensin-converting enzyme inhibitors (reduce smooth muscle hypertrophy and increase vasodilation), estrogen, and antioxidants. Diet and drug decisions are based on the level of dyslipidemia and number of other cardiac risk factors (see p. 128). Revascularization procedures may be employed (see Chapter 35).

34 Coronary Artery Disease

Location of Coronary Artery Blockage and Manifestations

Right Coronary Artery (RCA)

- Main supplier of right ventricle, the inferior wall of the heart, sinoatrial (SA) node, and the atrioventricular (AV) node
- EKG changes appear in leads II, IIIA, and a VF
- Occlusion leads to inferior (also called posterior) myocardial infarction (MI)
- Inferior MI has a high incidence of bradycardia and AV block

Left Coronary Artery (LCA)

- Main supplier of the anterior wall of the left ventricle, interventricular septum, and lateral walls of the left atrium and ventricle
- EKG changes appear in leads V3, V4, V5, V6, L1, and a VL
- Occlusion leads to massive anterolateral MI
- Creates major disruption in cardiac output, largest incidence of residual cardiac failure
- High mortality rate

Left Anterior Descending Artery (LAD)

- Main supplier of anterior wall of left ventricle, interventricular septum
- EKG changes in leads V1, V2, and V3
- Occlusion leads to anteroseptal MI
- High incidence of residual cardiac failure

Left Circumflex Artery

- Main supplier of lateral walls of left atrium and ventricle
- EKG changes appear in leads VL, I, V5, and V6
- Occlusion leads to lateral MI

Transmural MIs—Penetrate the complete myocardium and are large enough to create a Q wave, thus they are called Q wave MIs

Subendocardial MIs—Do not penetrate the entire myocardial wall, thus they do not create a Q wave and are called non-Q wave MIs

Overview

Coronary artery disease (CAD) includes conditions that diminish blood flow in the coronary arteries. Atherosclerosis and vasospasm are the most prevalent causes, with atherosclerosis being the most common. In CAD there is an imbalance between demand and supply of oxygenated blood to the myocardium, resulting in either transient ischemia (i.e., angina) or permanent damage to the myocardial cells (i.e., infarction). The left ventricle is most susceptible.

Coronary atherosclerosis remains the leading cause of death in the industrialized world. Over 1 million Americans have myocardial infarctions (MIs) each year, and it is estimated that there are 2 million Americans with silent ischemia.

Nonmodifiable risk factors for CAD include age, gender, race, and family history. Men are more often affected than women by an overall ratio of 4:1, although after age 70 the ratio is 1:1. In women the incidence greatly increases after menopause. With increasing longevity the incidence of CAD is expected to rise. Caucasian men have a higher incidence than African-American men and African-American women higher than Caucasian women. African Americans have an earlier onset and more severe disease. The nature of the relationship to CAD is unclear and may be related to the higher incidence of other risk factors in African Americans. Risk of CAD increases if a biological parent manifested CAD before the age of 55.

Modifiable risk factors that are most predictive of CAD are dyslipidemias (high total cholesterol, high low density lipoproteins [LDL], and low high density lipoproteins [HDL]), hypertension, diabetes, and cigarette smoking. Hyperhomocystinemia is emerging as an important risk factor. Other more controversial risk factors are obesity, sedentary lifestyle, heavy alcohol consumption, estrogen deficiency, and a personality characterized by hostility. Some research implicates infection and inflammation.

Pathophysiology

The coronary arteries (see p. 131) normally provide oxygen to meet the metabolic demands of the myocardium to perform its' work of impulse conduction and contraction.

In CAD, if plaque narrows the lumen by more than 75%, blood flow is impaired sufficiently to hamper metabolism when oxygen demand increases (e.g., exertion, etc.), resulting in ischemia. By-products of anaerobic metabolism (e.g., lactic acid) accumulate, causing substernal pain, or cross stimulate other nerves, causing radiation of pain. During ischemia episodes, conduction disturbances may lead to changes in the electrocardiogram (ECG). Reduction of oxygen demand reverses the ischemia. Predictable ischemia brought on by increased oxygen demand and relieved with reduction of demand is called *stable angina pectoris*.

If a complicated plaque ulcerates, inflammation occurs, platelets aggregate, and thrombi form, further diminishing the blood supply. Platelets release thromboxane A_1, a potent vasoconstrictor, causing spasms of the arteries. This leads to more platelet aggregation, more spasm, and a vicious cycle. Eventually, transient thrombotic occlusions of the coronary vessels occur unpredictably, often at rest, and with increased frequency, causing *unstable angina*, which is a preinfarction situation.

If an acute thrombus occludes the vessel completely, MI, or death of cells, occurs. Generally, there is a sequence of ischemia, injury, and infarction with a centrally infarcted area surrounded by an area of injury and then ischemia. Infarctions occur in various regions of the heart wall (i.e., anterior, posterior, inferior, and lateral) depending on the artery involved and penetrate myocardium to different depths. Subendocardial infarctions partially penetrate wall thickness, and transmural infarctions penetrate through the wall. Infarcted cells release intracellular substances into the blood, which may cause conduction disturbances.

Within 24 hours, inflammatory cells infiltrate the necrotic area and by 10 to 14 days weak scar tissue forms. Eventually, healing is complete by 6 weeks with nonfunctional scar tissue replacing normal tissue. Loss of functional tissue can lead to ventricular failure and cardiogenic shock, ventricular wall inertia with stasis of blood and mural thrombi, ventricular aneurysm, papillary muscle dysfunction and mitral regurgitation, dysrhythmias, and pericarditis. Dressler's syndrome, pericarditis, fever, and effusion may develop 1 to 4 weeks post-MI.

Myocardial cells in the vicinity of the infarcted area may lose their conductive and contractile functions for a period of time or they may undergo "remodeling" (i.e., a process mediated by the renin-angiotensin-aldosterone system that results in hypertrophy and abnormal contractile function both leading to ventricular failure). *Silent ischemia* or *infarction* may occur in a significant number of individuals, especially diabetics, the elderly, and postcardiac surgery patients because of autonomic dysfunction. *Prinzmetal's* or *variant angina* is a form of angina caused by coronary artery spasm, with or without atherosclerotic plaque, that occurs unpredictably and almost exclusively at rest.

Manifestations

Typically, angina is experienced as substernal chest discomfort, ranging from sensation of pressure or heaviness to moderately severe pain. The discomfort may radiate to the neck or the jaw, left shoulder down the inner aspect of the left arm, or occasionally the back or right arm. It is commonly mistaken for indigestion. The discomfort is precipitated by exertion, emotional stress, a heavy meal, extremes of temperature, sexual activity, smoking, and stimulants (e.g., cocaine). Other factors that may contribute are dysrhythmias, blood pressure extremes, left ventricular dysfunction, valvular problems, anemia, thyroid toxicosis, stimulant drugs, and lung disease. The discomfort is transient, usually 3 minutes. Discomfort lasting longer than 30 minutes suggests unstable angina or infarction. Pallor, diaphoresis, and dyspnea may occur.

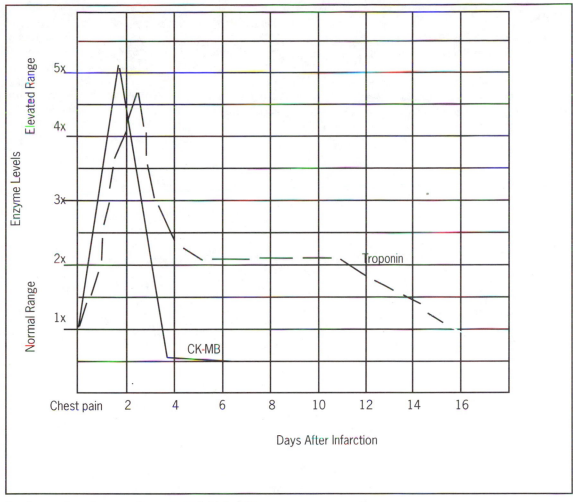

Cardiac marker changes after myocardial infarction.

The blood pressure and pulse are frequently elevated, though hypotension may be present. Dysrhythmias may occur and an S3 with ventricular dysfunction. On ECG, transient ST segment depression and T wave inversion are signs of subendocardial ischemia and ST segment elevation with transmural ischemia. The ECG lead where the changes occur indicates the location of the ischemia.

The first symptom of an MI is sudden, prolonged (>30 minutes), severe chest pain often described as heavy and crushing accompanied by dyspnea and diaphoresis. Radiation is similar to angina. It often causes a feeling of "gas" or unrelenting indigestion. Nausea and vomiting may occur. Initially, blood pressure drops, but blood pressure and pulse may transiently rise with sympathetic stimulation. Inflammation may cause fever, elevation of white blood cells and erythrocyte sedimentation rate, friction rubs, or murmurs. Serum glucose rises with stress.

ECG changes indicative of infarction are an initial peaked T wave. A depressed ST segment and T wave inversion indicates subendocardial ischemia, and ST segment elevation occurs with transmural ischemia or injury. A Q wave develops with transmural infarction. There is no Q wave with a subendocardial infarction. Gradually, ST segments and T waves return to normal, but Q waves persist.

Important cardiac markers released into the blood from necrotic cells are creatine kinase-MB band (CK-MB) (>3%, rises in 4 to 8 hours, peaks in 12 to 18 hours, and is normal in 3 to 4 days) and troponin I (>3.1 ng/ml, rises in 3 hours, and persists for 7 days).

Additional diagnostic tests used to localize areas of obstruction, ischemia, and infarction include stress testing, nuclear imaging with thallium (cold spots) or technician (hot spots), and coronary angiography.

Treatment

Preserving functional cardiac tissue by increasing oxygen supply and decreasing demand is the goal of treatment. Measures to increase perfusion are antihyperlipidemic medications; hemolytic, antiplatelet, and anticoagulating agents; and revascularization procedures. Vasodilators are generally ineffective because of nondistensible vessels. Medications that decrease oxygen demand are nitrates, beta blockers, calcium channel blockers, angiotensin-converting enzyme inhibitors, and angiotensin blockers. Lifestyle interventions include diet, exercise, smoking cessation, and stress management. Current research is addressing methods of stimulating myocardial cell repair after infarction (e.g., stem cell stimulation).

35 Hypertension

Classification of Blood Pressure for Adults Age 18 and Older*

Category	Systolic (mmHg)		Diastolic (mmHg)
Optimal†	<120	and	<180
Normal	<130	and	<85
High-normal	130 to 139	or	85 to 89
Hypertension‡			
Stage 1	140 to 159	or	90 to 99
Stage 2	160 to 179	or	100 to 109
Stage 3	≥180	or	≥110

*Not taking antihypertensive drugs and not acutely ill. When systolic and diastolic blood pressures fall into different categories, the higher category should be selected to classify the individual's blood pressure status. For example, 160/92 mmHg should be classified as stage 2 hypertension and 174/120 mmHg should be classified as stage 3 hypertension. Isolated systolic hypertension is defined as SBP of 140 mmHg or greater and DBP below 90 mmHg and staged appropriately (e.g., 170/82 mmHg is defined as stage 2 isolated systolic hypertension). In addition to classifying stages of hypertension on the basis of average blood pressure levels, clinicians should specify the presence or absence of target organ disease and additional risk factors. This specificity is important for risk classification and treatment.
†Optimal blood pressure with respect to cardiovascular risk is below 120/80 mmHg. However, unusually low readings should be evaluated for clinical significance.
‡Based on the average of two or more readings taken at each of two or more visits after an initial screening.

Recommendations for Followup Based on Initial Blood Pressure Measurements for Adults

Initial Blood Pressure (mmHg)*

Systolic	Diastolic	Follow Recommended†
<130	<85	Recheck in 2 years
130 to 139	85 to 89	Recheck in 1 year‡
140 to 159	90 to 99	Confirm within 2 months ‡
160 to 179	100 to 109	Evaluate or refer to source of care within 1 month
>180	>110	Evaluate or refer to source of care immediately or within 1 week depending on clinical situation

*If systolic and diastolic categories are different, follow recommendations for shorter time followup (e.g., 160/86 mmHg should be evaluated or referred to source of care within 1 month).
†Modify the scheduling of followup according to reliable information about past blood pressure measurements, other cardiovascular risk targets, or target organ disease.
‡Provide advice about lifestyle modifications.

Overview

Hypertension is a significant problem both in terms of its' prevalence and the severity of its' consequences. Hypertension is defined as a consistent systolic blood pressure (SBP) of 140 mmHg or greater, diastolic blood pressure (DBP) of 90 mmHg or greater, or taking antihypertensive medication. Approximately 50 million people have hypertension. Many are unaware of their hypertension and few are under good control.

Variation exists in the prevalence and consequences of hypertension among different age, gender, and racial and ethnic groups. There is an increasing incidence with increasing age. Hypertension tends to occur at an earlier age in African Americans. The incidence is higher in men than in women until the age of 55 then the risk is about equal until age 74, after which time women have a higher incidence than men. African Americans have a much higher prevalence, more severe hypertension, and diagnosis at a later stage than Caucasians. The greater severity is accompanied by a much higher rate of stroke mortality, heart disease, and hypertension-related end-stage renal disease. Hispanics have the same or lower prevalence of hypertension despite a high prevalence of obesity and diabetes.

Hypertension-related consequences of cardiovascular disease, stroke, and end-stage renal disease make hypertension a major public health concern. Cardiac disease and stroke are the first and third leading causes of death in the United States, respectively. Cardiac complications are the major causes of morbidity and mortality in essential hypertension. Hypertension is the major predisposing cause of stroke and is the second most common antecedent of end-stage renal disease.

Various methods of classification for hypertension based on pathology, severity, and associated risk factors are used to give direction to interventions. Most cases of combined systolic and diastolic hypertension in which no cause can be established are classified as *primary hypertension* (essential or idiopathic) and this constitutes 95% of hypertensive individuals (10% to 15% of the Caucasian population and 20% to 30% of African Americans). Primary hypertension may be controlled but the predisposition remains. *Secondary hypertension*, which constitutes 5% to 8% of hypertensive individuals, is caused by altered hemodynamics associated with a primary disease or condition that when removed results in cure of the hypertension if it has not been prolonged. *Isolated systolic hypertension*, an elevation of systolic pressure with a normal diastolic pressure, is common in the elderly and appears to be a significant cardiovascular risk factor.

A commonly recognized classification of hypertension according to level of blood pressure (Bp) elevation is delineated on p. 135. Since risk for cardiovascular disease in individuals with hypertension is determined not only by the level of Bp elevation but also by other risk factors and end-organ damage, a cardiovascular risk stratification classification for hypertension has been developed to guide treatment and is delineated on p. 137.

Hypertensive emergency is a severe level of hypertension with evidence of end-organ damage and needs to be treated within 1 hour. *Hypertensive urgency* is a severe level of hypertension without end-organ damage. It needs to be treated within a few hours.

Pathophysiology

Understanding the pathological mechanism involved in Bp elevation is necessary for understanding prevention and intervention strategies. Bp is a function of the cardiac output (CO) times the systemic vascular resistance (SVR) (Bp = CO x SVR). Elevation of Bp may be caused by increased CO, increased peripheral resistance, or both.

CO is increased by any condition that increases the heart rate or stroke volume (SV) (CO = Rate x SV). The heart rate is influenced by the autonomic nervous system. The SV is determined by preload and contractility. Preload is influenced by blood volume and sympathetic stimulation of the veins. Myocardial contractility is influenced by preload, sympathetic activation, condition of myocardial fibers, and the ionotropic environment. SVR is increased by increased blood viscosity, which is determined by the hematocrit, or reduced arteriolar diameter, which is determined by vascular compliance, the sympathetic nervous system, and local autoregulation.

Genetic and environmental causes may be responsible for primary hypertension. The genetic predisposition is thought to be polygenic with multiple defects. Hypotheses suggested in explaining causation of primary hypertension and exploited in interventions include sympathetic nervous system hyperactivity; increased renin-angiotensin-aldosterone, resulting in increased vascular tone and fluid retention, thus increasing preload; a defect in sodium excretion; and defect in vascular smooth muscle cell transport, resulting in intracellular accumulation of calcium that increases vascular reactivity.

In addition to family history, gender, and advancing age, environmental risk factors found to precipitate or aggravate hypertension are obesity; cigarette smoking; heavy alcohol intake (more than 3 drinks/day); high dietary sodium intake; low potassium, calcium, and magnesium consumption; and glucose intolerance.

Secondary hypertension is caused by primary diseases or conditions that increase CO or peripheral resistance such as catecholamine-secreting adrenal medullary tumors, excessive aldosterone secretion by the adrenal cortex in some disease states, renovascular disease with increased renin-angiotensin production, and iatrogenic causes such as medications (e.g., corticosteroids and estrogen).

High pressures within the arteries and arterioles stimulate hypertrophy and hyperplasia of smooth muscle cells and eventual fibromuscular thickening and endothelial injury. Inflammatory mediators increase permeability of the endothelium, allowing fluids and calcium to enter the wall and increasing reactivity and constriction. Endothelial injury caused by hypertension

Components of Cardiovascular Risk Stratification in Patients with Hypertension

Major Risk Factors

- Smoking
- Dyslipidemia
- Diabetes mellitus
- Age older than 60 years
- Sex (men and postmenopausal women)
- Family history of cardiovascular disease (women under the age of 65 or men under the age of 55)

Target Organ Damage/Clinical Cardiovascular Disease

- Heart diseases (left ventricular hypertrophy, angina/prior myocardial infarction, prior coronary revascularization, heart failure)
- Stroke or transient ischemic attack
- Nephropathy
- Peripheral arterial disease
- Retinopathy

Risk Stratification and Treatment*

Blood Pressure Stages (mmHg)	Risk Group A (No risk factors; no TOD/CCD)†	Risk Group B (At least one risk factor not including diabetes; no TOD/CCD)	Risk Group C (TOD/CCD and/or diabetes, with or without other risk factors)
High-normal (130 to 139/85 to 89)	Lifestyle modification	Lifestyle modification	Drug therapy§
Stage 1 (140 to 159/90 to 99)	Lifestyle modification (up to 12 months)	Lifestyle modification‡ (up to 6 months)	Drug therapy
Stages 2 and 3 ($\geq$160/$\geq$100)	Drug therapy	Drug therapy	Drug therapy

For example, a patient with diabetes and a blood pressure of 142/94 mmHg plus left ventricular hypertrophy should be classified as having stage 1 hypertension with target organ disease (left ventricular hypertrophy) and with another major risk factor (diabetes). This patient would be categorized as Stage 1, Risk Group C, and recommended for immediate initiation of pharmacologic treatment.

* Lifestyle modifications should be adjunctive therapy for all patients recommended for pharmacologic therapy.

† TOD/CCD indicates target organ disease/clinical cardiovascular disease.

‡ For patients with multiple risk factors, clinicians should consider drugs as initial therapy plus lifestyle modifications.

§ For those with heart failure, renal insufficiency, or diabetes.

Reprinted courtesy of the National Institutes of Health.

may also cause or aggravate atherosclerosis further, diminishing lumen patency and vessel distensibility. Eventually, structure and functions of the end organs (i.e., the heart, aorta, kidneys, eyes, brain, and lower extremities) are compromised with resulting ischemia, edema, and even hemorrhage. Elevation of hydrostatic pressure within arteries can cause tissue edema.

Cardiac complications include left ventricular hypertrophy, coronary artery disease, angina pectoris/ischemia, left ventricular failure, myocardial infarction, and sudden death. Vascular complications include aneurysm formation and arterial insufficiency. Renal complications are parenchymal damage, nephrosclerosis, renal artery sclerosis, insufficiency, and failure. Retinal complications (i.e., retinopathy) include retinal vascular sclerosis, exudation, and hemorrhage. Cerebral vascular complications include transient ischemic attacks (TIAs), stroke/brain attack, aneurysm, and hypertensive encephalopathy.

Manifestations

Initially, elevation Bp is usually asymptomatic. An early symptom might include early morning headache as a result of night time cerebral edema. It diminishes during the day. Manifestations tend to be related to end-organ damage, including retinopathy, visual disturbance, papilledema, carotid bruits, distended neck veins, left ventricular hypertrophy, angina, heart failure, myocardial infarction, abnormalities of heart rhythm, murmurs, third and fourth heart sounds, lung crackles and bronchospasm, pulmonary edema, abdominal bruits, pulsations, diminished peripheral pulses, proteinuria, hematuria, abnormal creatine clearance, and hypertensive encephalopathy (headache, irritability, confusion, and altered mental status due to cerebral vasospasm).

Treatment

Lifestyle modifications to prevent hypertension or lower Bp include weight reduction; alcohol limitation; aerobic exercise; limitation of sodium intake; maintenance of calcium, potassium, and magnesium intake; and stress management. If these measures fail to control Bp, pharmacological measures will be implemented. Pharmacological measures are aimed at decreasing the fluid volume, decreasing the cardiac output, and vasodilation.

36 Congestive Heart Failure

Manifestations of Left Ventricular Failure

Signs
- Increased heart rate
- Pulsus alternans (alternating strong/weak)
- S3 and S4 heart sounds
- Displaced or forceful apical impulse
- Left ventricular heave
- Crackles
- Cheyne-Stokes respiration
- Decreased O_2 saturation
- Shortness of breath

Symptoms
- Fatigue
- Dyspnea
- Orthopnea
- Paroxysmal nocturnal dyspnea
- Nocturia
- Dry, hacking cough (decreased cardiac output can cause mental status disturbance, activity intolerance, cool pale extremities with increased capillary refill time, decreased urine output; chest pain possible)

Manifestations of Right Ventricular Failure

Signs
- Right ventricular heave
- Murmurs
- Peripheral edema/tight shoes
- Weight gain
- Dependent edema
- Ascites
- Anasarca
- Increased jugular pressure, hepatojugular reflux
- Hepatomegaly

Symptoms
- Fatigue
- Dependent edema
- Right upper quadrant pain
- Anorexia and bloating
- Nausea

Overview

Congestive heart failure (CHF) is a pathophysiologic syndrome in which the heart is unable to pump an adequate cardiac output (CO), resulting in perfusion of body tissues that is inadequate to meet metabolic needs. In addition to inadequate CO, there is an elevation of pressure in the left ventricle (LV) because blood is not moving forward. Pressures are reflected backward through the pulmonary veins, causing increased pulmonary pressure and pulmonary congestion. CHF refers primarily to left ventricular failure (LVF). However, the increased pulmonary pressure resulting

from LVF increases pressure against which the right ventricle must pump, eventually resulting in right ventricular failure (RVF). LVF is the most common cause of RVF. Elevation of pressure from RVF is reflected back through the veins, causing systemic congestion. Pulmonary disease may be a primary cause of RVF.

CHF is associated with numerous types of cardiovascular disease (CVD), especially hypertension (HTN) and coronary artery disease (CAD). More than half of the deaths from heart disease are due to end stage CHF. One and a half percent to 2% of the American population is afflicted with CHF. There is a 65% 6-year mortality rate for women and an 80% mortality rate for men. CHF results in 700,000 hospital admissions each year and is the most common admitting diagnosis after age 65. It is associated with long hospital stays and sizeable cost is estimated to be $102 billion a year. Research has demonstrated that better control of CHF can substantially reduce health care expenditures. The prevalence of CHF is expected to continue to rise because of declines in mortality from other CVD and because of the aging population. Age is the most common risk factor for CHF.

The causes of CHF may be divided into two subgroups: (1) underlying cardiac diseases and (2) causes that precipitate the onset of CHF in those with underlying cardiac problems. In addition to aging, the other most common risk factors for CHF are CAD, a more common cause in Caucasians, and HTN, a more common cause in African Americans. Other risk factors include cardiomyopathy, diabetes, valvular heart disease, and renal failure. Twenty percent of survivors of myocardial infarction, a common cause of CHF, will be incapacitated by CHF within 6 years. Precipitating causes of decompensation in CHF include anemia, infection, hyperthyroidism, hypothyroidism, exacerbation of HTN, dysrhythmias, endocarditis, and hypervolemia. Noncompliance with diet or medications can precipitate CHF episodes.

Pathophysiology

CHF results from complex interaction among factors that affect contractility, preload (i.e., ventricular volume at end of diastole, estimated by LV end diastolic pressure), and afterload (forces opposing LV ejection estimated by arterial blood pressure) and the subsequent neurohumoral and hemodynamic compensatory responses to falling CO. These responses ultimately exacerbate and perpetuate the problem.

CO is determined by stroke volume (SV) multiplied by heart rate. SV is determined by preload, contractility, and afterload. An increased preload stretches myocardial fibers, increasing the strength of contraction; however, excessive stretch results in decreased contractility. Increased contractility will increase SV but, if excessive, oxygen demand results in decreased contractility. Any increased afterload will decrease SV. Heart rate, which is influenced by the autonomic nervous system, will increase the CO until it is excessive (i.e., >160 beats/minute) in which case the duration of diastole is shortened, reducing ventricular filling and SV.

Several compensatory mechanisms to decrease CO are activated. Initially, the sympathetic nervous system (SNS) is stimulated, causing increased heart rate, increased contractility, vasoconstriction, and antidiuretic hormone (ADH) secretion. Venous constriction and ADH increase preload. These mechanisms help restore CO until limits are exceeded, then excessive myocardial oxygen demand and preload will result in decreased contractility and decompensation.

Falling CO with subsequent decreased renal perfusion also activates the renin-angiotensin-aldosterone system (RAAS), resulting in vasoconstriction and fluid retention. This increases the preload and CO until the preload is excessive and decompensation occurs. Angiotensin II and aldosterone have been implicated as causes of damage to the myocardium.

Ventricular hypertrophy occurs as a compensatory mechanism, but the myocardium eventually outgrows its' oxygen supply and increases the oxygen demand, resulting in decreased contractility. Recently, endogenous vasodilators (e.g., atrial natriuretic factor [ANF]) and other peptides have been identified, and their role in compensation of CHF and treatment is being defined.

Ventricular failure can be defined as *systolic dysfunction*, *diastolic dysfunction*, and *mixed systolic/diastolic dysfunction*.

Systolic dysfunction is characterized by diminished CO (ejection fraction [EF] <40%) due to decreased contractility. Activation of the SNS and RAAS ultimately, excessively increases preload and afterload, further decreasing contractility. A viscous cycle is established. Increased pressure in the LV causes pulmonary venous congestion. The most common cause of decreased contractility is ischemic heart disease. Cardiac dysrhythmias, dilated cardiomyopathy, chronic alcohol abuse, and myocarditis also decrease contractility.

Diastolic dysfunction has the classic findings of CHF with abnormal diastolic but normal systolic function/normal EF. It is characterized by resistance to ventricular filling resulting from abnormal relaxation of the myocardial muscle and increased pressure in the LV at the end of diastole. It is caused by conditions that stiffen the myocardium, such as ischemic heart disease with scarring, hypertrophic and restrictive cardiomyopathies, or pericardial disease. Increases in heart rate decrease filling time, thus exacerbating diastolic dysfunction. The pulmonary congestion that results from LVF may ultimately lead to RVF and systemic congestion.

An acute life-threatening complication of CHF is pulmonary edema, a situation in which the alveoli and airways become flooded with fluid containing red blood cells. Gas exchange is severely compromised and progressive acidosis develops. Other complications of CHF include cardiogenic shock, pleural effusion, LV thrombus, dysrhythmias, and impaired liver function.

Manifestations

The clinical manifestations of CHF reflect both decreased perfusion of body tissues resulting from decreased CO (forward effects) and pulmonary congestion that results from the increased LV pressure (backward effects). The manifestations of right ventricular dysfunction reflect the systemic congestion. Table 1 compares the manifestations of LVF and RVF. Table 2 lists the manifestations of pulmonary edema. A physical examination can often establish the diagnosis of CHF. A chest x-ray may show cardiomegaly, pulmonary congestion, edema, and pleural effusion. Arterial blood gases may indicate the alterations in gas exchange that result from CHF. An echocardiogram can estimate the ejection fraction. The New York Heart Association classification system, which is based on the severity of the symptoms, is commonly used as part of diagnosis.

Treatment

In addition to treating the underlying cause of the CHF and implementing lifestyle modifications (e.g., reducing dietary salt, exercising), pharmacological therapy involves using angiotensin-converting enzyme (ACE) inhibitors, diuretics, and ionotropic agents for systolic dysfunction. Some calcium blockers are used in diastolic dysfunction, slowing the heart rate; thus, they support diastolic filling. Beta blockers have an increasing role because of decreased symptoms and decreased mortality. Intravenous ionotropics are used in pulmonary edema. An intra-aortic balloon pump is sometimes needed for cardiogenic shock.

Common Dysrhythmias

	P Wave	P-R Interval	QRS
Sinus Bradycardia Slow discharge of SA node, R<60/minute, regular rhythm, may cause decreased CO/hypotension Etiology: physical training, sleep, hypothermia hypothyroid, vagal stimulation (suctioning), increased intracranial Sick Sinus Syndrome (SSS) (elderly), certain drugs (beta-blockers)	Normal	Normal	Normal
Sinus Tachycardia Rapid discharge of SA node, >100/minute, regular rhythm may cause decreased CO/hypotension, myocardial ischemia Etiology: hypotension, hypovolemia, fever, anemia, hypoxia, hyperthyroid, heart failure, certain drugs (e.g., Theophyllin [Roxane Laboratories, Inc, Columbus, OH])	Normal	Normal	Normal
Premature Atrial Contraction (PAC) Originate from ectopic atrial foci, usually normal conduction Rate varies, irregular rhythm, impulse conduction through AV node may be delayed or nonconducted May be prelude to supraventricular tachycardia Etiology: stimulants, hyperthyroid, infection, COPD, heart disease	Abnormal	Variable	Normal
Paroxysmal Supraventricular Tachycardia (SVT) Originate from ectopic focus above bundle of His, "re-entry" rate from 100 to 300/minute, regular rhythm If R>180/minute, then decreased CO/hypotension, myocardial ischemia Etiology: exertion, emotion, stimulants, rheumatic heart disease	Abnormal or hidden	Variable	Normal
Atrial Flutter Ectopic atrial focus "re-entry Atrial R 250 to 400/minute, usually slow ventricular response AV block, usually fixed 2:1, 3:1 High rate could decrease CO Etiology: CAD, valve problem, hyperthyroid, some drugs	Saw tooth shaped	Variable	Normal

CO = cardiac output, MI = myocardial infarction, CAD = coronary artery disease, SA = sinoatrial, AV = atrioventricular

(continued on p. 144)

Overview

Cardiac dysrhythmias are disruptions in the normal formation or conduction of electrical impulses that stimulate and coordinate atrial and ventricular myocardial contractions providing for an effective cardiac output. There is a wide variety of types and causes of dysrhythmias. Because coordinated electrical function of the heart is directly related to the coordinated myocardial contraction necessary for normal cardiac output, dysrhythmias may have serious consequences.

There are two basic types of dysrhythmias: *tachydysrhythmias*, which are the most common, and *bradydysrhythmias*. There are two fundamental causes of dysrhythmias: disorders of impulse formation or automaticity and disturbances of impulse conduction. There are two major groups of dysrhythmias: *supraventricular dysrhythmias*, which arise above the ventricles, and *ventricular dysrhythmias*, which arise in the ventricles. Ventricular dysrhythmias are more dangerous because the ventricles are the main pumping chambers.

Causes of dysrhythmia may relate to structural abnormalities of the heart (e.g., inflammation or scarring after a myocardial infarction) or to an abnormal physiological environment for cardiac cells (e.g., ischemia/hypoxia, electrolyte imbalance, or the presence of some drugs). Neuroendocrine hormones, such as epinephrine, acetylcholine, and thyroxine, can impact dysrhythmias. Most patients with serious dysrhythmias have underlying cardiac disease but some have a normal heart. Individuals with underlying cardiac pathology tend to tolerate dysrhythmias less well than those who do not, though a life-threatening dysrhythmia in an individual with a normal heart can result in sudden cardiac death.

Dysrhythmias can range from asymptomatic, occasional missed beats to symptomatic to sudden cardiac death. They are dangerous to the extent that they reduce cardiac output, impairing perfusion to the myocardium and brain. Less serious dysrhythmias, if they compromise the cardiac output, tend to deteriorate into life-threatening dysrhythmias. Thus, prompt recognition and intervention are essential.

Pathophysiology

The two fundamental pathophysiological mechanisms underlying dysrhythmias are disordered impulse formation or automaticity and disordered impulse conduction.

There are a variety of types of impulse formation problems. Cardiac cells normally capable of automaticity (i.e., sinoatrial [SA] node, atrioventricular [AV] node, and His-Purkinje system) may produce dysrhythmias if their rates of discharge change. The SA node, which is normally the pacemaker for the heart, may discharge at a rate slower or faster than normal (i.e., 60 to 100 beats per minute [bpm]), producing sinus bradycardia or sinus tachycardia. Pacemakers from the secondary sites may escape the control of the SA node and discharge before the SA node in one of two ways. If the SA node discharges at a rate slower than the rate of secondary pacemakers, electrical discharges from the secondary sites may automatically discharge at their intrinsic rates (i.e., AV node at 40 to 60 bpm or the His-Purkinje system at 30 to 40 bpm), producing "escape" beats or rhythms. Also, the secondary pacemakers may begin to discharge at a rate faster than the SA node escaping its' control.

Dysrhythmias may be produced if tissues that ordinarily do not express automaticity (i.e., atrial and ventricular muscle) develop spontaneous phase 4 depolarization and discharge at a rate faster than the SA node. Then early beats, such as atrial premature beats or ventricular premature beats, may be "triggered" at these ectopic foci and may begin a run of dysrhythmias that replaces normal sinus rhythm. Ectopic beats may originate at a single focus or multiple foci. There are situations in which so many ectopic foci are discharging from many different sites that there is no organized contraction of the heart chamber—only a quivering of the atrial or ventricular muscle (i.e., fibrillation).

Disturbances of conduction can occur in the SA node or the AV node, in the intraventricular conduction system, and within the atria and ventricles. They are responsible for SA exit blocks, AV conduction blocks, and establishing reentry circuits (see below). Impulse conduction through the AV node can be impaired to varying degrees. If conduction is slowed but not stopped, it is first degree block. If some impulses pass through and others do not, it is second degree block, and if no impulses pass through, it is third degree block.

Re-entry, also called *recirculating activation*, is a generalized mechanism underlying many dysrhythmias, such as premature beats, supraventricular tachycardias, and atrial flutter. Re-entry establishes localized, self-sustaining circuits of repetitive cardiac stimulation. Re-entry occurs in a branched Purkinje fiber when there is a unidirectional block in one of the branches. Since the block only prevents the impulse from traveling down through the branch, the impulse from the other branch passes up the unidirectionally blocked fiber in a retrograde fashion. It may then pass back down through the unblocked branch, creating a re-entrant activation of that branch. The impulse may continue to cycle, creating a circuit that causes repetitive ectopic beats and initiates pathological rhythms.

Manifestations

Dysrhythmias are detected because they produce symptoms or because they are detected during monitoring. Most of the symptoms of dysrhythmias are related to a decreased cardiac output. Sometimes they are felt as palpitations, a fluttering sensation, or skipped beats. Both bradycardias and tachycardias, because of the diminished diastolic filling time of the ventricles, can reduce cardiac output. Symptoms of diminished cardiac output include fatigue, lightheadedness, confusion, poor peripheral perfusion, dyspnea, syncope, and sudden cardiac death. Abrupt slowing of the rate can cause convulsions. Dysrhythmias can also precipitate congestive heart failure, angina, and infarction.

A noninvasive method for detecting dysrhythmias is the electrocardiogram (ECG). Twelve leads are placed on different areas of the chest wall and limbs to evaluate electrical activity from different perspectives. An ECG may be determined at a single point in time or continuously by continuous ambulatory monitoring (Holter monitor) or via telemetry. An invasive method of evaluating dysrhythmias is intracardiac electrophysiologic (EP) studies, which require cannulation of veins or arteries.

	P Wave	P-R Interval	QRS
Atrial Fibrillation Total disorganization, atrial electrical activity without effective atrial contraction Atrial R 300 to 600/minute, irregularly irregular ventricular, may be rapid; if rapid, decrease CO, mural thrombi/emboli Etiology: usually heart disease, also hyperthyroid, infection	Chaotic	Can't be measured	Normal
Junctional/Nodal Arrhythmia Originates in AV node, may move retrograde, producing abnormal P wave before or after QRS Indicate problem with SA node; if rapid, decrease CO	Abnormal or hidden	Variable	Normal
First-Degree AV Block Every impulse is conducted, but conduction is prolonged Etiology: CAD, drugs (digoxin, beta blockers), rheumatic fever	Normal	>.20 second	Normal
Second-Degree Block—Type I AV conduction time is gradually prolonged until an atrial impulse is nonconducted and QRS is dropped, then repeats Ventricular rate may be slower Etiology: usually myocardial ischemia, drugs	Normal	Progressive lengthening	Normal width one not conducted
Second Degree—Type 2 Atrial impulses dropped, without antecedent lengthening P-R Certain number of impulses are not conducted 2:1. 3:1 block Often progresses to third-degree block; if slow pulse, decrease CO Etiology: CAD, MI, digoxin	Occurs in multiples	Normal or prolonged	Widened Preceded by two or more P waves
Third Degree—Complete AV Block No atrial impulses conducted, atria and ventricle contract separately, result is decreased CO and heart failure Etiology: calcification of conduction system, CAD, cardiomyopathy	Normal	Variable	Normal or widened
Premature Ventricular Contraction (PVC) From single or multiple ectopic focus in ventricle Premature, distorted QRS, R = 60 to 100/minute, irregular Bigeminy, triplets, >3 is ventricular tachycardia May decrease CO, indicates ventricular irritability Etiology; ischemia, stimulants, hypokalemia, stress, fever	None	Not measurable	Wide and distorted
Ventricular Tachycardia Run of three or more PVCs, ventricular focus or foci fire repeatedly, take control as pacemaker, R = 110 to 250/minute May cause profound decreased CO, immediate intervention May progress to ventricular fibrillation	Usually none	Not measurable	Wide and distorted
Ventricular Fibrillation Severe derangement, firing multiple ventricular foci No effective ventricular contraction, terminal if untreated Etiology: ischemia, infarction, CAD, cardiomyopathy	None	Not measurable	Wide and distorted

Treatment

Medications are a common method of intervention for significant dysrhythmias. Symptomatic bradycardias and AV conduction blocks may also be treated with pacemakers. Carotid massage, cardioversion (i.e., controlled defibrillation), and pacemakers may be used to treat supraventricular tachydysrhythmias. Immediate intervention by defibrillation (e.g., conventional or implanted) is necessary for life-threatening ventricular dysrhythmias. Radiofrequency catheter ablation uses high frequency electromagnetic energy to destroy points of origin or pathways necessary for the propagation of some dysrhythmias. Avoidance of stimulants such as caffeine and tobacco and stress management are other important measures.

38 Cardiomyopathies

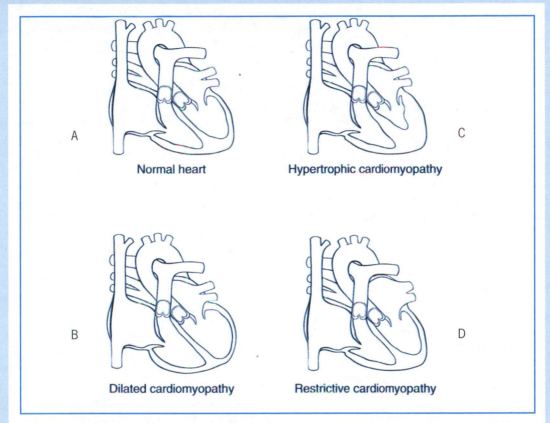

A — Normal heart

C — Hypertrophic cardiomyopathy

B — Dilated cardiomyopathy

D — Restrictive cardiomyopathy

Diagram showing the major distinguishing pathophysiologic features of the types of cardiomyopathies. (A) The normal heart. (B) In the dilated type of cardiomyopathy, the heart has a globular shape and the largest circumference of the left ventricle is not at its base but midway between the apex and base. (C) In the hypertrophic type, the wall of the left ventricle is greatly thickened and the cavity reduced, but the left atrium may be dilated because of poor diastolic relaxation of the ventricle. (D) In the restrictive type, the left ventricular cavity is of normal size, but again, the left atrium is dilated because of the reduced diastolic compliance of the ventricle.

Overview

Cardiomyopathy (CMP) is a term used to describe a diverse group of cardiac diseases that primarily effect the structure and function of the myocardium (i.e., the heart muscle). Two major divisions of CMP are ischemic and nonischemic. This chapter deals only with nonischemic CMP.

Ischemic CMP refers to the type of myocardial dysfunction that occurs in coronary artery disease (see Chapter 34). *Nonischemic CMPs* are classified into three groups based on their pathophysiologic effects on the heart: dilated, hypertrophic, and restrictive. While some CMPs may be secondary to specific causes (e.g., infiltrative disorders), most are idiopathic (i.e., the cause is not known).

Dilated Cardiomyopathy

Overview

Dilated CMP accounts for more than 90% of all CMPs and results in 20,000 deaths per year. It can occur at any age, but its peak incidence is in the fourth or fifth decade. African-American men have 2.5 times higher risk than Caucasians and women. Half the cases of dilated CMP are idiopathic, and the remainder are secondary to some known cause. Certain chemotherapeutic agents, particularly doxorubicin and daunorubicin, cause serious myocardial damage. A disproportionate number of individuals with dilated CMP are alcoholics. Damage may be due to direct toxic effects or due to nutritional deficiencies. Dilated CMP is seen more frequently in cocaine addicts than ever before. Peripartum CMP is seen 3 to 4 months after pregnancy. Another group of dilated CMP may be the consequence of previous viral, bacterial, or parasitic infections. Autoimmune, thyrotoxicosis, diabetes, and hypersensitivity reactions to some medications have been associated.

Pathophysiology

Dilated CMP is characterized by cardiomegaly due to ventricular dilation and by impaired myocardial contractility and mixed systolic and diastolic dysfunction, a condition in which poor systolic function (weakened muscle function) is further compromised by dilated ventricular walls that are unable to relax. A decreased ejection fraction/CO, increased end diastolic pressure with pulmonary congestion, and stasis of blood with mural thrombi are the result. The walls of the ventricle do not become thickened as in congestive heart failure, which is thought to be due to diffuse inflammation and rapid degeneration of myocardial fibers and fibrosis. Deterioration is rapid after the onset of symptoms, and 20% to 50% of patients die within 1 year. The majority of deaths occur within 5 years.

Manifestations

Clinical manifestations of dilated CMP develop insidiously. Patients present with signs and symptoms of congestive heart failure. The most common symptoms are dyspnea and fatigue. A dry cough, orthopnea, and paroxysmal nocturnal dyspnea occur. Palpitations are common, and exertional chest pain indistinguishable from angina occurs in some patients. Dizziness may result from dysrhythmias. A decrease in activity tolerance occurs. Signs may include increases or decreases of blood pressure, tachycardia, S3 and S4 heart sounds, and murmurs of mitral or tricuspid regurgitation. Pulmonary congestion results in increased respiratory rate, crackles, and abnormal blood gases. There may be edema; weak pedal pulses; and cool, pale extremities with poor capillary refill. Hepatomegaly and jugular venous distention may occur. Systemic and pulmonary emboli are common complications. Left heart failure is the cause of death in 75% of the patients. Sudden death from dysrhythmia may occur.

The best diagnostic tool is the echocardiogram, which shows dilated ventricles, global diminished ventricular wall motion, and an ejection fraction of less than 45%.

Treatment

Few causes of dilated CMP are reversible (e.g., nutritional, alcohol related). Treatment is mainly supportive and similar to the treatment of congestive heart failure (e.g., decreasing afterload and enhancing contractility).

Patients with terminal end-stage dilated CMP may require heart transplantation. Fifty percent of heart transplants are done for dilated CMP.

Hypertrophic Cardiomyopathy

Overview

Hypertrophic CMP, also known as *idiopathic hypertrophic subaortic stenosis* (IHSS), is less common than dilated CMP. It is more common in men and is often seen in active, athletic individuals. It appears to have an autosomal dominant genetic basis.

Pathophysiology

The hallmark of hypertrophic CMP is massive ventricular wall thickening with disproportionate thickening of the intraventricular septum. This results in a hyperdynamic state with increased contractility and increased ejection fraction. There is loss of ventricular wall compliance and impaired diastolic relaxation (i.e., diastolic dysfunction). The thickened septum may obstruct left ventricular outflow through the aorta. The decreased ventricular filling and obstruction to outflow may result in decreased cardiac output. Any condition that increases the contractility also increases the obstruction (e.g., cardiotonic medications like digoxin and exertion).

Manifestations

Major clinical manifestations are exertional dyspnea, fatigue, syncope, angina, and left heart failure. If the hypertrophied muscle outgrows its blood supply, a myocardial infarction may occur. Palpitations are common and often related to dysrhythmias. Common dysrhythmias are supraventricular tachycardia, atrial fibrillation, ventricular tachycardia, and ventricular fibrillation. Any of these dysrhythmias may lead to loss of consciousness or sudden cardiac death, which is the most common cause of death. Diagnosis is made by electrocardiogram (ECG) and echocardiogram. Increased voltage (height) and duration (width) of QRS complexes indicate ventricular hypertrophy on ECG. Dysrhythmias are also frequently seen. The primary diagnostic tool is the echocardiogram, which reveals the classic feature—asymmetrical left ventricular hypertrophy. It may also demonstrate abnormal wall motion and diastolic dysfunction.

Pathophysiological Characteristics of Cardiomyopathies

Type of Cardiomyopathy	Associated Conditions	Anatomic Derangement	Physiologic Derangement	Manifestations
Dilated or congestive	Infection Alcohol Pregnancy Some drugs	Cardiomegaly—ventricular dilation without hypertrophy Chamber volume increased Decreased contractile muscle fibers Diffuse necrosis Mitral valve incompetence	Poor systolic function Diminished contractility Decreased ejection fraction Increased end diastolic (residual) volume Blood stasis Mural thrombi	Fatigue Weakness Dyspnea Palpitations Left ventricular failure Dysrhythmias
Hypertrophic	Autosomal dominant inheritance	Disproportionate thickening of interventricular septum Aortic outflow obstruction in some cases Chamber volume is decreased Mitral valve incompetence	Increased contractility Decreased compliance Poor diastolic function	Dyspnea Angina Syncope Palpitations Dysrhythmias Left ventricular failure Sudden death
Restrictive	Infiltrative diseases (e.g., amyloidosis)	Rigid, noncompliant myocardium Mild cardiomegaly Fibrotic myocardium Atrioventricular valve incompetence	Impeded ventricular filling Diastolic dysfunction Decreased compliance	Right ventricular failure Dysrhythmias

Adapted from Huether, S., & McChance, K. (2000). *Understanding pathophysiology* (2nd ed.). St. Louis, MO: C. V. Mosby Co.

Treatment

The goals of treatment are to reduce the ventricular stiffness, improve the ventricular filling, and relieve the left ventricular outflow obstruction by decreasing the contractility and cardiac rate with beta blockers. Verapamil has also been successful. Surgical resection of the hypertrophied tissue, *ventriculomyotomy* and *myectomy*, may relieve symptoms in those who don't respond to medications.

Restrictive Cardiomyopathy

Overview

Restrictive CMP is the least common of the CMPs. Although the specific etiology is unknown, it is usually associated with an infiltrative disease of the myocardium. Secondary causes include amyloidosis, sarcoidosis, hemochromatosis, glycogen storage disease, myocardial fibrosis, and radiation to the thorax.

Pathophysiology

Myocardial fibrosis, hypertrophy, and infiltration produce stiffness of the ventricular wall, which results in diminished compliance and decreased ventricular diastolic filling with high diastolic filling pressures to maintain cardiac output.

Manifestations

The most common clinical manifestation of restrictive CMP is heart failure, particularly right-sided heart failure. The most common symptom is exercise intolerance because the ventricle cannot increase the rate without further compromising the diastolic filling. Angina, fatigue, syncope, and dyspnea on exertion are also common. Signs of both right- and left-sided heart failure may be present and peripheral edema, hepatomegaly, ascites, and jugular venous distention may be present. Pulmonary congestion, or crackles, may be evident. The most common dysrhythmia that may be produced is atrial fibrillation. Diagnosis is made by chest x-ray, which shows cardiomegaly and pulmonary congestion or ECG, which shows tachycardia and reveals tachycardia and dysrhythmia. An echocardiogram may reveal thickened ventricular walls, small cavities, and an enlarged atria. Endomyocardial biopsy and a computed tomography scan may aid diagnosis.

Treatment

There is no specific treatment for restrictive CMP other than treating the underlying disease. Interventions may be aimed at improving the diastolic filling by controlling the heart rate and treatment of congestive heart failure. A heart transplant may need to be considered.

39 Inflammatory Heart Disease

Clinical Manifestations of Pericarditis

History
- Chest pain—Pleuritic is relieved by sitting; substernal radiates to neck, shoulders, back, and epigastrium
- Dyspnea

Physical Examination
- Pericardial friction rub
- Fever

Diagnostic Tests
- Leukocytosis
- Electrocardiogram (ECG) may show S-T and T wave changes
- Chest x-ray may show cardiac enlargement
- Echocardiogram may show pericardial effusion

Pericardial Effusion
- Pain may or may not be present, dyspnea, cough, friction rub
- If tamponade, tachycardia, tachypnea, narrow pulse pressure
- Pulsus paradoxus (>10 mmHg fall in systolic pressure with inspiration)
- Increased central venous pressure, edema, ascites
- Diagnostic tests: chest x-ray, ECG, echocardiogram, magnetic resonance imaging (MRI)

Constrictive Pericarditis
- Progressive dyspnea, fatigue, weakness, chronic edema
- Hepatomegaly; ascites, jugular venous distention
- Atrial fibrillation
- Diagnostic tests: chest x-ray, echocardiogram, computed tomography (CT) scan, MRI

Pericarditis

Overview

Pericarditis, which is inflammation of the pericardium, may be a primary condition or result from secondary disease. Viral infections are the most common cause and often follow an upper respiratory infection. Males under 50 years old are most commonly effected. Bacterial pericarditis is rare. Other causes include systemic disease such as autoimmune and connective tissues diseases (e.g., rheumatoid arthritis, systemic lupus erythematosus, or rheumatic fever), uremia, neoplasm, and trauma (e.g., radiation, chest injury, open heart surgery, or pacemaker insertion). It may also result from diseases of adjacent structures, myocardial infarction, and pulmonary disease. Pericarditis may spread from or to the myocardium.

Pathophysiology

In pericarditis, the pericardial membranes become inflamed and roughened and they rub together. A transudate (protein free) or an exudate (proteinaceous) may develop and may fill the pericardial sac (i.e., *peri-*

cardial effusion). The fluid may be serous (heart failure), purulent (bacterial infection), serosanguineous (neoplasm, uremia), or hemorrhagic (ruptured aneurysm or trauma). If fluid accumulates slowly, it may not be clinically significant; however, when fluid accumulates rapidly, *cardiac tamponade* (i.e., compression of the heart) may occur, impairing venous return, filling the heart, and causing systemic congestion and decreased cardiac output. Cardiac failure, cardiogenic shock, and death can result.

Chronic inflammation can gradually lead to *constrictive pericarditis* in which pericardial membranes become thickened and fibrous and adhere, encasing the heart in a hard shell that restricts cardiac filling, and causing systemic congestion and reduced cardiac output.

Manifestations

See Clinical Manifestations of Pericarditis on p. 148.

Treatment

Treatment is specific to the underlying cause (e.g., antibiotics for infection) and to reduce inflammation and its' sequelae. Small effusions are treated with nonsteroidal anti-inflammatory drugs (NSAIDs) and corticosteroids if the inflammation is refractory to the NSAIDs. A pericardiocentesis may be needed for large effusions or a pericardial fenestration for continuous drainage. In constrictive pericarditis, a pericardectomy, or removal of the pericardium, may be needed.

Infective Endocarditis

Overview

Infective endocarditis, formerly known as *bacterial endocarditis*, is an infection of the endocardium, or inner lining of the heart, and most often involves the valves. Prior to the era of antibiotics, it was a lethal disease. It is now relatively rare, though there are approximately 5,000 to 8,000 new cases in the United States each year. Two forms of endocarditis are described: subacute and acute. The subacute form has a longer course, a more insidious onset, less toxicity, and causative organism of low virulence, commonly *Streptococcus viridans.* It responds well to treatment. The acute form has a shorter course, more rapid onset, more toxicity, and more virulent organism, commonly *Staphylococcus aureus.* It can cause death within days or weeks if untreated.

Infective endocarditis occurs when turbulent blood flow in the heart allows causative organisms to grow on damaged valves or other endothelial surfaces. Conditions predisposing individuals to endocarditis have changed with the decreasing incidence of rheumatic heart disease and recognition and treatment of mitral valve prolapse. Risk factors include congenital and degenerative heart diseases that damage valves and endothelial surfaces. Individuals with artificial valve replacement may develop endocarditis. Organisms may gain entry to the blood stream during intrusive procedures such as dental procedures, gynecological examinations, and placement of urinary catheters. Intravenous drug abusers are at high risk.

Organisms other than bacteria can be involved (e.g., gram-negative bacilli, fungi, and yeast), particularly in the immunocompromised individual.

Pathophysiology

Pathogenesis of infective endocarditis first involves *endothelial damage,* which attracts platelets and stimulates thrombus formation. This facilitates the adherence of organisms that entered the blood stream and survived body defenses, allowing their colonization. Some very virulent organisms do not require the initial endothelial damage. The mass of fibrin, leukocytes, platelets, and microorganism is called a *vegetation.* This process commonly involves valves and surrounding endothelium. The valves may become scarred and perforated. Valvular incompetence and invasion of the myocardium may result in heart failure. Emboli may break free from the vegetative growth, travel in the blood stream to distant organs, and form abscesses.

Manifestations

See Clinical Manifestations of Endocarditis on p. 151.

Treatment

Prophylactic treatment involves administration of antibiotics prior to invasive procedures. With infection of valves, antibiotics are started and continued for 4 to 6 weeks. Deteriorated valves are surgically replaced if necessary.

Myocarditis

Overview

Myocarditis is a focal or diffuse inflammatory process involving the myocardium and resulting from a variety of etiological agents including pathological organisms (mainly viruses but also fungi, parasites, and rickettsiae), radiation, toxins, systemic diseases (e.g., systemic lupus erythematosus, rheumatic fever), and immune reactions. It often follows an upper respiratory infection. It is frequently associated with pericarditis and endocarditis.

Pathophysiology

The pathogenesis of myocarditis is poorly understood because there is a period of several weeks (in some forms, a decade) between exposure to the infecting organism and development of manifestations. Infiltration of organisms, blood cells, toxins, and immune substances around coronary arteries and between muscle fibers can result in fiber dysfunction and degeneration that may impede contractility and conduction and may cause dilation of the heart or

Clinical Manifestations of Endocarditis

History

- Fever
- Anorexia, weight loss
- Back pain
- Night sweats
- Embolization to coronary arteries could cause myocardial infarction

Physical Examination

- New or significantly changed heart murmur
- Petechial lesions of skin, conjunctiva, oral mucosa

Diagnostic Tests

- Positive blood cultures
- Elevated erythrocyte sedimentation rate (ESR)
- ECG changes: prolonged P-R interval, conduction blocks

Clinical Manifestations of Myocarditis

History

- May be asymptomatic
- Dyspnea, fatigue, syncope
- Palpitations, chest discomfort

Physical Examination

- Cardiac enlargement
- Faint heart sounds, friction rub
- Pericardial effusion, congestive heart failure

Diagnostic Tests

- ECG changes, ischemia
- Leukocytosis, atypical lymphocytes, ESR
- Echocardiogram, myocardial biopsy

diminished wall motion. Though commonly benign, it can result in heart failure, dysrhythmias, and mural thrombi. It has been theorized that dilated cardiomyopathy is a manifestation of myocarditis.

Manifestations

See Clinical Manifestations of Myocarditis above.

Treatment

Specific treatment is not yet established. Treatment usually consists of managing any cardiac decompensation. Immunosuppressive agents are used in some cases after the infective stage of the disease to reduce myocardial inflammation and prevent damage.

Rheumatic Heart Disease

Overview

Acute rheumatic fever (ARF) is an acute, febrile, inflammatory disease caused by a delayed immune response to a pharyngeal infection by the group A beta hemolytic streptococcus. In its acute form, it results in inflammation of the joints, skin, nervous system, and heart. Inflammation in the heart may involve the pericardium, endocardium, and myocardium. If the streptococcal infection is untreated, resulting damage to the heart can result in *rheumatic heart disease* (RHD), a chronic condition characterized by destruction, scarring, and deformity of the heart valves. Antibiotic treatment of streptococcal infections within 9 days usually prevents ARF.

Initial and recurrent episodes of ARF are most common in childhood between the ages of 5 and 15 as a complication of streptococcal pharyngitis. Recurrent attacks may occur. The incidence of ARF has declined in recent years with socioeconomic and medical improvements. However, because overcrowding and poor hygiene are risk factors for ARF, the disease continues to be a concern in underprivileged populations. It has a tendency to run in families.

Pathophysiology

Rheumatic fever causes inflammation in all three layers of the heart, but the primary lesions involve the endocardium. Inflammation causes swelling of the valve leaflet and erosion along the edges. Vegetation are deposited on the erosions, valve elasticity is lost, and leaflets become adherent. Valvular dysfunction, most commonly mitral stenosis, develops. Fibrinoid, necrotic deposits called *Aschoff's bodies* develop in the myocardium. Pericardial inflammation is characterized by serosanguineous effusion. Cardiomegaly and heart failure may develop with chronic rheumatic heart disease. Conduction disturbances and atrial fibrillation are common.

Treatment

Penicillin or erythromycin is used to treat the rheumatic fever and is used continuously to prevent recurrence. Salicylate, which is used as an anti-inflammatory agent; corticosteroids; and bed rest are used with serious inflammation. The valves may need to be surgically repaired or replaced.

40 Valvular Problems

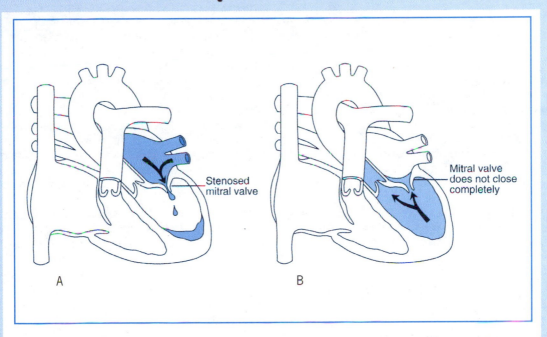

A

B

Valvular stenosis and regurgitation. (A) Hemodynamic effect of mitral stenosis. The stenosed valve is unable to open sufficiently during left atrial systole, inhibiting left ventricular filling. (B) Hemodynamic effect of mitral regurgitation. The mitral valve does not close completely during left ventricular systole, permitting blood to re-enter the left atrium.

Labels in figure: Stenosed mitral valve; Mitral valve does not close completely

Valvular Problems

Overview

There are four heart valves: two atrioventricular valves (i.e., mitral and tricuspid) and two semilunar valves (i.e., aortic and pulmonic). It is the coordination of the opening and closing of these valves with the pressure gradients created during the phases of the cardiac cycle that determines the forward flow of the blood. During systole, the aortic and pulmonic valves are normally open and the mitral and tricuspid valves are closed. During diastole, the mitral and tricuspid valves are open and the aortic and pulmonic valves are closed.

Disorders of the endocardium damage the heart valves, impeding cardiac function to various degrees. The types of valvular disease are defined according to the valve affected and the type of functional alteration

(i.e., stenosis [due to a narrowed orifice] and regurgitation [due to incomplete closure]). Though any of the valves may be affected, those on the left side of the heart are more commonly affected. Valvular problems may be congenital or acquired. At one time, most acquired valvular disease in the United States was a result of rheumatic fever, but other causes are more common today (e.g., atherosclerotic heart disease in the elderly).

Pathophysiology

A stenotic valve is a valve whose orifice has been restricted, thus impeding the forward flow of blood. The work load for the heart chamber "in front of" the valve increases because the pressure needs to increase to overcome the resistance to outflow (increased afterload) and the chamber hypertrophies.

In valvular regurgitation (also called *incompetence* or *insufficiency*), a regurgitant or incompetent valve is a valve that does not close completely, thus permitting backward flow of blood into the chamber "in front of" the valve. This increases the volume of blood the heart must pump, the work load of both the atrium and ventricle, and additional workload for the heart. It also causes cardiomegaly. Increased volume leads to chamber dilation, and increased work load leads to hypertrophy of the heart muscle.

The dilation and hypertrophy that occur are compensatory mechanisms to support the pumping ability of the heart. Eventually, contractility and the ejection fraction may diminish, the end diastolic pressure increases, and the ventricles fail. Abnormal valves also predispose to cardiac infection and thrombus formation. Cardiac dysrhythmias, particularly atrial fibrillation and flutter and atrioventricular blocks, may occur.

Mitral valve prolapse syndrome is a form of valvular disease more prevalent in young women in which the valve leaflets balloon upward into the left atrium during systole. It has a high incidence, suggesting that it may be a normal variant rather than pathological. It is usually associated with minimal morbidity or mortality, though severe sequelae are potentially possible (e.g., mitral regurgitation, ventricular failure, thromboemboli, and sudden death). Studies suggest that there is a genetic component. It is often associated with connective tissue disorders, and there may be a relationship to hyperthyroidism.

Manifestations

The diagnostic work-up for valvular problems may include a chest x-ray that provides information about chamber size. An electrocardiogram may show hypertrophy and dysrhythmia. An echocardiogram provides information about the morphology and function of the valves, the left ventricular function, the direction of blood flow, and the size of the atria and ventricles. A transesophageal echocardiogram (TEE) improves the image.

The severity of the valve dysfunction and capacity of the heart to compensate determine the degree of incapacity and the manifestations. The manifestations relate both to the compensatory mechanisms and diminished cardiac dysfunction.

Most individuals with mitral stenosis have underlying rheumatic heart disease. Initially, it is asymptomatic with symptoms occurring only when the orifice is reduced by 50%. Symptoms, often precipitated by atrial fibrillation that develops in 80% of the individuals, include those of left heart failure (e.g., dyspnea, orthopnea, paroxysmal nocturnal dyspnea [PND], and dry cough), increased respiratory infection, and hemoptysis. As the stenosis progresses, there will be symptoms of diminished cardiac output (e.g., fatigue, syncope, chest pain). Eventually, with increasing pulmonary hypertension, there will be manifestations of right sided heart failure (e.g., anorexia, hepatomegaly, ascites, edema, jugular venous distention [JVD]). The individual may experience palpitations if atrial fibrillation develops. Atrial enlargement may lead to hoarseness. On physical examination, there is a low pitched, rumbling, mid-diastolic murmur at the apex with an accentuate S1 and a diastolic snap.

The manifestations of mitral regurgitation, related to overfilling of the atrium and increased workload for the left atrium and ventricle, depend on how abruptly it develops. Chronic mitral regurgitation may be asymptomatic for years with slow development of left ventricular failure with exertional dyspnea, fatigue, syncope, palpitations, and atypical chest pain. Physical examination reveals a loud, high pitched, blowing, pansystolic murmur radiating to the axilla. A midsystolic click and S3 may be present. Arial fibrillation is common. The left atrium and ventricle are dilated and hypertrophied. Acute mitral regurgitation may have a fulminant course of pulmonary edema and shock.

Aortic stenosis tends to develop gradually with ventricular hypertrophy overcoming the impedance to outflow. Eventually, hypertrophy leads to ischemia and clinical manifestations develop, including reduced systolic blood pressure and narrowed pulse pressure.

Treatment

Valvular dysfunction may be treated with cardiotonic medications, fluid volume control, blood pressure control, and prophylactic antibiotics prior to invasive procedures. Surgical repair or prosthetic valve replacement may be necessary. The valve may be replaced with a mechanical or a biological prosthesis. The mechanical prosthesis predisposes to the risk of thromboembolism and requires chronic anticoagulation. A biological prosthesis (e.g., porcine, bovine, cadaver) does not require chronic anticoagulation, but it does require eventual reoperation.

Clinical Manifestations of Valvular Stenosis and Regurgitation

Manifestation	Aortic Stenosis	Mitral Stenosis	Aortic Regurgitation	Mitral Regurgitation	Tricuspid Regurgitation
Cardiovascular outcome*	Left ventricular failure	Right ventricular failure	Left heart failure	Left heart failure	Right heart failure
General symptoms	Fatigue	Fatigue, weakness		Fatigue, weakness	Peripheral edema (with heart failure)
Respiratory effects	Dyspnea on exertion	Dyspnea on exertion, orthopnea, paroxysmal nocturnal dyspnea, predisposition to respiratory infections, hemoptysis, pulmonary hypertension, edema	Dyspnea with effort	Dyspnea; occasional hemo ptysis	Dyspnea
Central nervous system effects	Syncope, especially on exertion	Neural deficits only associated with emboli e.g., hepatomegaly)	Syncope	None	None
Gastrointestinal effects	None	Ascites; hepatic angina with hepatomegaly	None	None	Ascites, hepatomegaly (with heart failure)
Pain	Angina pectoris	Chest pain	Chest pain (anginal)	None	Palpitations
Heart rate, rhythm	Bradycardia, dysrhythmias (with heart failure)	Palpitations (atrial fibrillation)	Palpitations, water-hammer pulse	Palpitations	Atrial fibrillations
Heart sounds	Systolic murmur	Diastolic murmur, accentuated first heart sound, opening snap	Diastolic and systolic murmurs	Murmur throughout systole	Murmur throughout systole
Most common cause	Congenital, rheumatic fever	Rheumatic fever	Bacterial endocarditis;- aortic root disease	Floppy valve; coronary artery disease	Congenital

*Untreated disease

Reprinted with permission from Huether, S.,& McChance, K. (2000). Understanding pathophysiology (2nd ed.). St. Louis, MO: C. V. Mosby Co.

41 Vascular Disorders

Comparison of Arterial and Venous Problems—Clinical Manifestations

Chronic Arterial Insufficiency
- Intermittent claudication
- Calf pain with popliteal artery occlusion
- Hip pain with aortoiliac artery occlusion
- Rest pain in advanced cases
- Diminished, absent, or asymmetrical pulses
- Bruits
- Skin is shiny, thin, fragile, and taut
- Loss of hair
- Cool temperature
- Trophic nail changes
- Pale, blanched appearance when leg is elevated
- Dependent rubor
- Minimum edema

Acute Arterial Occlusion
- Sudden appearance of:
    Pain
    Pallor
    Pulselessness
    Paresthesia
    Poikilothermy
    Paralysis

(continued on p. 158)

Aneurysm

Overview

An aneurysm is a localized dilation of a blood vessel or cardiac chamber wall because of congenital or acquired weakness of the muscle. Because of the constant pressure the aorta sustains, it is particularly susceptible. The abdominal aorta is involved 75% of the time and the thoracic aorta 25%. Peripheral arteries are less often affected. A popliteal artery aneurysm is third in order of frequency. Ventricular aneurysms may occur in the heart, and cerebral aneurysms in the brain. Aneurysms are potentially life threatening because rupture and hemorrhage or thromboembolism may occur.

Two major classifications of aneurysm are *true aneurysms* and *false aneurysms* or *pseudoaneurysms*. With a true aneurysm, at least one wall of the artery is intact. True aneurysms are further subdivided based on shape into *saccular aneurysm*, a bulge with a narrow neck connecting it to one side of the artery, and a *fusiform aneurysm*, circumferential and relatively, uniformly shaped. A false aneurysm involves the dissection of all the layers of the arterial wall (e.g., from trauma, infection, or disruption of a suture line), causing bleeding that is contained, or tamponaded, by surrounding tissues. Aortic dissection, sometimes incorrectly referred to as *dissecting aneurysm*, occurs when a tear in the inner layer of an arterial wall allows blood to collect between layers of the wall.

Risk factors include congenital weakness of the arterial wall, atherosclerosis, hypertension, dyslipidemias, diabetes, smoking, advanced age, trauma, and infection. Syphilis, once a major cause, and other infections can also be factors. There is a familial tendency, probably genetic, in the development of abdominal aneurysms. Popliteal aneurysms occur almost exclusively in males. Myocardial infarction is the cause of ventricular aneurysms.

Pathophysiology

Atherosclerosis is the cause of most degenerative arterial disease. Plaque formation results in the deposit of lipids, fibrin, and debris below the intima, in the media, causing degenerative changes that lead to loss of elasticity, weakness, and dilation. Smoking, hypertension, high serum lipids, insulin resistance, all of which damage the arterial walls, can initiate plaque formation. High pressure within the vessel contributes to the weakness, dilation, and risk of rupture. With turbulent blood flow, thromboembolism may occur. The dilation of a vessel may compress surrounding structures and cause inflammation. Aneurysms can impede blood flow distally. Growth of aneurysms is unpredictable, but the larger the size, the greater the risk of rupture. (An aneurysm is considered present when the diameter of the aorta is greater than 4 cm). Rupture of an abdominal aortic aneurysm into the peritoneal cavity causes death in minutes if untreated. Retroperitoneal bleeding can produce local tamponade, allowing more time for intervention. Cerebral aneurysms can cause focal neurological deficits due to compression of tissue or ischemia. Bleeding may occur into the subarachnoid space. Aneurysms may leak slowly rather than rupture.

Manifestations

Aneurysms are commonly asymptomatic and are only discovered during routine or coincidental physical examination or x-ray. See p. 155 for clinical manifestations.

Treatment

The goal of treatment is to prevent rupture. The only effective treatment for aneurysms is surgery. Surgery is performed any time in a symptomatic individual or when the diameter is >5 cm in an asymptomatic individual. Blood pressure needs to be monitored and controlled. With rupture, immediate surgery is required.

Chronic Arterial Occlusive Disease

Overview

Chronic arterial occlusive disease is a slowly progressive disorder in which partial or total arterial occlusion, predominantly in the lower extremities, deprives the extremities of oxygen and nutrients. The primary cause is atherosclerosis. It usually occurs in the sixth through eighth decade of life but at an earlier age in diabetics and is a factor in the high incidence of nontraumatic amputation in this population. It occurs more frequently in males and has a familial tendency. The most important risk factors are smoking, hypertension, diabetes, and dyslipidemia. Other risk factors include obesity and sedentary lifestyle.

Pathophysiology

Atherosclerotic plaque leads to thickening of the intima and media of arterial walls impinging on the lumen. Primarily larger arteries and bifurcations are affected, thus involvement is usually segmental with normal areas between obstructed areas. The arteries most commonly affected are the aortoiliac, femoral, popliteal, tibial, and peroneal. The diminished perfusion leads to progressive oxygen deprivation (i.e., ischemia) of the tissues supplied. The by-products of anaerobic metabolism (e.g., lactic acid) stimulate pain receptors. This mostly occurs in the larger muscles (e.g., thighs, calves, buttocks) during exercise when an oxygen debt is incurred. With cessation of exercise and clearing of metabolic products, the pain subsides. Later pain at rest occurs with more severe ischemia.

Ischemia leads to atrophy of tissues and poor healing capacity, infection, and tissue necrosis. Ischemic ulcers, gangrene, and amputation are the most significant complications.

Manifestations

See p. 156 for clinical manifestations.

Treatment

Treatment goals are to slow the progression, improve the perfusion, and prevent trauma. Reperfusion efforts may include percutaneous transluminal angioplasty, stenting, arthrectomy, arterial bypass surgery often with patch graft angioplasty, endarterectomy (rarely), and use of antiplatelet medications.

Varicose Veins and Chronic Venous Insufficiency

Overview

Varicose veins (i.e., varicosities) are distended, tortuous, palpable superficial veins of the lower extremity. Primary varicosities, a condition that has a familial tendency, are those in which superficial veins are dilated with or without incompetent valves. Secondary varicosities can result from any condition in which there has been a prolonged increase in venous pressure (e.g., from a previous deep vein thrombosis [DVT] or obstruction to venous return that occurs in pregnancy), resulting in venous distention, pooling of blood, and valvular incompetence. Risk factors, in addition to DVT and

Chronic Venous Insufficiency
- Dull discomfort worsened by standing
- Progressive edema
- Thin, shiny, atrophic skin
- Cyanotic
- Brownish pigmentation
- Eczema, weeping dermatitis
- Thick, fibrous subcutaneous tissues
- Pain with ulceration
- Varicosities
- Recurrent ulcerations just above the ankle on medial or anterior aspect

Superficial Thrombophlebitis
- History of trauma or intravenous line
- Dull pain
- No significant swelling
- Induration, redness, tenderness, and warmth

Deep Vein Thrombosis
- Pain in calf or thigh, though sometimes there is no pain
- History of recent surgery, inactivity, oral contraceptives, neoplasia, congestive heart failure
- Edema, tenderness, or vein
- Slight fever, tachycardia
- Local warmth, redness
- <20% have positive Homans' sign

pregnancy include occupations requiring long periods of standing, obesity, and external pressure from tumors.

Chronic venous insufficiency (CVI) is inadequate venous return over time. It generally develops secondary to DVT or superficial venous insufficiency. The increased venous dilation and pressure lead to changes in the skin and subcutaneous tissues.

Pathophysiology

Increased venous pressure and pooling of blood cause the veins to enlarge, stretching the valves that normally prevent the back flow of blood. The valves become incompetent, blood flow is reversed, and venous pressure and distention are further increased. There is an increase in capillary hydrostatic pressure, causing fluid and pigment to leak out with discoloration and edema developing. Stasis pigmentation, subcutaneous induration, dermatitis, and superficial thrombophlebitis can occur. The increased tissue pressure from edema can cause circulation to become so sluggish that metabolic demands of cells for oxygen and nutrient is not met and this can lead to cell death and venous stasis ulcers.

Manifestations

See above for clinical manifestations.

Treatment

Conservative treatment of venous incompetency includes rest with affected leg elevation, compression stockings, avoidance of prolonged standing, and exercise. With inadequate response to conservative treatment or recurrent thrombophlebitis, surgical intervention to remove the vein is indicated. Unsightly superficial varicosities may be treated with sclerotherapy.

1. Which of the following heart valves is opened at the beginning of systole?

(A) The mitral valve and the aortic valve

(B) The aortic valve and the pulmonic valve

(C) The mitral valve and the tricuspid valve

(D) The aortic valve and the mitral valve

2. The community health nurse visits an elderly patient who tells her that he has been vomiting and has diarrhea. She is concerned about the possibility of his developing a decreased cardiac output and hypotension. Which of the following would be the earliest sign that his body is compensating for a diminishing cardiac output?

(A) The duration of systole is increasing.

(B) His feet are swelling.

(C) His heart rate is increasing.

(D) His urine output is decreasing.

3. In evaluating the patient's lipid profile, the nurse notes which of the following factors as most directly linked to atherosclerosis?

(A) High very low density lipoproteins (VLDL)/triglycerides (TG) and high high density lipoproteins (HDL) cholesterol

(B) High low density lipoprotein (LDL) cholesterol and low HDL cholesterol

(C) Low LDL cholesterol and high HDL cholesterol

(D) Low VLDL/TG and high LDL cholesterol

4. In the physical examination of an individual, which of the following factors would be evidence of atherosclerotic plaque?

(A) A bounding pulse

(B) An S3 heart sound

(C) An arterial bruit

(D) A low blood pressure

5. Which of the following individuals is less likely to have classic angina pain?

(A) A young male

(B) An elderly male

(C) An alcoholic

(D) A diabetic

6. Which of the following would be indications that an individual has had an myocardial infarction (MI)?

(A) Decreased hemoglobin, elevation of white blood cells, and S-T segment elevation

(B) Decreased serum glucose, elevation of CK-MB enzymes, and S-T segment depression

(C) Elevation of serum troponin, elevation of blood sugar, and S-T segment elevation

(D) Elevation of CK-MB enzymes, decreased white blood cells, and S-T segment elevation

7. Which type of headache might be an early indication of hypertension?

(A) Progressively worsens as the day goes on

(B) Severe with visual disturbances

(C) Early morning headache that gets better as the day goes on

(D) Throbbing headache accompanied by nausea and vomiting

8. Which of the following is an indication of end-organ damage in hypertension?

(A) Positive Homans' sign

(B) Productive cough

(C) Abdominal bruits

(D) Ptosis (drooping) of the eyelid

9. Which of the following statements is true regarding the role of preload in congestive heart failure?

(A) Decreasing the preload is a compensatory mechanism for decreased cardiac output.

(B) Venous constriction will diminish the preload.

(C) An increase in the blood pressure will cause an increase in the preload.

(D) An excessive preload can cause decompensation in heart failure.

10. Which of the following signs and symptoms indicates right-sided heart failure?

(A) Paroxysmal nocturnal dyspnea

(B) Crackles heard in the lungs

(C) Peripheral edema

(D) Frothy, blood tinged sputum

11. What does the absolute refractory period refer to?

(A) The period in which the cardiac cells will respond to the slightest stimulus.

(B) The period in which the myocardial cells will not respond to any stimulus.

(C) The period in which only the atrioventricular (AV) node will respond to a stimulus.

(D) The period when only a very strong stimulus will result in depolarization.

12. The patient's electrocardiogram shows a rate of 56 beats per minute. What should the nurse do?

(A) Call the physician immediately.

(B) Further assess the patient.

(C) Administer oxygen via nasal prongs.

(D) Prepare atropine for administration.

13. An irregularly irregular cardiac rhythm characterized by absence of a P wave and an erratic, undulating baseline is called what?

(A) Atrial fibrillation

(B) Atrial flutter

(C) Paroxysmal atrial tachycardia

(D) Premature atrial contraction

14. Which of the following is a characteristic of a second degree atrial ventricular block type 1?

(A) No atrial impulses are conducted. The atria and ventricles contract separately.

(B) Every impulse is conducted, but conduction (P-R interval) is prolonged.

(C) Atrial impulses are dropped without antecedent prolongation of the P-R interval.

(D) A-V conduction is gradually prolonged until an atrial impulse is nonconducted and a QRS complex is dropped.

15. Pericardial effusion that can occur in pericarditis has which of the following hemodynamic consequences?

(A) Decreased cardiac output and systemic venous congestion

(B) High blood pressure and pulmonary congestion

(C) Decreased cardiac output and pulmonary congestion

(D) Low blood pressure and pulmonary hypertension

16. Which type of valvular heart disease causes obstruction of the systolic ejection of blood from the left ventricle into the aorta?

(A) Mitral stenosis

(B) Mitral regurgitation

(C) Aortic stenosis

(D) Aortic regurgitation

17. A 19-year-old athlete went out for his first day of football practice. He experienced sudden cardiac death. He had no prior symptoms of cardiac disease. The cause of death was determined to be cardiomyopathy. Which form of cardiomyopathy was it most likely to be?

(A) Dilated cardiomyopathy

(B) Hypertrophic cardiomyopathy

(C) Restrictive cardiomyopathy

(D) Dystrophic cardiomyopathy

18. Which of the following is a correct statement regarding dilated cardiomyopathy?

(A) It is the least common form of cardiomyopathy.

(B) The ventricular myocardium is hypertrophied.

(C) The manifestations are like congestive heart failure.

(D) It is a form of diastolic dysfunction.

19. Which of the following is a manifestation of chronic venous insufficiency?

(A) Dry, necrotic ulcers in the feet

(B) Thick, deformed toe nails

(C) Edema

(D) Hair loss

20. Which of the following may contribute to deep vein thrombosis?

(A) Dehydration, oral contraceptives, and high intake of calcium

(B) Immobility, diabetes, and digoxin

(C) Dehydration, immobility, and oral contraceptives

(D) Hypertension, immobility, and dehydration

1. The correct answer is B.

During the preceding diastolic period, the blood in the aorta and pulmonary artery has run off, so the pressure in these vessels drops. As the ventricles begin to contract at the beginning of systole, the pressure in the ventricles increases in the aorta and pulmonary artery, thus forcing the aortic and pulmonic valves open. Blood moves forward during systole into the aorta and pulmonary artery; therefore, these two valves must be open.

2. The correct answer is C.

Hypovolemia leads to a decrease in preload that then leads to a decrease in cardiac output. The falling output causes a fall in pressure that is sensed by osmoreceptors in the aortic arch and carotid bifurcation, which then causes activation of the cardioaccelerator center in the brainstem. The increased sympathetic outflow stimulates an increase in heart rate and contractility, thus increasing the cardiac output (CO = R x SV). The sympathetic nervous system is the earliest compensatory mechanism to be activated.

3. The correct answer is B.

The lipoprotein that has been identified in atherosclerotic plaque is LDL, the cholesterol-carrying lipoprotein. HDL is the lipoprotein that clears cholesterol from the blood.

4. The correct answer is C.

The bulging of the arterial plaque into the lumen of the blood vessel creates turbulent blood flow, which results in bruits and thrills on physical examination. It may also cause a diminished pulse, and the blood pressure may rise because of the loss of distensibility of the artery.

5. The correct answer is D.

Because of autonomic neuropathy, diabetics often have silent ischemia. Women also tend to not have classic angina symptoms but rather shoulder or abdominal discomfort rather then the typical substernal chest pain.

6. The correct answer is C.

When infarcted myocardial cells die, they release intracellular substances into the blood that serve as a cardiac marker of MI. The stress response to an MI results in elevation of blood sugar and an elevation of the S-T segment, indicating infarction or transmural ischemia.

7. The correct answer is C.

With hypertension, some cerebral edema develops at night when the individual is lying down. When the individual is upright during the day, venous drainage from the head decreases the edema and the headache improves. Severe headache with visual disturbances may occur with more severe levels of blood pressure.

8. The correct answer is C.

Hypertension damages blood vessels, especially at bifurcations, thus initiating atherosclerotic plaque development. The turbulent blood flow created by the irregularity of the arterial walls causes bruits in the renal arteries, aorta, and iliac arteries. None of the other choices are indications of end-organ damage.

9. The correct answer is D.

An increase in preload will improve myocardial contractility and cardiac output to a point because an increase in venous return/blood volume in the ventricle will cause increased tension in the myocardial fibers. If the preload is excessive, however, the actin and myosin if the myocardial fibers are spread too far apart and the strength of contraction will be diminished.

10. The correct answer is C.

When the right side of the heart does not adequately pump blood forward into the lungs, it will back up into the systemic venous circulation and leak into the tissues as edema.

11. The correct answer is B.

During depolarization and most of repolarization, the membrane potential has not been reestablished, so no stimulus will cause another depolarization. During the later part of repolarization, membrane potential has been reestablished enough to enable another stimulus to cause depolarization. This the relative refractory period.

12. The correct answer is B.

A pulse rate of 56 constitutes bradycardia. Individuals who are sleeping or individuals who are physically fit normally have low pulse rates. With a low pulse rate the individual should be evaluated for indication of low cardiac output, such as altered mental status, poor peripheral perfusion, weakness, and low urine output.

13. The correct answer is A.

In atrial fibrillation, totally disorganized electrical activity of the atrial myocardium results in no effective contraction, only fibrillation. The electrocardiogram reveals an erratic, undulating baseline with no P wave present. Ectopic atrial foci produce between 400 and 700 impulses per minute. In atrial flutter "saw toothed" flutter waves are present and in paroxysmal atrial tachycardia and premature atrial contraction P waves are present.

14. The correct answer is D.

D describes a second-degree block type 1. Choice A refers to a third-degree block.

15. The correct answer is A.

Pericardial effusion prevents adequate diastolic relaxation, thus impeding venous return and preventing adequate filling of the ventricles so it diminishes cardiac output and causes systemic congestion.

16. The correct answer is C.

The aortic valve is situated between the left ventricle and the aorta. Stenosis, which is a narrowing of the opening, impedes the flow of blood. Choice B refers to a first-degree block type 1, and choice C refers to a second-degree block type 2.

17. The correct answer is B.

Hypertrophic cardiomyopathy often occurs in young, athletic males. The first indication may be sudden death when exertion causes the hypertrophied septum to contract and it blocks the aortic output.

18. The correct answer is C.

In dilated cardiomyopathy, which is the most common form of cardiomyopathy, the thin left ventricular myocardium is unable to contract adequately during systole, resulting in the blood backing up into the lungs.

19. The correct answer is C.

The increase in venous hydrostatic pressure, which develops when fluid accumulates in the veins, causes fluid to lead out into the tissues and causes edema. The other three choices refer to the manifestations of arterial insufficiency.

20. The correct answer is C.

Dehydration increases the blood viscosity and immobility leads to stasis of blood. Certain oral contraceptives increase the coagulability of blood. Diabetes, hypertension, and high intake of calcium do not increase the risk of clotting.

PART VIII

Gastrointestinal System

Eileen M. Crutchlow, EdD, APRN-C

42 Anatomy and Physiology of the Gastrointestinal System

The gastrointestinal (GI) track includes the mouth, pharynx, esophagus, stomach, and small and large intestines. These structures together with the salivary glands, the pancreas, and the biliary system (discussed elsewhere) comprise the GI system. It provides nutrients to the body by moving, storing, and absorbing nutrients; secreting digestive juices; and digesting food.

In the mouth, food is broken down, moistened by saliva, becomes a semisolid mass, and is swallowed. Reflex muscular movements propel the food bolus into the pharynx through the laryngopharynx into the esophagus, which is a muscular tube about 25 cm long. Strong muscular contractions and mucous secreted from epithelial cells in the lining move the bolus along. At the lower end of the esophagus near its junction with the stomach is the lower esophageal sphincter (LES). This site remains tonically constricted to prevent reflux of acidic gastric contents.

The bolus moves into the stomach, a reservoir that holds food, and digestion proceeds. The stomach is divided into anatomical areas: the cardia, which connects it to the esophagus; the fundus, the uppermost portion; the body, the largest section; the antrum, the lower section; and the pylorus, which connects the stomach to the duodenum. Here the pyloric sphincter, a muscular opening that controls gastric emptying, limits the reflux of bile from the small intestine back into the stomach. There are gastric glands in the stomach containing specialized cells that act to either promote the digestive process or protect structures involved. These cells are chief cells, producing an inactivated form of the digestive enzyme pepsin, which converts proteins into proteoses and peptones; parietal cells, producing hydrochloric acid and intrinsic factor needed for vitamin B_{12} absorption; mucous cells, producing an alkaline mucous protecting the stomach lining; and gastrin cells, which monitor pH. A 1 mm thick layer of mucous protects the stomach lining from digestive juices.

The nutrient bolus passes from the stomach into the small intestine, which is 5 m long and divided into three sections: the duodenum, measuring 22 cm; the jejunum, measuring 2 m; and the ileum, comprising the remaining length. Circular folds line the inner walls and contain millions of finger-like projections called *intestinal villi* that have both digestive and absorption functions. Intestinal villi are themselves covered by their own finger-like projections called *microvilli*. The microvilli have a covering called the *brush border* containing digestive enzymes. This subdividing serves to expand the surface area of the 5 m long small intestine about 600 times. Intestinal glands found between the villi secrete fluid into the intestine for absorption by the villi. Goblet cells secrete mucous. Specialized cells found at the beginning of the duodenum secrete thicker mucous to protect that site from the gastric contents entering the small intestine. Peristaltic contractions propel the nutrient bolus through the small intestine toward the large intestine. The sphincter separating the two structures (i.e., the ileocecal valve) prevents contents in the large intestine from moving back into the small intestine.

The large intestine, which is about 1.5 m long, contains no villi. It too is divided into sections: the cecum, to which the appendix is attached; the colon, which is subdivided into the ascending, transverse, and descending, which together form a frame around the small intestine; the sigmoid colon; the rectum; and anus. The large intestine absorbs water and electrolytes and contains goblet cells, which produce mucous and endocrine cells and secrete hormones.

The GI track's wall consists of four layers: mucosa, which is involved in absorption and secretion; submucosa, which contains loose connective tissue, blood vessels, nerves, and lymphatic tissue; muscular layer, which consists of circular and longitudinal fibers responsible for peristaltic movements; and serosa. The outer covering called the *visceral peritoneum* secretes a fluid that keeps the outer surface of the alimentary tube moist.

Sympathetic and parasympathetic fibers innervate the GI track. Parasympathetic fibers increase digestive actions. Branches of the vagus nerve innervate the esophagus, stomach, pancreas, gallbladder, small intestine, and proximal large intestine. Nerves arising in the sacral region of the spinal cord innervate the distal large intestine. Sympathetic fibers decrease digestion, causing contraction of sphincters and other muscles to block movement of digestive products through the alimentary canal.

Gastrin, which is secreted by the mucosa of the stomach antrum in response to food entering the stomach, increases stomach motility and constriction of the LES. Cholecystokinin, which is secreted by the mucosa of the jejunum in response to the presence of fats, acts on the gallbladder to pour bile into the small intestine to aid in digestion and absorption of fatty foods. Secretin, which is secreted by the mucosa of the duodenum in response to the entrance of gastric juices from the stomach, inhibits the GI tract. Gastric inhibitory peptide, secreted by the mucosa of the small intestine in response to the presence of fats and carbohydrates, slows stomach motility and emptying.

Peristalsis is the process of mixing food with digestive juices and moving it toward the anus. Peristalsis, or propulsion, is initiated by distension of the intestinal wall. New food arriving in the stomach stays close to the esophagus in the fundus. Older food moves to the walls of the stomach body where constant pressure is placed on it. Moving next into the antrum strong contractions mix the food, gastric secretions, and fluids into a thick, white substance called *chyme*. The liquefied and partially digested mixture moves into the small intestine, where the major part of absorption and digestion occur. Peristaltic waves, involving regular and irregularly spaced segments of contracting intestine, are intensified by the ingestion of food. They move chyme through the intestine and spread out the mucosa, facilitating the absorption of nutrients. Chyme passes through the ileocecal valve into the colon, where water and electrolytes are absorbed, and the fecal mass is stored awaiting defecation. It takes about 3 to 5 hours for the chyme to pass from the pyloric sphincter to the ileocecal valve.

Segmental mixing movements in the outpouchings of the colon wall expose the contents of the large intestine to mucosa for the absorption of water. About 500 ml of chyme enters the colon each day—400 ml of water are absorbed and 100 ml of feces is left for elimination. It

- Gastroscopy—A fiberoptic endoscope is inserted through the esophagus and the stomach up to the jejunum to visualize mucosal irregularities, varices, ulcers, perforations, or tears. It can be used to obtain brushings of gastric mucosa to identify the presence of *H. pylori*.

- Mesenteric angiography—Used with conscious sedation to localize and possibly perform therapeutic embolization of a bleeding site that does not respond to conservative therapy and cannot be visualized by endoscopy.

- Peroral pneumogram—After ingested barium has reached the cecum, air is passed into the rectum to allow for evaluation of the terminal ileum. This can be performed concurrently with an upper GI series.

- Sigmoidoscopy—A fiberoptic endoscope is inserted through the rectum to visualize the mucosa of the sigmoid colon. It can detect obstruction, carcinoma, inflammatory disease, and other irregularities.

- Upper GI series—Fluoroscopic study used to evaluate the upper GI tract. Films are taken at timed intervals to observe barium as it passes through structures. Different contrast media are used depending on the diagnoses being considered. It can identify, for example, hiatal hernias, esophageal varices, carcinomas, GI perforations, and GI reflux.

Laboratory Tests

- Ca 50 (carbohydrate antigen)—Tumor marker used to plot progression of many types of tumors, but it is especially useful for those of the GI tract.

- Carcinoembryonic antigen (CEA)—An antigen released during rapid proliferation of epithelial cells particularly of the GI tract. Although not diagnostic, frequent measurement can help to guide management and evaluate success of treatment measures. Levels will rise 3 months before clinical symptoms of recurrent colorectal cancer are present.

- Colorectal cancer allelotyping for chromosomes 17p and 18q—Blood and tissue samples are used to determine the presence of cellular p53 and DCC genes located on chromosomes 17p and 18q, respectively. These genes are known to suppress the development of tumors in various locations. In the process of a normal cell becoming a colorectal cancer cell, predictable changes take place, including the suppression of these genes.

- Fecal fat—Stool samples are taken following ingestion of a diet with a predetermined amount of fat to measure the amount passed. It is used to diagnose conditions associated with poor fat absorption (i.e., pancreatic disorders, Crohn's disease, hepatobiliary diseases).

- Fecal antigen assay—One test of choice to verify eradication of the *H. pylori* bacteria following treatment for the disease.

- *Helicobacter pylori*—Quick office serology for IgA and IgG antibodies to *H. pylori*.

- Ki-67 proliferation marker—Marker used to help determine prognosis and outcomes in patients with specific types of cancers, including colorectal cancer. Proliferation refers to the numbers of cells involved in a cycle and the time it takes to complete a cycle. Aggressive, rapidly growing tumors have a poorer prognosis. This can also aid in managing inflammatory bowel conditions.

- Urea breath test/C-Urea—Breath samples are taken 10 to 30 minutes after ingestion of radiolabeled urea to stimulate *H. pylori* bacteria to release labeled carbon dioxide if it is present. It is noninvasive and one of the studies of choice to verify eradication of the disease following treatment.

- Vitamin B_{12} absorption test (Schilling test)—A 24-hour urine is collected following oral ingestion of Co-B_{12} and unlabeled intramuscular B_{12}; 5 days later the test is repeated with active intrinsic factor added to the oral dose. Intrinsic factor is secreted by the parietal cells in the stomach antrum, and normal ileal absorption is needed for adequate amounts of vitamin B_{12} to be absorbed into the body. Ileal disease or resection, Crohn's disease, pancreatitis, postgastrectomy, and cystic fibrosis are some conditions that will affect this process.

Digestive Juices and Action

Source	Type	Action
Salivary glands	Bicarbonate	Moistens food
	Salivary lipase	Digests fat
Stomach	Hydrochloric acid	Digests protein
		Kills bacteria
	Pepsin	Digests protein
	Gastric lipase	Digests fat
	Intrinsic factor	Aids in absorption of vitamin B_{12} in the small intestine
	Mucous	Protects stomach lining
Liver	Bile acids	Dissolve fats
	Cholesterol	Excreted in bile
	Phospholipids	Aid in absorption of fats
	Immunoglobulins	Act as antibodies
Pancreas	Bicarbonate	Protects digestive enzymes
		Neutralizes acid
	Water	Carries enzymes
	Amylase	Digests starch and glycogen
	Lipases	Digest fats
	Proteases	Digest protein

takes about 18 hours for food to pass through the large intestine.

Carbohydrate digestion begins in the mouth by action of salivary amylase and continues in the stomach and small intestine under the action of pancreatic amylase. The brush borders of the intestine secrete maltase, sucrase, and lactase to aid in the process. Digested carbohydrates are absorbed as glucose and galactose across the intestinal epithelium, as fructose absorbed by facilitated diffusion, and as monosaccharides via the blood stream to the liver.

Lipids are acted on in the small intestine by the action of enzymes from the liver and pancreas. Without enzymes to emulsify lipids into a form that can be acted upon by pancreatic lipase, fat absorption is decreased by about 25%. This seriously effects the absorption of fat-soluble vitamins A, D, E, and K.

Protein digestion begins in the stomach by the action of pepsin and continues in the small intestine by the action of the pancreatic juices and the brush border-secreting peptidases. Digestion breaks protein down into different types of amino acids that are transported via different carrier systems into the blood stream and to the liver.

43 Gastritis

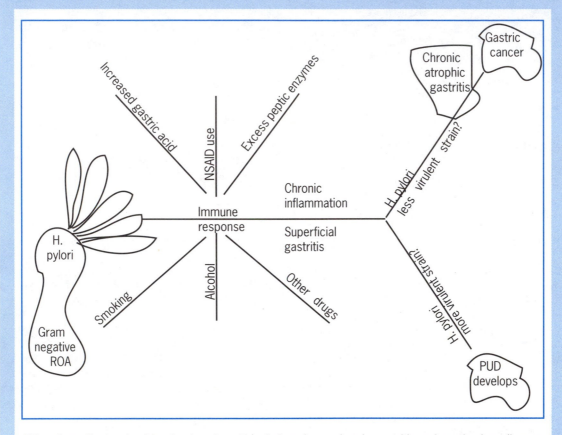

This schematic drawing hypothesizes how *H. pylori* produces chronic gastritis and peptic ulcer disease (PUD). The organism invades the mucous layer of the gastric mucosa, causing an anti-inflammatory response. Other factors can also cause an inflammatory response. Any one can enhance or maintain another, producing a chronic superficial gastritis. A more virulent strain of *H. pylori* goes on to cause PUD. A less virulent strain maintains the gastritis, which eventually causes mucosal atrophy and epithelial metaplasia—the precursor to gastric cancer.

Overview

Gastritis is an inflammation of the mucosa of the stomach. It has many causes, can occur as either an acute or chronic problem, or can be related to a specific condition of which it is a symptom.

Chronic Gastritis

Pathophysiology

Chronic gastritis is defined as the presence of chronic mucosal inflammatory changes that lead to the development of mucosal atrophy and epithelial metaplasia. Typical inflammatory changes found include lymphocytic and plasma cell infiltrate in the lamina propria and inflammation of mucosal pits. There are also loss of glands and mucosal atrophy.

The most common pathogen responsible for gastritis in Western countries is the gram negative rod *Helicobacter pylori* (*H. pylori*). This organism can be transmitted by a number of routes. As it has been identified in dental plaque, an oral route is one mode thought to occur by kissing or sharing utensils, food, or drink; gastric-oral via vomitus; or fecal-oral via poor hand washing techniques. It is believed to be transmitted in childhood and remains dormant until later in life when an unknown factor causes it to become active. Only about 15% of those infected with the organism actually develop gastritis with prevalence increasing with age. In some areas of the world it is almost endemic. For example, it has been found in almost 80% of Puerto Ricans; however, most remain asymptomatic all their lives. Fifty percent of American Caucasians over age 60 have been found to have the pathogen, and it has a greater prevalence in non-Caucasians, in immigrants from developing countries, and in those with low income.

When activated, *H. pylori* begins as an acute infection with nausea and/or vomiting and abdominal pain that appears to resolve in a few days. The organism does not disappear, however, but rather remains and produces an enzyme called *urease* that decomposes the by-product of protein metabolism, urea, to produce ammonia. Ammonia neutralizes gastric acid, allowing the organism to thrive. Safely tucked beneath the gastric mucosa adjacent to the gastric epithelial cells it colonizes, producing an inflammatory response. Some organisms burrow deeper into the gastric glands, causing the glands to atrophy. It is thought that chronic gastritis is a result of the ammonia and other by-products of the organism damaging the mucosal surface. The majority of people infected with *H. pylori* are asymptomatic, but the infection is strongly associated with the development of peptic ulcer disease (PUD). Those infected are at risk for adenocarcinoma and low grade B-cell gastric lymphoma (MALToma) as the proliferation of lymphoid tissue within the gastric mucosa is a precursor for gastric lymphoma.

Pernicious anemia gastritis, also a form of chronic gastritis, is an autoimmune disorder of the stomach's fundic glands that results in an absence of free hydrochloric acid in the stomach and malabsorption of vitamin B_{12}. It is caused by an autoantibody response to gastric gland parietal cells, leading to destruction of the glands, mucosal atrophy, and loss of the acid and intrinsic factor they produce. Inflammation destroys the acid-secreting parietal cells and the zymogenic cells that produce intrinsic factor. The loss of intrinsic factor leads to the development of pernicious anemia. Parietal cell antibodies are present in about 90% of patients. Without the acid-inhibiting gastric G cells, a severe hypergastrinemia develops, producing an intestinal

metaplasia in which gastric epithelium is replaced by columnar and goblet cells of the intestinal variety. Metaplasia of this type of cell is known to give rise to the development of gastric carcinoma. Patients with pernicious anemia have a three-fold increase in the incidence of adenocarcinoma and should have regular endoscopies.

Acute Gastritis

Pathophysiology

Acute erosive gastritis is a transient inflammation of the gastric mucosa that, while short lived, can result in either a mild or severe bleeding state. It is most commonly caused by nonsteroidal anti-inflammatory drugs (NSAIDs) or excessive ingestion of alcohol, but it is also seen in critically ill patients as part of a stress response.

NSAIDs such as aspirin, ibuprofen, and naproxen are widely used to treat musculoskeletal and other chronic pain disorders. They act by suppressing the synthesis of prostaglandins. One source of prostaglandin production is from the gastric epithelial cells, which produce them to protect the stomach mucosa from gastric acid. Without prostaglandins the mucosa is susceptible to the effect of the gastric acid. The condition is often asymptomatic with complaints, if any, being anorexia, nausea, vomiting, and epigastric pain. Vomiting of material resembling coffee grounds or the discovery of blood in a nasogastric tube aspirate is the most common initial manifestation of a problem. On endoscopy superficial injury to the mucosa is found, including small hemorrhages, petechiae, and erosion. These lesions can vary in size and number and may be located at a single site or scattered throughout the stomach. The extent of the injury is not related to the amount of bleeding. Only the mucosa is affected; the submucosa and muscularis mucosae are not penetrated as is the case with PUD. Endoscopy hemostasis techniques are not effective in treating the gastritis because the bleeding is usually diffuse.

A stress-induced gastritis will usually occur within the first 18 hours of the onset of the illness episode. Critically ill patients who experience respiratory failure, are put on mechanical ventilation, or develop a coagulopathy are at high risk. While not causing death, the development of gastritis is associated with a high mortality rate.

Alcoholic gastritis accounts for 20% of all upper gastrointestinal (GI) bleeding in that population. As alcohol is a gastric irritant that stimulates gastric acid secretion, the individual must completely stop drinking alcohol for any kind of recovery to be possible.

Other causes of gastritis are acute bacterial infections, viral infections with cytomegalovirus (CMV) commonly seen in those with human immunodeficiency virus (HIV) or after organ transplant, fungal infections with

Multiple, small (<1 cm), superficial erosions occur, which may be transient and asymptomatic or cause mild symptoms and superficial bleeding.

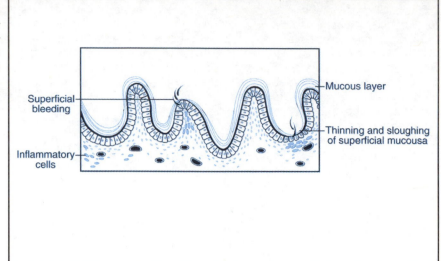

Mucosa atrophies and parietal and chief cells are lost. They are replaced by intestinal epithelium (intestinal metaplasia), a precursor to gastric cancers.

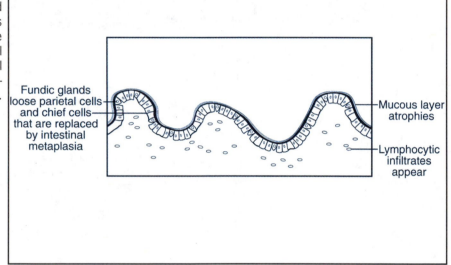

H. pylori bacteria located on the superficial layer of the gastric mucosa. If left untreated, this will progress to an acute then chronic gastritis.

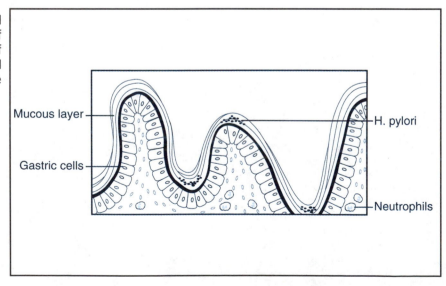

candida seen in immunocompromised patients, and granulomatous gastritis caused by a variety of systemic diseases such as Crohn's disease, tuberculosis (TB), and sarcoidosis.

Management

Antibiotics are used to treat *H. pylori* and are 85% effective. After treatment, antibody levels remain high for another 6 to 12 months despite eradication of the organism. Relapse is associated with reinfection with the organism. Treatment for pernicious anemia is discussed in Part III. NSAID-induced gastritis can be reduced by discontinuing the medication, reducing the dosing amount, and/or scheduling the lowest effective dose. Taking the medication with meals is helpful to some patients. Symptoms can be further controlled by using sucralfate or an H2 receptor antagonist. Endoscopy should be performed if symptoms persist.

For stress-induced gastritis, treatment is aimed at prevention by administering sucralfate or H2 receptor antagonist prophylaxis routinely to those patients who fall in the categories of those likely to suffer from stress-induced gastritis.

Peptic Ulcer Disease

Factors Affecting the Mucosa

Aggressive Factors

- Pepsin—Causes proteolytic and mucosal damage
- Bile—Mucosal damage with motility or abnormal gastric anatomy disorders
- Alcohol—Increases production of gastric acid
- Tobacco—Decreases production of bicarbonate, a protective factor
- Caffeine—Acts with histamine to stimulate the production of gastric acid
- *H. pylori*—Invades gastric mucosa, producing an inflammatory response allowing erosion and ulceration to develop
- Nonsteroidal anti-inflammatory drugs (NSAIDs)—Cause topical irritation and inhibit the production of prostaglandins

Protective Factors

- Mucous—Forms protective barrier over the epithelial lining
- Bicarbonate—Helps neutralize stomach acid
- Mucosal blood flow—Provides well oxygenated environment for the gastric and duodenal mucosa
- Prostaglandins—Enhance mucosal blood flow, inhibit gastric acid secretion, inhibit histamine release, inhibit parietal cells from producing H+, and are active in daily repair of gastric epithelium
- Genetics—Enhance or retard development of peptic ulcer disease (PUD); three-fold increase in those with a first-degree relative with the disease

Medications Used in Treatment of PUD

Antacids

- Decrease symptoms, promote healing, reduce recurrences
- Capacity to neutralize stomach acid varies with product, amount taken, and individual response
- Available over the counter (OTC)
- Liquids more effective than tablets

(continued on p. 174)

Overview

Despite a decreasing incidence since the 1950s, peptic ulcer disease (PUD) remains a serious health concern. In developing countries it is common to find children with it, but in the United States it is rarely seen until after age 15. About 500,000 new cases are diagnosed each year in the United States; another 4 million individuals experience recurrence of the disease. Fifteen percent of the United States population is thought to be diagnosed with it at some point in their lives. PUD has a slightly higher frequency in males and peaks at age 50 then again at about age 75.

Pathophysiology

Chronic ulcers can be found anywhere in the gastrointestinal (GI) tract and are named according to their location or etiology (i.e., gastric or stress ulcers). The term *PUD* however refers to those occurring in the stomach or duodenum. An ulcer begins as a superficial erosion of the mucosa that is then subjected to the presence of pepsin and hydrochloric acid. The acid erodes the tissue as it attempts to heal itself and forms scar tissue at the base of what is now a developing ulcer.

There are aggressive and defensive factors within the stomach and duodenum that balance each other to maintain a state of homeostasis. Aggressive forces are acid producers while defensive forces are mucosal protectors. All people produce acid that is needed for digestion, but they can be separated into high, medium, or low acid producers. However, people who are high acid producers do not develop PUD at any greater rate than low acid producers. It is when the imbalance is between the aggressive and protective factors that an ulcer develops. Once considered a chronic disease, PUD is now thought to be caused by three major factors: *Helicobacter* (*H.*) *pylori*, nonsteroidal anti-inflammatory drugs (NSAIDs), and Zollinger-Ellison syndrome.

H. Pylori

This microorganism is found in 95% of patients with duodenal ulcers and 75% with gastric ulcers. It is transmitted by an oral-oral or fecal-oral route. There are various strains of the organism, with some more virulent than others. Those acquiring a less virulent strain tend to develop gastritis rather than actual PUD. Infection with *H. pylori* does not always cause PUD to develop. What triggers the organism's attack on the mucosal lining is not known. It gains access to the gastric mucosa through the epithelial cells protecting it. In the mucosa, the bacteria releases toxins, stimulating an inflammatory response that causes tissue injury and the release of antibodies that can be detected in the blood. The organism mainly invades the gastric mucosa, but it is unclear how it causes duodenal ulcers to form. Perhaps the duodenum also has patches of gastric cells, which allows it to colonize, or excessive production of gastric acid in the stomach causes erosions that allow the organism to take hold. The majority of people infected with *H. pylori* are asymptomatic but their risk of developing gastric cancer is 3 to 6 times higher than noninfected people.

NSAIDs

These medications act by inhibiting the enzyme cyclooxygenase (COX), preventing the production of prostaglandins. COX has two forms and each has a different function. COX-1 helps maintain homeostasis of the gastric mucosa, while COX-2 is responsible for the inflammatory response from an injury stimulus. Both NSAIDs and aspirin inhibit the effects of COX-2. If COX-1 is inhibited, ulcers will form because the protective mechanism cannot work. Individuals routinely taking NSAIDs produce less mucous and bicarbonate, have a 20% prevalence of gastric ulcers and a 5% prevalence of duodenal ulcers, and have three times the rate of serious complications than do non-NSAID users. Risk is greatest during the first 3 months and in those who also smoke, drink alcohol, or take steroids. Newer COX-2-inhibitor NSAIDs, such as Celebrex (Pharmacia, Peapack, NJ) and Vioxx (Merck, Whitehouse Station, NJ), are less likely to cause ulcers as they spare the gastric mucosa while still affecting prostaglandin synthesis. As most NSAIDs can be purchased over the counter (OTC), it is important to always inquire about their use when taking a health or medication history. The elderly are especially at risk because, with arthritic and other musculoskeletal conditions, they tend to be NSAID users.

Zollinger-Ellison Syndrome (Gastrinomas)

This syndrome consists of hypersecretion of gastric acid, PUD, and nonbeta-islet cells tumors of the pancreas. The gastrinomas tumors, 50% to 75% of which are malignant with a 40% rate of metastasis, produce the hypersecretion. This syndrome accounts for about 1% of PUD, has a genetic predisposition, and is seen in 40 to 75 year olds.

Duodenal Ulcers

Most PUD occurs here with 95% located in the first portion of the duodenum and 90% located within 3 cm of the junction of the pyloric and duodenal mucosa. They are usually small and rarely become cancerous. The mechanisms for development are most likely high gastric acid production and *H. pylori* infection. Risk factors include smoking, alcoholic cirrhosis, and chronic renal disease. There is also a familiar tendency to developing them and no evidence that psychological factors play a role. Patients with duodenal ulcers experience sharp, burning, or gnawing epigastric pain in a fasting state that can awaken them from sleep. Eating or using antacids neutralizes the acid and relieves the pain.

Gastric Ulcers

While less common than duodenal ulcers, gastric ulcers have a higher mortality rate. The ulcer is deep, penetrates beyond the mucosal layer, and tends to involve surrounding tissue. They are thought to be caused by a breakdown of mechanisms that normally protect the gastric mucosa coupled with changes in the output of gastric acid. While acid production remains at normal or slightly below normal levels, gastric emptying is sluggish, allowing acid to bathe the area for a prolonged period of time predisposing to ulcer development. Direct injury contributes to gastric ulcers as with the regurgitation of bile secondary to delayed gastric emptying or NSAID use. While *H. pylori* does attack the gastric mucosa, it is less likely to be involved here than in the duodenum. Smoking and steroid use also predispose to gastric ulcers. Pain from gastric ulcers is less

Types

Absorbable

- Rapidly and completely neutralize gastric acid
- Sodium and calcium bicarbonate strongest
- Are absorbed into blood and can upset acid-alkaline balance, producing alkalosis

Nonabsorbable

- Fewer side effects
- Combine with stomach acid and stay in stomach, relieving symptoms
- Can interfere with absorption of other drugs (i.e., digitoxin, iron)

Aluminum hydroxide

- Commonly used
- Can decrease blood phosphate levels
- Should not be taken by those on dialysis, those with kidney disease, or alcoholics

Magnesium hydroxide

- More effective than aluminum hydroxide
- Can cause diarrhea in large doses

Other Ulcer Drugs

Sucralfate

- Forms protective coat in base of ulcer
- Alternative to antacids
- Few side effects

H2 antagonists

- Reduce acid and digestive enzymes in the stomach
- Once or twice daily dosing
- Available OTC

Omeprazole and lansoprazole

- Inhibit acid secretion
- Long lasting
- Promote greater healing in less time than H2 antagonists

Antibiotics

- To treat *H. pylori*
- Combination therapy with bismuth subsalicylate, tetracycline, and metronidazole or amoxicillin
- Omeprazole and an antibiotic are also used

Misoprostol

- Used in prevention of gastric ulcers when NSAIDs must be used

---

severe than with duodenal ulcers but is produced, not relieved, by food or antacids because eating causes acid to be secreted.

Complications

About 25% of those with PUD will experience one of the following complications:

1. Hemorrhage—Most commonly found in those with *H. pylori* who are taking NSAIDs. The ulcer erodes through a blood vessel with the amount of bleeding dependent upon the size of the involved vessel. Small vessels present with chronic, slow bleeding as evidenced by dark, tarry stools positive for occult blood; hematemesis; and anemia. A large vessel will present as the sudden onset of major bleeding, hypotension, and tachycardia and has a high mortality rate. Treating *H. pylori* significantly decreases a recurrence of hemorrhage.

2. Perforation—An ulcer can erode through the wall of the stomach or duodenum, allowing its contents to leak into the peritoneal cavity and causing peritonitis. This presents with acute onset of severe abdominal pain, rebound tenderness, fever, and hypotension.

3. Obstruction—As gastric ulcers heal they produce scars that can be large enough to obstruct the gastric outlet, preventing food from passing through into the duodenum. This presents with a feeling of being bloated or full, weight loss, a palpable abdominal mass, and vomiting after eating.

Management

Nonpharmacological management consists of stopping or at least reducing the use of aspirin and NSAIDs and not smoking. Pharmacotherapy consists of H2 receptor antagonists to decrease acid production by up to 90%; proton pump inhibitors, which are the most powerful inhibitors of acid secretion; antacids to neutralize acid; and antibiotics to treat *H. pylori*. "Triple therapy" of bismuth, nitroimidazole, and amoxicillin or tetracycline is most effective. There is no evidence to support using milk or not eating spicy foods in the treatment of PUD.

45 Irritable Bowel Syndrome

Manning Criteria

A least 6 months of recurrent symptoms of the following:

- Abdominal pain or discomfort that is (at least one of the following):

    Relieved by defecation

    Associated with a change in stool frequency

    Associated with a change in stool consistency

and

- Two or more of the following, at least 2 days per week:

    Altered stool frequency (greater than three bowel movements a day or less than three movements a week)

    Altered stool form (lumpy/hard or loose/watery)

    Altered stool passage (straining, urgency, or feeling of incomplete passage)

    Passage of mucous

    Bloating or feeling of abdominal distension

Differences Between Inflammatory Bowel Disease and Irritable Bowel Syndrome

	Inflammatory Bowel Disease		*Irritable Bowel Syndrome*
	Ulcerative colitis	Crohn's disease	
Epidemiology	Abrupt onset Peak ages 15 to 30/60 Caucasian>African American Female>Male	Insidious onset 15 to 40 Female>Male	Late teens/early adulthood Female>Male
Pathology	Possible autoimmune infection may precipitate familial tendency Continuous, irregular superficial inflammation of mucosal layer of colon and rectum	Possible autoimmune infection may precipitate genetic predisposition Skipping ulcerations involving mucosal and submucosal layers along the entire GI tract; 50% involve small intestine/colon Strictures/fistulas common	Cause unknown Bowel has increased response to stimuli and visceral hypersensitivity Altered perception of CNS

(continued on p. 178)

Overview

Irritable bowel syndrome (IBS) is a chronic functional gastrointestinal (GI) disorder characterized by periods of exacerbation often associated with stress. In the United States it is more common in women usually beginning in late adolescence or early adulthood. It is the most common GI disorder found in the primary care setting, accounting for 50% of all visits to gastroenterologists. The vast majority of patients are able to function with little or moderate difficulty, while only 5% are seriously debilitated by the disorder.

Pathophysiology

IBS is a chronic condition causing abdominal pain that is relieved by defecation. It is associated with changes in bowel habits, either constipation or diarrhea, and abdominal distension. Bowel movements (BMs) frequently begin normally but with each successive movement progress to diarrhea accompanied by abdominal pain, urgency, flatus, and a feeling of incomplete evacuation. Pencil thin stools may be present if spasms are occurring in the rectosigmoid region. No blood is found in the stool. Pain may be in any quadrant of the abdomen but its location is fairly consistent for an individual. The pain is sharp or burning and does not radiate. Patients do not report being awakened from sleep with pain or feeling a need to defecate, a pertinent negative classically associated with functional bowel disorder. Weight loss does not occur.

The etiology of IBS is unknown and there are no findings with laboratory, endoscopic, or radiological studies. The condition is diagnosed by excluding other conditions, most notably the inflammatory bowel disorders, and by the Manning Criteria (see p. 176), a pattern of symptoms that must be present for at least 3 to 6 months. While there are no findings on exam, it is postulated that patients with IBS experience a heightened response to stimuli such as meals or stress with increased intestinal motility and prolonged contractions in discrete areas of the intestine. Patients also have low sensation and pain thresholds in the smooth muscle of the ileum and colorectum, causing them to respond to stimuli to which people without IBS do not respond.

Patients generally complain of much discomfort, but the severity of the symptoms experienced is not proportionate to the degree of motility and contraction actually occurring in the gut. More recently it has been found that the syndrome has constipation variant and diarrhea variant subsets. Those with constipation variant IBS appear to have an abnormality in vagal (cholinergic) function. Those with diarrhea variant IBS may have a sympathetic adrenergic dysfunction.

Intolerance of selected foods is common, particularly gas-forming foods and those containing sorbitol, lactose, or gluten. Those with diarrhea variant IBS have difficulty with fatty foods and are generally intolerant of fast food. Women, on entering menopause, will report that symptoms were first noted in relation to their menstrual cycle but had thought them to be a normal component and did not recognize them as a separate entity.

While no direct effect of psychological stress has been documented, the correlation of symptoms with the occurrence of stressors has been noted. Because of the close connection of the central nervous system (CNS) and the GI tract it can be expected that those with significant psychological distress will have some GI complaints. This, however, does not support a causal relationship between the two events.

Stressful life events—whether they are related to family, work, economic, or environmental factors—frequently precede an exacerbation of the disorder. Those with mild symptoms generally manage these events without outside help but will report symptoms of IBS when questioned. Those with moderate symptoms have a higher incidence of anxiety and somatization disorders and often present with recurrent GI complaints that cannot be satisfactorily managed without attending to the associated emotional problems as well. The small percent severely impaired by IBS have a much higher incidence of major depression and panic attacks and are usually being treated for these disorders. The IBS symptoms may be thought to be a part of the emotional disorder but cannot be managed by treating the emotional disorder only. It has also been found that women with a history of physical or sexual abuse, when questioned, report a greater incidence of IBS than do women who have no such history.

Management

Treatment is aimed at management of symptoms using antidiarrheals, laxatives, and antispasmodics as appropriate. Diet should provide adequate fluids and fiber while eliminating foods that produce symptoms. Cognitive-behavioral therapy to identify triggers and stress reduction techniques also help. Relaxation training such as yoga or meditation can help individuals decrease smooth muscle tension and autonomic arousal. Some may benefit from short-term psychotherapy. Those more severely stressed may need long-term psychotherapy and medication.

Signs and Symptoms

Abdominal pain	Intermittent, mild crampy tenderness	Crampy or steady Periumbilical or right lower quadrant (RLQ)	Sharp, burning; may be diffuse or left lower quadrant (LLQ)
Mass present	No	Common	No
Bleeding	Common	Occasionally	No
Diarrhea	Frequent watery stools with blood and mucous	Chronic, recurrent, may have some blood	Intermittent, predominant Symptom varies with individual
Perianal lesions	No	One third develop perianal abscesses or fistulas	No
Weight loss	With severe diarrhea	Common	No
Fever/malaise	During severe exacerbation	With exacerbation and abscess formation	No
Psychological	As result of long-standing disease	As result of long-standing disease	Exacerbation with stressful situations
Course/prognosis	75% to 80% relapse after first attack; most have mild to moderate disease Routine colonoscopy with biopsy after having the disease for 7 to 8 years because of increased colon cancer risk	Recurrent, progressive Typically need surgery after 7 years to treat/ repair fistulas or abscesses; shortened life span	Chronic, intermittent Rare functional limitations

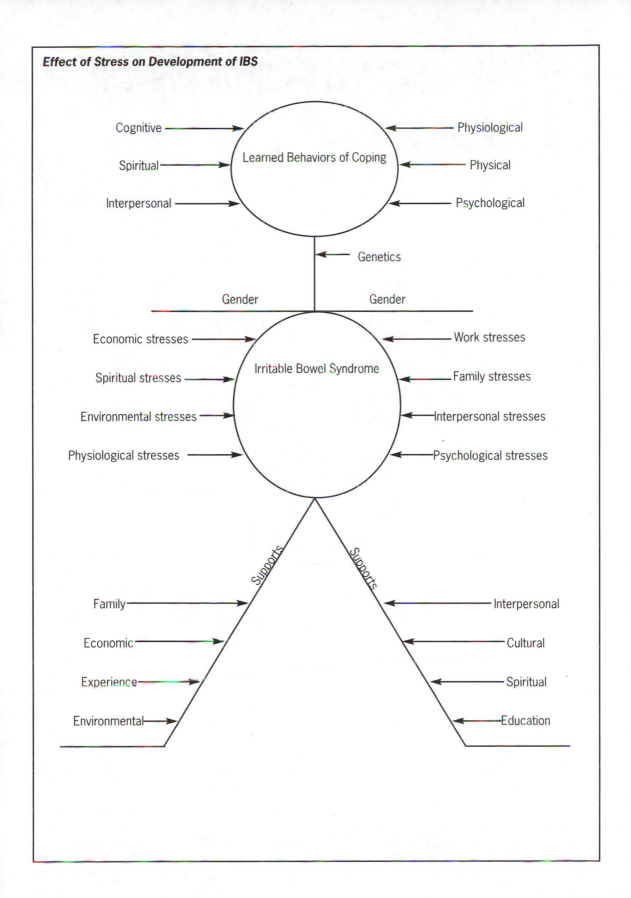

Effect of Stress on Development of IBS

Cognitive → Learned Behaviors of Coping ← Physiological

Spiritual → ← Physical

Interpersonal → ← Psychological

Genetics

Gender — Gender

Economic stresses → Irritable Bowel Syndrome ← Work stresses

Spiritual stresses → ← Family stresses

Environmental stresses → ← Interpersonal stresses

Physiological stresses → ← Psychological stresses

Supports — Supports

Family → ← Interpersonal

Economic → ← Cultural

Experience → ← Spiritual

Environmental → ← Education

Inflammatory Bowel Disease: Part I

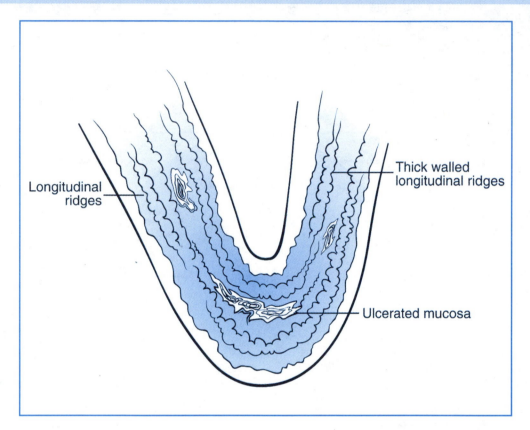

Longitudinal ridges

Thick walled longitudinal ridges

Ulcerated mucosa

Ulcerative colitis: This segment of colon shows long ridges of thickened wall separated by depressions of ulcerated mucosa.

Overview

Inflammatory bowel disease (IBD) includes two disorders: ulcerative colitis (idiopathic proctocolitis) and Crohn's disease (regional enteritis). Both conditions are chronic and characterized by periods of exacerbation and remission. Exact etiology is unknown, but a genetically associated autoimmune disorder activated by an infectious process is suspected. The changes produced by IBD result when immunocyte cells located in the mucosal layer are stimulated to release inflammatory mediators such as histamine, prostaglandins, leukotrienes, and cytokines. These act on the secretory and smooth muscle cells of the gastrointestinal (GI) tract, altering its functions and neuronal activity. GI salt and water transportation and the absorption and excretion of nutrients, salt, water, and electrolytes are affected. Onset of IBD occurs in late adolescence/young adulthood or around age 60. It occurs more commonly in whites than African Americans/Asians, Jewish than non-Jewish, and women than men.

Ulcerative Colitis

Pathophysiology

Ulcerative colitis, the more common of the two inflammatory disorders, is a chronic recurrent disease primarily involving the colon. The inflammatory action is confined to the mucosal layer of the gut and produces a progressive loss of epithelium with resulting surface erosion and ulceration. The pattern of ulceration begins in the rectum then extends proximally in a continuous fashion and can involve the entire colon. The disease is confined to the rectosigmoid region in most patients. Less than 20% have involvement of the entire colon. Necrosis of epithelial tissue can result in abscess formation with adjacent abscesses joining to form large areas of ulceration. Seventy-five percent of people have repeat attacks after an initial episode.

Onset may be acute with episodes of diarrhea and abdominal pain that generally increase in frequency and severity. Bloody diarrhea is the hallmark of the disease with the amount varying according to the location and extent of the disease. Patients experience rectal discomfort, tenesmus, incomplete emptying, and urgency with active disease. There may be spasm and stasis of stool, resulting in constipation with distal colon inflammation. Most patients have mild disease with few if any physical findings. Endoscopic findings are subtle, showing only mucosal edema, loss of normal vascular patterns, and erythema. Moderately ill people present with symptoms that may include slight weight loss, abdominal tenderness, and low grade fever. Severely ill patients experience weakness, dehydration, tachycardia, and significant abdominal tenderness. Endoscopic findings demonstrate mucosal granularity, friability, ulceration, bleeding, pseudopolyps, and mucopurulent exudate. Absent bowel sounds and abdominal distension suggest a perforation or megacolon.

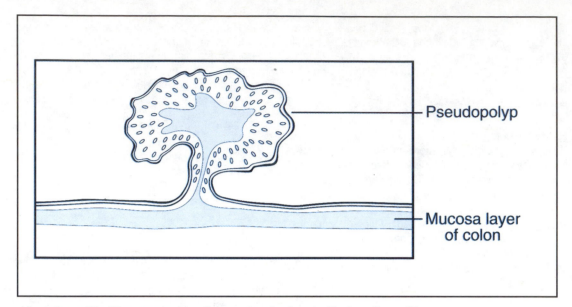

Ulcerative colitis: Microscopic view of a pseudopolyp found with ulcerative colitis.

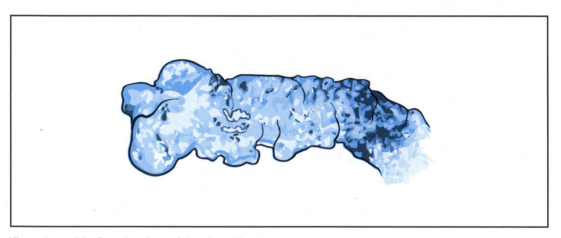

Ulcerative colitis: Pseudopolyps of the sigmoid colon.

47 Inflammatory Bowel Disease: Part II

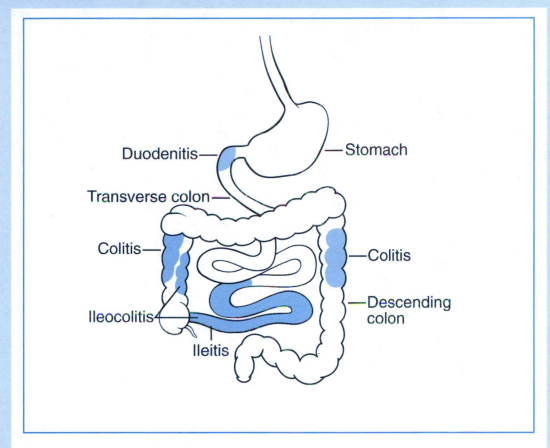

Duodenitis — Stomach

Transverse colon —

Colitis —

Colitis

Descending colon

Ileocolitis

Ileitis

Shaded areas are those frequently affected by Crohn's disease.

Crohn's Disease

Pathophysiology

Crohn's disease is an insidious, slow-developing, chronic, progressive disorder that involves the full thickness of the bowel wall. The pattern of ulceration is linear and penetrating, skipping over regions of normal tissue. Typically occurring in the distal colon, 40% of cases involve the small intestine alone and 30% the proximal ascending colon alone. Ulceration and inflammation can, however, involve any segment of the GI tract from mouth to anus with a characteristic "skipping" pattern of sharply demarcated areas of diseased and normal bowel segments adjacent to each other.

Endoscopy shows focal mucosal ulcers resembling canker sores, edema, and loss of normal mucosal texture. As the disease progresses, ulcers coalesce in a linear manner along the long axis of the bowel with relatively disease-free areas between the ulcerative streaks. Noncaseating granulomas and fissures, which develop into fistulas, are common. Transmural ulceration and inflammation can result in submucosal thickening and may involve the adjacent mesentery and lymph nodes. Fissure formation and submucosal thickening produce a characteristic "cobblestone" appearance. Strictures, abscess or fistula formation, perforation, adhesions, track formation, and small intestine obstruction are frequent complications. Bleeding from deep ulcerations may occur and can be insidious or massive.

Patients present complaining of low grade fever, abdominal pain, a number of liquid bowel movements per day, abdominal tenderness, malaise, weight loss, and fatigue. The diarrhea is nonbloody and intermittent. Abdominal pain is described as either crampy or steady in the right lower quadrant (RLQ) or periumbilical region and is often postprandial. A mass may be present in the lower abdomen because of inflamed and thickened loops of intestine. Recurrent bouts of diarrhea and progressive disease produce weight loss and anemia from inadequate absorption of iron, folate, vitamin B_{12}, and other vitamin deficiency.

Narrowing of the small bowel may occur as a result of inflammation and spasm, producing intestinal obstruction. Fistula formation can result in abscess formation with fever, chills, leukocytosis, and a tender abdominal mass. Fistulas can occur between the colon and small intestine or bladder or vagina with invasion of these structures by colonic bacteria. One third of patients develop anal and/or perianal fistulas, while one third develop systemic manifestations including inflammatory disorders of the eye, skin, mucous membranes of the mouth or renal disorders especially nephrolithiasis from increased oxalate absorption associated with steatorrhea.

Management

When the cause of a disorder is unknown, management must be aimed at providing symptomatic relief. All management techniques aim to manage symptoms and to bring about a remission, which then is carefully protected. It is far easier to maintain remission than to achieve one.

Pharmacological therapy seeks to control diarrhea and discomfort with antidiarrheals and antispasmodics. The underlying problem of inflammation is treated with aminosalicylates, anti-inflammatory and immunosuppressive medicines, and enemas. Antibiotic therapy is used for abscess formation and bacterial contamination of the gut. It takes a combination of therapeutics to achieve remission, and patients must be strongly cautioned to continue with therapy in order to prevent repeat flare-ups.

Adequate nutritional status is critical for patients with IBD. Because it is absorbed by the jejunum, an elemental diet may also effect remission in up to 90% of patients with colon or distal small bowel involvement. Once remission is achieved, a low residue diet with any possible trigger foods eliminated works best. Nutritional supplements like Ensure (Abbott Laboratories, Columbia, OH) or Sustacal (Bristol Myers, Evansville, IN) may be needed for healing and repair. Nutritional therapy for ulcerative colitis is less effective, with a low residue diet and multivitamin supplemental therapy working best.

Surgery is used for about 30% of patients with ulcerative colitis because of dysplasia, hemorrhage, strictures, perforation, or cancer. The only procedures that cure ulcerative colitis are ileostomy and total proctocolectomy, which is generally unacceptable to most patients.

Lifestyle changes needed include education about and commitment to a therapeutic regimen that supports remission. Although there is no psychological basis for IBD, the problems that chronicity brings may be helped with psychotherapy and/or support group involvement.

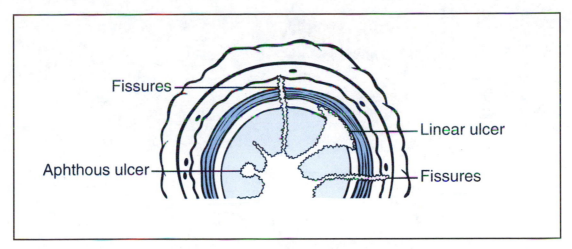

Mucosal and transmural lesions of Crohn's disease.

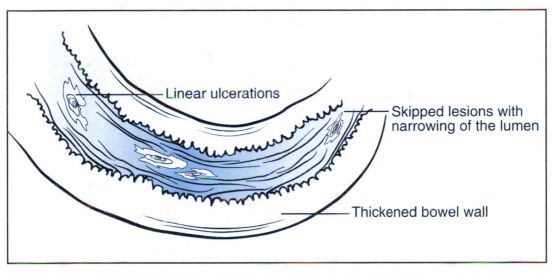

Crohn's disease of the ileum showing narrowing of the lumen, bowel wall thickening, serosal extension of mesenteric fat ("creeping fat"), and linear ulceration of the mucosal surface.

48 Diverticulitis

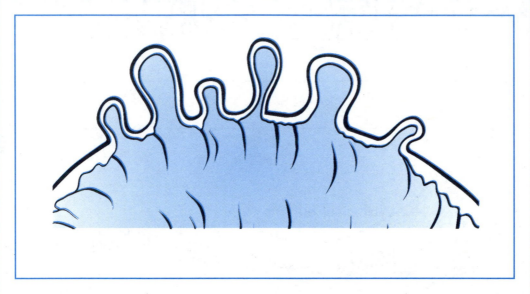

Diverticula are small pouches of mucosa that bulge outward into the mesentery through weak spots in the muscle wall of the colon. This figure shows a cross-section of the colon and multiple diverticula.

Overview

By age 80 more than 50% of the United States population has acquired the condition called *diverticulosis* in which individual outpouchings (i.e., diverticula) in the mucosa and submucosa of the muscular wall of the large intestine herniate through weak sites. Most cases are asymptomatic and are discovered incidental to endoscopy or barium enema. It is believed to be caused by a diet low in fiber, resulting in chronic constipation. Because of dietary factors it is a condition seldom found in developing countries where a more fibrous diet is the norm.

Pathophysiology

Most diverticula occur in the distal sigmoid colon in the presence of long-standing constipation. From the prolonged effort of moving small, hard stools along, the muscular layer becomes hypertrophied, rigid, thick, and fibrous. High intraluminal pressure is needed to propel stool through the colon but this same pressure can force the mucosa through a preexisting area of weakness in the wall, producing a diverticula. Most individuals are asymptomatic and require no treatment except for a high fiber diet or fiber supplements such as bran. Some may complain of abdominal pain lasting hours to days and relieved by passing flatus or feces. As these events are often accompanied by either diarrhea or constipation, a constellation of symptoms also found with the condition of irritable bowel, it is speculated that there may be a relationship between the two diseases.

There are two common complications of diverticulosis: bleeding and diverticulitis.

Bleeding of a diverticular sac occurs because of the proximity to branches of the colonic intramural arteries. Typically, it occurs in an older individual taking nonsteroidal anti-inflammatory drugs (NSAIDs). The person is asymptomatic and experiences an episode of acute bleeding with no warning. The individual complains of abdominal cramping followed by the passage of a large quantity of bright red or maroon blood mixed with clots. Depending on how much blood is passed there may be symptoms of shock. Bleeding can persist for hours or days before a spontaneous remission occurs. Eighty percent of persons with diverticular bleeding have a single episode and require no further treatment. Persistent or recurrent bleeding requires angiography or scintigraphic studies to identify the site followed by surgery to repair it.

Diverticulitis is the most common complication of diverticulosis. It develops when either an obstruction, usually fecal matter, or a perforation leads to inflammation. Intra-abdominal infection can range from mild to severe complete with abscess formation, development of sinus tracks, and/or peritonitis. More commonly, a microperforation occurs, resulting in a localized inflammation and infection with complaints of mild to moderate aching, and abdominal pain usually in the left lower quadrant (LLQ). Patients have low grade fever, LLQ tenderness, constipation, nausea, vomiting, a palpable mass, and leukocytosis. If the perforation is larger or the inflammation more severe, symptoms can vary accordingly.

Management

Treatment depends on the severity. Mild disease is treated conservatively with antibiotics and a low residue diet. Severe cases require hospitalization, a nasogastric (NG) tube, intravenous (IV) fluids, and IV antibiotics. Some persons may require surgery to remove the diseased colon, form a temporary colostomy until the infection and inflammation have cleared, when the colostomy is reversed and the colon reconnected. Local abdominal abscesses are treated with a percutaneous catheter for drainage and antibiotic therapy. Recurrent attacks occur in about one third of patients and require elective surgery for removal of the affected site and anastomosis of the colon.

This figure shows the protrusion of the mucosa and submucosa through the muscle wall.

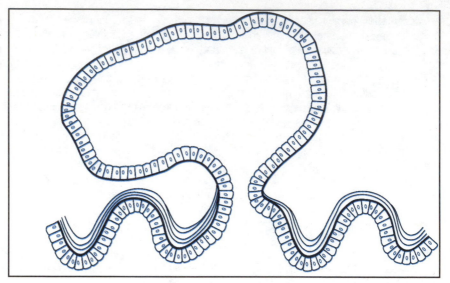

This figure is a view of the diverticulum from inside the colon itself.

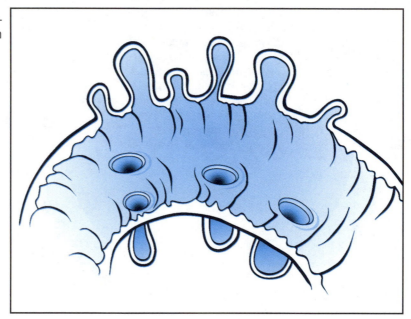

Intestinal Obstruction and Paralytic Ileus

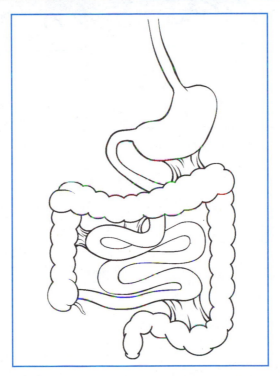

Adhesions, or bands of connective tissue, sometimes form after abdominal surgery. This figure shows that structures that have not yet twisted or looped are still under tension from pulling.

Intestinal Obstruction

A blockage in either the small or large intestine will stop the movement of abdominal contents through the intestine. The severity of symptoms is related to the site and degree of obstruction. Most obstructions block the intestinal lumen, resulting in distention and dehydration, which is the loss of large amounts of fluids. Symptoms include crampy periumbilical pain as peristaltic waves try to force abdominal contents through the obstructed site. The pain initially comes in waves and lasts seconds to minutes but eventually becomes constant and severe. Severe vomiting occurs within minutes of the onset of pain, causing dehydration and electrolyte imbalance. Similar but less severe symptoms occur when the obstruction site is in the distal colon. Vomiting does not occur for several

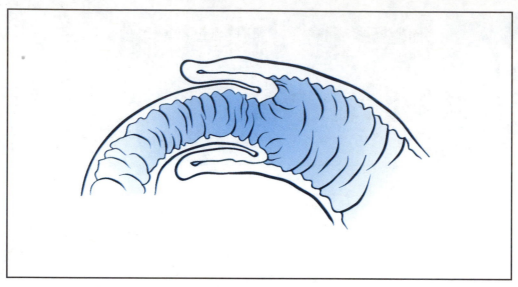

Intussusception: The telescoping of one section of intestine into another structure, producing an obstruction.

hours after the onset of pain, but abdominal distension is more pronounced.

Adhesions, which are bands of connective tissue that form after abdominal surgery, are the most common cause of intestinal obstruction. They can pull, twist, loop, or compress a section of bowel, causing an obstruction. Hernias develop when a loop of bowel protrudes through a weak abdominal wall. Inguinal hernias are common in men; femoral and umbilical hernias occur in both sexes. The peritoneum along with a loop of bowel is pushed through the opening, preventing the passage of abdominal contents. Stasis and edema increase the size of the loop, leaving it trapped (incarcerated) and the blood supply threatened or compromised. When drainage leads to infarction of the bowel loop, it is said to be *strangulated*. A volvulus, or twisted bowel, usually occurs in the sigmoid colon. The degree of twist determines how much, if any, abdominal content can pass along. Intussusception is the telescoping of one section of bowel into another segment, producing an obstruction. It may result from a tumor that is pulling the bowel wall it is attached to into the segment with it or because vigorous peristalsis drags it through. The latter is more common in children. Neoplasms of the colon are a rare cause of intestinal obstruction but,

if left undetected, they can grow to a size that partially or completely occludes the lumen, causing an obstruction.

Initial treatment in all cases is aimed at restoring fluid and electrolyte balance. Nasogastric suctioning will relieve vomiting and abdominal distension. Surgery is needed to relieve the obstruction.

Paralytic Ileus

This disorder is a neurogenic and peristaltic failure of the intestine. It is seen most commonly in patients hospitalized with acute pancreatitis, appendicitis, or gastroenteritis. It is also more likely to be seen in those patients with any of the following: abdominal surgery, peritoneal irritation, hemorrhage, severe medical illness. It is also likely to be seen in those taking medications that can affect intestinal activity (i.e., anticholinergics, opioids). Patients complain of abdominal distension; mild, diffuse, continuous abdominal pain; nausea; and vomiting. Bowel sounds are absent as are signs of peritoneal irritation. Treatment focuses on the underlying problem. Patients are maintained on intravenous fluids, on a nothing-by-mouth diet, and have a nasogastric tube until bowel sounds return, which is when oral fluids can be resumed.

50 Gastroenteritis: Part I

Differentiating Types of Diarrhea

Type	Characteristics	Incidence/ Intubation	Duration
Acute			
Gastroenteritis: Norwalk virus (most common in adults)	Most common type; small bowel secretory form; seen in family/school outbreaks especially during winter and summer; water-borne, person-to- person, and foodborne; pro-drome of malaise then abrupt onset of	Norwalk: 1 to 2 days	Norwalk: 1 to 2 days
Rotavirus (most common in children)	of diarrhea, nausea/vomiting (N/V), abdominal cramps, headache, low grade fever; resolves spontaneously; in adults is mild illness with diarrhea predominating; can be serious in children with vomiting predominant	Rotavirus: 3 to 4 days	Rotavirus: 24 to 96 hours
Bacterial			
Salmonella	From contaminated food or water; can be passed by asymptomatic carrier	3 to 10 days	3 to 6 weeks
Shigella	Contaminated food and water	1 to 2 days	3 to 7 days
Campylobacter jejuni	Most common of bacterial causes	1 to 3 days	1 week
Staphylococcus	No prodrome; no fever; severe N/V; severe diarrhea, abdominal cramps; moderately common	1 to 6 hours after ingesting contaminated foods, especially meats	12 to 36 hours
	All bacterial causes produce watery stools containing mucous, pus, and leukocytes; all occur after eating foods, especially meats, that also made others sick; and there is a high relapse rate		

(continued on p. 193)

Overview

Acute gastroenteritis (AGE) is one of the most common illnesses afflicting people, second only to the common cold. It is the most common gastrointestinal (GI) disorder worldwide. An infectious illness common during childhood, it spreads rapidly through sites where people gather, such as daycare centers, schools, nursing homes, and prisons. Diarrhea, which often accompanies it, is the leading cause of death in young children in developing countries.

Pathophysiology

Gastroenteritis is an inflammation of the lining of the stomach and intestine accompanied by fever, nausea, vomiting, watery diarrhea, and abdominal cramping. It is usually caused by viruses or bacteria. Incubation is several hours to 1 to 3 days with a duration of 12 to 60 hours. Associated viruses are generally transmitted by fecal-oral route in crowded areas with poor hygiene. The diarrhea and vomiting that accompany it are discussed next and in Chapter 51.

Rotaviruses are the most common cause of infectious diarrhea in children under 3 years of age in whom it can be a serious, even life-threatening, illness whereas in adults it produces only mild symptoms or is completely asymptomatic. Enteric adenovirus, also transmitted by a fecal-oral route, is the second leading cause of diarrhea in children under age 3. Norwalk virus, which is highly infectious, affects all age groups and is passed either by a fecal-oral route or via contaminated water or food. It is the chief cause of outbreaks in adult communities, such as nursing homes and prisons, but it can also affect children.

Viruses act by invading and killing cells of the intestinal villi, disturbing the structural integrity of the region so that foods cannot be completely digested. Instead food molecules act as osmotic agents, pulling large amounts of water, electrolytes, and intestinal fluids to themselves, which are passed along as watery diarrhea. Normally, the host's immune system quickly responds, and as the lifetime of mature intestinal cell is only about 3 to 5 days, the illness is usually self-limiting. Infected cells slough away and are replaced by new cells with antibodies to the invaders. If the individual, especially the young child, can be supported through the illness episode, he or she can emerge with a defense against the organism should it invade again at some future time.

Bacterial causing AGE includes *campylobacter jejuni*, which is found in unwashed or undercooked chicken and other meats or from surfaces, such as cutting boards and countertops, that have been contaminated by these products. A bacterial source is usually suspected when other individuals who have shared the same food or water source as the patient become ill at the same time with similar symptoms. Illness within 12 hours of ingestion is likely due to a bacterial source. The host's response is dependent on prior exposure to the organism, age, and nutritional and immune status.

Bacteria entering the body must overcome its normal defensive mechanisms. They must survive stomach acidity and normal bacteria in the gut; however, most do not. Some bacteria secrete endotoxins into food so that, even if the organism dies, its toxin is left behind to cause illness (e.g., *Staphylococcus aureus* growing in unrefrigerated foods containing mayonnaise). Surviving bacteria find their way into the gut by either attaching themselves to intestinal epithelium where they secrete their endotoxin or by invading intestinal mucosa, producing cellular inflammation and death. Endotoxins act on cells, enhancing fluid secretion and retarding fluid and electrolyte absorption from the gut.

Management

Treatment is aimed at prevention through careful hygiene and replacing fluids lost during the acute phase and immediately thereafter. In severe cases in very young or old patients, oral rehydration therapy with specially formulated fluids or intravenous therapy may be needed to reestablish fluid and electrolyte balance.

Diarrhea

Overview

Diarrhea is defined as a change from normal bowel habits evidenced by increased frequency, amount, and water content of stools.

Pathophysiology

Diarrhea has many causes, some inconvenient and some serious, but all are associated with an increase in the water content of the stools. This increase is caused by an increase in the amount of fluid secreted, a decrease in the amount of fluid absorbed, or an alteration in the motility of the bowel.

An increase in the amount of fluid secreted (i.e., secretory diarrhea) occurs when increased amounts of fluids are transported out of epithelial cells. Caused by inflammation, an enterotoxin, or hormonal changes, secretory diarrhea will continue even if the individual fasts. The amount of fluids absorbed will be decreased when there is either an abnormality in the absorptive surface of the intestinal mucosa or when some unabsorbed material in the intestinal lumen acts as an osmotic force drawing water to itself. Fasting will improve this condition. When the motility of the bowel increases, intestinal contents have less contact time with the mucosal surface so that adequate fluids cannot be absorbed. This can occur as a result of a vagotomy or with hypergastrinemia.

When the diarrhea originates in the small bowel, stools are large, loose, and provoked by eating either a meal or a specific food. It is often accompanied by pain in the right lower quadrant (RLQ) or periumbilical region. When it originates in the large bowel, usually the left or rectosigmoid colon, small, loose stools are passed frequently accompanied by crampy left lower quadrant (LLQ) pain and tenesmus.

Acute diarrhea is usually infectious in origin and accompanied by abdominal cramps, fever, chills, nausea, and vomiting. Chronic diarrhea is defined as the passage of more than 200 grams of loose stool per day for more than 3 weeks. This is associated with some type of chronic condition with the diarrhea being symptomatic.

Management

Treatment of mild diarrhea is symptomatic and includes rehydration, a low fiber diet, and antidiarrheals. Chronic diarrhea requires diagnosis of the cause followed by corrective and supportive therapy.

Type	Characteristics	Incidence/Intubation	Duration
Traveler's diarrhea	Small bowel, secretory diarrhea caused by action of a toxin contaminating food or water; watery diarrhea with stools; contains blood, pus, and leukocytes	Found in persons who are in or have returned from a tropical environment	1 to 2 days
Chronic			
Inflammatory bowel	Bloody stools, abdominal pain, weight loss, fever, arthralgias Extraintestinal symptoms involving skin, joints, liver, and/or heart		
Irritable bowel	Motility disorder; alternating bouts of constipation and diarrhea Loose stools after bout of abdominal pain which defecation relieves; early morning evacuation; tenesmus; rectal urgency; mucous on stool surface		
Giardiasis lamblia	Can have an acute or gradual onset with explosive diarrhea; abdominal discomfort; distension; watery, foul smelling stools; flatulence; anorexia; nausea; weight loss	Most common parasitic diarrheal infection in United States and overseas; endemic to Rocky Mountains; history of drinking water contaminated by human waste; hikers and campers are at high risk	Days to months
Chronic pseudo-membranous enterocolitis	Osmotic diarrhea caused by taking antibiotics, especially clindamycin or ampicillin, that kill normal bacteria present in the colon present to metabolize carbohydrates that have not been absorbed; when not metabolized this material draws water to itself, producing a profuse, watery diarrhea and abdominal pain; allows a clostridium difficile superinfection to occur	3 days up to 6 weeks	3 to 10 days
Lactase deficiency	Onset is usually in adulthood with bloating, abdominal cramps, and diarrhea after ingesting more than customary intake of milk or milk products, which raises the lactose load; can cause failure to thrive in children	Seen in Asians, Africans, and Jews and can occur in infants	

Differentiating Types of Vomiting

Type	Characteristics	Other Findings/Diagnostics
Gastroenteritis (viral or bacterial)	Most common cause in all age groups; acute onset; may be accompanied by diarrhea, mild fever, crampy abdominal pain, and muscle aches; may be associated with ingestion of contaminated food	Hyperactive bowel sounds; minimal abdominal tenderness on palpation
Gastritis	Acute or chronic nausea/vomiting (N/V) occurs after eating; can be induced by alcohol ingestion or drugs or be associated with ulcers that result from irritation, spasm, and edema of the pyloric muscle	
Pancreatitis	Repeated episodes of N/V, abdominal pain that radiates to the back; associated with excessive alcohol intake	Elevated serum amylase
Appendicitis	Anorexia, N/V early symptoms in most patients; pain precedes vomiting	Elevated leukocytes
Binge drinking	Excessive alcohol consumption; early morning N/V and dry heaves	
Esophageal obstruction	Vomiting of undigested food, odorless, early AM or after meals	Endoscopy
Pyloric obstruction	In children: persistent projectile vomiting of large amounts of food, especially in infants <3 months; in adults: associated with tumor or scar formation from an ulcer	Palpable mass; weight loss

(continued on p. 196)

Overview

Nausea and vomiting are common problems with a variety of causes. Nausea is defined as an unpleasant sensation described as "feeling sick" or "queasy." It is frequently followed by vomiting.

Pathophysiology

Vomiting may be induced by stimulation of any of the following: afferent vagal or splanchnic fibers stimulated by biliary or gastrointestinal distension, peritoneal or mucosal irritation, or infection; the vestibular system affected by motion or infection; the higher central nervous system (CNS) affected by sights, smells, or emotions, or the chemoreceptor trigger zone in the area of the medulla, which is affected by drugs, chemotherapeutic agents, uremia, toxins, acidosis, hypoxia, or radiation therapy.

Vomiting is a symptom. The cause of vomiting may be indicated by the type and pattern of vomiting (see pp. 194 and 196). Acute vomiting without significant abdominal pain is likely due to drugs, infectious gastroenteritis, or food poisoning. Acute vomiting with abdominal pain is indicative of peritoneal irritation, intestinal obstruction, or pancreatic and/or biliary disease. Persistent vomiting may be due to pregnancy, gastric outlet syndrome, psychogenic causes, or sys-temic disorders. Vomiting immediately after eating is associated with bulimia. Vomiting undigested food within a few hours of eating may be caused by gastric outlet syndrome or gastroparesis. Problems caused by vomiting include dehydration, electrolyte imbalance, metabolic acidosis, and aspiration.

Management

Acute vomiting is treated with rest and rehydration. Dehydration and electrolyte imbalances are treated accordingly. Persistent and psychogenic vomiting is managed by treating the underlying cause.

Type	Characteristics	Other Findings/Diagnostics
Lower bowel	Abdominal distension with none or very small amount of stool; green bile in vomitus; breath may have fecal odor	Decreased/absent bowel sounds
Labyrinthine disorders	N/V accompanied by vertigo, tinnitus, and motion sickness	Nystagmus
ICP	Sudden forceful vomiting not accompanied by nausea; headache; symptoms get progressively worse over hours or days	Positive neurological findings; changes in mentation; motor function
Morning sickness	N/V occurring in early morning during first trimester of pregnancy that usually ends by the fourth month	Last menstrual period >6 weeks ago Elevated human chorionic gonadotropin (HCG) level
Bulimia	Self-induced vomiting after binge eating; usually in young women with poor self-image and preoccupation with being thin; may be accompanied by laxative abuse	
Metabolic etiologies	Seventy-five percent of those with diabetic ketoacidosis Ninety percent of those with Addison's crisis	Check blood sugar levels
Drug induced	Associated with cancer treatment either drug (especially cisplatin) or radiation therapy, producing severe N/V caused by serotonin released from cells activating receptors an stimulating the vomiting center and chemoreceptor trigger zone; with opiate drug withdrawal, vomiting begins 36 hours after last dose, accompanied by sweats, chills, and restlessness; peaks at 72 hours	

Cancers of the Gastrointestinal Tract

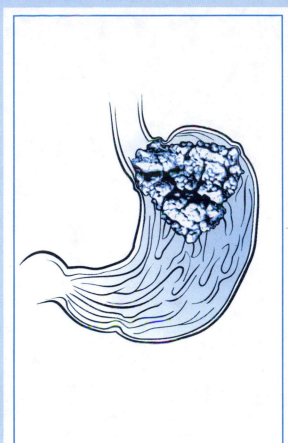

Carcinoma of the stomach arising from the gastric mucosa (see arrow) and extending into the esophagus. Risk factors include the following:

Dietary

- Smoked foods
- Pickled foods
- Nitrates (contained in preservatives of prepared meats and in some drinking water supplies)
- High salt intake

Nondietary

- Chronic gastritis with intestinal metaplasia due to either *H. pylori* or pernicious anemia
- Altered anatomy after subtotal gastrectomy

Esophageal Cancer

Overview

Esophageal tumors are almost always malignant, and their incidence is rising at an alarming rate. Any individual over age 40 complaining of dysphagia is considered to have an esophageal malignancy until proven otherwise. Five-year survival rates are only about 5%.

Pathophysiology

Two types of cancer predominate. Squamous cell carcinoma, associated with the use of tobacco and alcohol, is more common in African-American males. Patients usually seek help because of progressive dysphagia for solids then liquids by which time the tumor is already inoperable. Adenocarcinoma arises from columnar epithelium tissue and is associated with

Barrett's esophagus, which is a complication of chronic gastric esophagitis. This is found more commonly in Caucasians in the distal one third of the esophagus. Patients seek help for persistent heartburn that progresses to dysphagia. The tumor gradually narrows the lumen of the esophagus, infiltrates the surrounding tissues, and can invade the trachea, causing a tracheoesophageal fistula.

Management

Surgery is the treatment of choice for tumors of the lower one third of the esophagus, while radiation is the treatment for the upper two thirds. Surveillance of known/suspected cases of Barrett's esophagus is paramount.

Stomach Cancer

Overview

Gastric cancer, one of the most common cancers worldwide, is more prevalent in developing countries among lower socioeconomic groups in urban settings. Japan, China, South America, and Eastern Europe have a high incidence, while the United States and Canada have a low incidence. Immigrants acquire the same risk as natives, pointing to environmental factors in its development. Rare before the age of 40, the mean age at the time of diagnosis is 63. Cancers in the antrum and body have been declining, while those of the cardia and gastroesophageal junction are increasing at an alarming rate. Causes are thought to be chronic *H. pylori* infection; genetic predisposition; and dietary, especially diets with foods high in nitrates, smoked, salted, or pickled foods and rich in complex carbohydrates (e.g., fava beans).

Pathophysiology

Gastric cancers have several morphological types including polypoid intraluminal masses, ulcerating masses, diffuse and spreading through the submucosa, and superficial confined to the mucosa or submucosa with or without lymphatic involvement—the only type with a good prognosis. Most individuals, up to 90%, do not seek help until the disease is very advanced, having relied on over-the-counter (OTC) medications for what had been mild but persistent abdominal complaints they mistook for indigestion. Tumors of the cardia and gastrointestinal (GI) junction present with dysphagia and weight loss caused by anorexia and early satiety. Advanced cases also complain of persistent abdominal pain and have iron deficiency anemia from occult blood loss. Half of those with advanced disease have a palpable mass. Diagnosis is made by endoscopic cytology brushings and biopsy of suspected lesions.

Management

All patients are surgical candidates unless there is clear evidence of metastasis or the individual is considered a poor surgical risk. Chemotherapy is used for nonsurgical candidates, radiation therapy to treat complications such as obstruction, and stent placement and nutritional support provide some palliative care. Eighty-five percent of patients will experience recurrence within 2 years of surgery. A look at preventing the disease points to dietary changes, the need to monitor and eradicate *H. pylori*, and carefully monitoring those with a strong family history.

Colorectal Cancer

Overview

Adenocarcinoma, also called *colorectal cancer*, is the second leading cause of cancer death and the most common type of cancer of the large bowel. With the exception of Japan, it is most prevalent in industrialized countries. Six percent of Americans will develop it in their lifetime; 40% will die from it. Both sexes are equally affected, and 90% are diagnosed after age 50. Since the promotion of early detection, 5-year survival rates have risen to 60% but are much lower for low income groups, especially African-American males.

Adenomas are precursors of most colorectal cancers. While the reason for this is unknown, strong environmental and genetic links are recognized. Dietary factors include high calorie, high fat, and high red meat content and alcohol consumption. Other lifestyle factors include obesity, lack of exercise, and long-term exposure to cigarette smoke. It is estimated that one half of colorectal cancers could be prevented by lifestyle modifications alone. There are clearly established links between the development of this cancer and familial adenomatous polyposis, nonpolyposis colorectal cancer, and nonadenomatous polyposis. A history of inflammatory bowel disease also increases risk with a duration of 10 to 15 years of active disease and extensive involvement of the disease being the important factors. Colorectal cancers associated with inflammatory bowel diseases arise from the ulcer craters and are difficult to detect.

Pathophysiology

Benign adenomatous polyps, which are precursors of colorectal cancer, are generally detected and excised on screening exams. All have some degree of dysplasia as determined by cytology atypia and architectural abnormality. Those classified as mild dysplasia have few characteristics of cancer; those classified as severe dysplasia have many cancer characteristics but remain noninvasive. A malignant polyp contains cancer cells and is invasive. It appears to take about 10 to 15 years for a benign polyp to become malignant with genetic mutations occurring in a predictable order. Ras oncogene mutations are seen in 50% of adenocarcinomas and 75% have alterations in the tumor suppression genes, especially those involving chromosomes 17 and 18. Several other types of benign polyps can be found, but these do not become malignant.

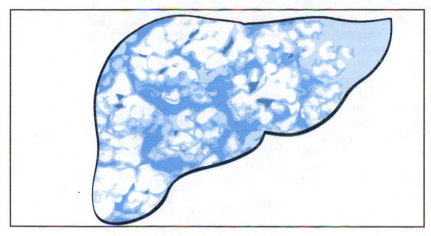

Hepatocellular carcinoma of the liver. Risk factors include the following:

- Hepatitis B carrier state from infancy
- Alcoholism
- Chronic liver disease

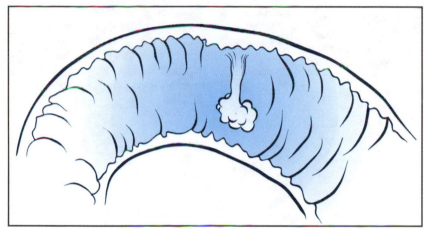

Adenomatous polyp of the colon.

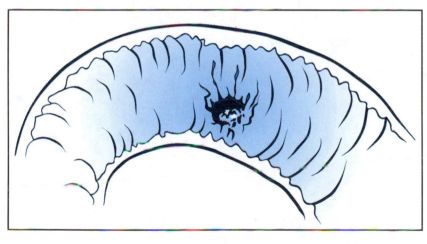

Adenocarcinoma of the colon. Risk factors include the following:

- Adenomatous polyps
- Inflammatory bowel disease

Most colorectal cancers present as ulcerative, infiltrating, or nodular lesions in either the rectum, sigmoid, or descending colon. Metastasis occurs via either lymphatic invasion to the mesentery lymph nodes or through the portal system to the liver and eventually through systemic circulation to the lung and other body sites. Tumor staging is based on the depth of invasion and extent of lymphatic involvement. Stage I tumors have a 97% 5-year survival rate; Stage IV tumors a 4% survival rate. The loss of DCC or p53 tumor suppressor genes indicates poor prognosis as do findings of differentiated histology, abnormal deoxyribonucleic acid (DNA) content, and invasion into adjacent structures or elevation of CEA, which is the plasma carcinoembryonic antigen. Tumor size does not predict prognosis.

Adenomatous polyps are generally asymptomatic. Symptoms of cancerous tumors are dependent on their size and location. Cancer of the right colon presents with occult bleeding, iron deficiency anemia, and some complaints of pain. A mass may be palpable in the right lower quadrant (RLQ). Tumors here and in the cecum do not generally cause obstruction because the lumen is large and stools are soft in this area of the bowel.

Cancers of the transverse colon usually present as an obstruction. Those of the left and sigmoid colon present with rectal bleeding and symptoms of bowel obstruction (e.g., crampy abdominal pain, change in bowel habits, and changes in stool size and consistency). Cancers of the rectum produce small amounts of bright red bleeding, urgency, and increased stool frequency with a change in size and consistency. Advanced cancers produce perianal pain, hematuria, urinary frequency, and vaginal fistulas. They can perforate into the peritoneum, producing a local abscess or peritonitis.

Management

Detection screening exams and lifestyle changes have a major impact on the development and cure rates of colorectal cancer. Surgical resection is the only potentially curative treatment for those diagnosed with the disease. Chemotherapy and radiation improve prognosis. Chemotherapy is the treatment of choice for those with metastasis. Individuals with diagnosed adenomas require surveillance colonoscopy every 3 years.

53 Liver and Biliary Anatomy and Physiology

Diagnostic Studies

- Endoscopic retrograde cholangiopancreatography (ERCP)—Using a flexible fiberoptic endoscope, a contrast medium is instilled into the duodenal papilla or ampulla of Vater to view the hepatic tree and pancreatic ducts. After viewing, the endoscope can be used to drain cysts, remove stones from the common bile duct, or place stents across biliary or pancreatic structures.

- Hepatic angiography—Assessment of hepatic vasculature commonly used prior to transplantation, to place a transjugular intrahepatic portosystemic shunt (TIPS), or following trauma.

- Hepatobiliary scan (HIDA)—A radionuclide study that shows hepatic parenchyma; extrahepatic bile ducts; gallbladder; normal passage into the intestine; and the size, shape, and position of the liver. A series of images permits visualization of the gallbladder and determines the patency of the biliary system. It is used to evaluate biliary leaks, cholecystitis, and biliary atresia; to differentiate obstructive from nonobstructive jaundice; and to evaluate upper abdominal pain.

- Liver biopsy (percutaneous liver biopsy)—Insertion of a needle through the abdominal wall into the liver to obtain tissue samples to diagnose or confirm liver disease and responses to therapy and to evaluate transplant allografts.

Laboratory Tests

- Hepatitis screen—Five major types of hepatitis have thus far been identified with additional types being considered. Because they present with common symptoms, a hepatitis screen can be used to determine the presence, type, stage, and progress of the disease. Each type of hepatitis has specific markers that rise and fall in a predictable pattern. Markers specify the type of hepatitis (i.e., HAV for hepatitis A; HBcAB or HBsAG for hepatitis B; anti-HCV for hepatitis C; HDAg for hepatitis D; and IgM anti-HVE for hepatitis E). The form of immunoglobulin found indicates that an infection is in the early stages (i.e., IgM or later stages IgG). Use of the prefix "anti" explains that the body has produced an antigen to the virus. Lastly, because some types of the hepatitis virus have various layers or components, different names are used to represent the identified component (i.e., HBcAg means the hepatitis B core antigen, anti-HBs means the antibody to the hepatitis B surface antigen). Once the particular type of hepatitis is known, the specific kind and pattern of hepatitis markers for that virus can be consulted.

Hepatitis A markers:

- HAV-ab (hepatitis A antibody)

  IgM—Acute infection

  IgG—Postinfection, previous exposure, immunity

Hepatitis B markers

- Anti-HB (hepatitis B core antibody)—Rises within 2 weeks of contracting virus, rises again during chronic phase, and remains present for life. *(continued on p. 203)*

The liver, which is the largest organ in the body, is located below the diaphragm in the upper right quadrant of the abdomen. It has a dual blood supply with one third of the total being oxygenated blood under high pressure arriving from the hepatic artery. The remaining two thirds of the total comes via the portal vein and brings blood rich in nutrients under low pressure from the stomach, intestines, spleen, and pancreas. These two sources mix as they begin to flow through the liver and collect in the left and right hepatic veins, which then drain into the inferior vena cava.

The functional unit of the liver is the lobule in which hepatocyte cells are organized around a central vein in a spoke-like fashion to form a hexagon. At the corners of the hexagon are the portal tracts where branches of the hepatic artery, portal vein, and lymphatic vessels converge. Blood flows from these tracts through vascular spaces called *sinusoids* toward the central vein. Lining the walls of the sinusoids are various one layer thick cells: hepatocytes, which are responsible for carbohydrate and fat metabolism, blood detoxification, and initial bile formation; bile duct cells, which add to the composition of bile and propel it; endothelial cells, which help filter blood; perisinusoidal cells, which aid in lipid and vitamin A metabolism, production of proteins, and liver regeneration; and Kupffer's cells, which are phagocytes. Because the outer portion of the hexagon has initial contact with well oxygenated, nutrient rich blood it is less vulnerable to injury and circulatory disturbances than cells located near the central vein.

Via these structures and processes the liver converts fructose and galactose to glucose; removes excess glucose from the blood in response to insulin; makes and stores glycogen, which reconverts into glucose when circulating glucose levels fall; builds and breaks down phospholipids, triglycerides, and cholesterol as needed; manufactures bile to send to the gallbladder for use as needed; makes ketone bodies as needed; removes excess amino acids from the blood and deaminates them or converts them to other amino acids; stores iron, copper, and vitamins including B_{12}; synthesizes plasma proteins needed for blood clotting such as albumin, which holds water in the blood vessels, fibrinogen, and prothrombin; digests bacteria and toxic substances to cleanse the blood; detoxifies substances such as urea from amino acid metabolism; converts ammonia to urea for excretion by the kidneys; produces the bases for nitrogen containing compounds needed to make deoxyribonucleic acid (DNA) and ribonucleic acid (RNA); and forms lymph.

The liver is capable of renewing itself. Hepatocytes generally live up to 120 days but can survive for months or years. They can proliferate rapidly in response to injury and cell loss.

Bile duct epithelial cells can also do this. Hyperplasia of hepatocytes will occur in response to significant metabolic alterations in carbohydrate or lipid metabolism. Hypertrophy can occur when there is a need for increased chemical transformation as with drug detoxification. Cell death is characterized by shrinkage, cytoplasmic condensation, nuclear loss, and disappearance of individual hepatocytes as they slide down the sinusoids and are carried away via blood into the central vein. The liver loses cells and mass with age so that by age 90 about two thirds of the hepatic mass is lost. Fat accumulates, cells shrink, and functions are compromised.

Liver cells may be injured by drugs, alcohol, chemicals, or viruses. The result is cellular death, accumulation of fat within liver cells, or a combination of the two. With mild injury liver cells can regenerate, but repeated episodes of even mild disease are cumulative and can lead to scarring and permanent damage. Chronic progressive diseases have the same effect. With severe disease and the death of large numbers of liver cells, it may be impossible for regeneration to occur. Postnecrotic scarring can change liver architecture to such a degree that normal functioning is impossible. Some substances, especially alcohol, but also obesity, diabetes, and malnutrition can produce excessive accumulations of fats in the liver. This probably results from an imbalance between the amount of fats arriving and the ability of the liver to mobilize very low density lipoproteins as triglycerides. With abstinence and good nutrition this condition can be reversed.

Bile is formed when blood passes through the liver. There bilirubin, the yellow-orange colored, iron-free heme present from red blood cell (RBC) breakdown, is removed from it. Bilirubin is combined with water and other substances excreted by the liver (i.e., bile salts, lecithin, cholesterol, and minerals) to form bile. Bile travels in the opposite direction as blood and collects in bile canaliculi located at the periphery of the hexagon. These collecting ducts gradually increase in size and eventually end in the left and right hepatic ducts that join to form the common hepatic duct. This duct and the cystic duct of the gallbladder together form the common bile duct. Bile is constantly secreted, concentrated, and stored in the gallbladder. Bile contains no enzymes but acts as a digestive detergent, emulsifying fat into small globules so that more surface area can be acted upon by pancreatic enzymes.

The pancreas is located across the abdomen behind the stomach with its head fitting into the curve of the duodenum where the pancreatic duct empties. It operates as a dual gland. As an exocrine gland, the pancreas releases the following digestive enzymes: amylase, which breaks down carbohydrates; trypsin and chymotrypsin, which break down protein; and lipase, which breaks down fat. As an endocrine gland, small clusters of cells called *Langerhans' cells* discharge secretions into the blood. Langerhans' cells are composed of different types of cells: alpha cells, which secrete glucagon; beta cells, which secrete insulin when blood glucose levels rise after eating; and delta cells, which secrete somatostatin, which inhibits the secretion of both glucagon and insulin.

Jaundice is a condition in which the skin, tissues, and conjunctiva become yellow because of the excess bilirubin in the blood. This may be caused by an obstruction such as a tumor, a gallstone in the duct, or a congenital defect. It may also be present in liver dis-

- Anti-HBc, HbeAb (hepatitis b antibody)—Indicates resolution of infection; if found in the presence of chronic hepatitis B surface antigen, it indicates an asymptomatic healthy carrier.
- HBs-AB (hepatitis B surface antibody)—Represents clinical recovery and immunity to virus; if present with hepatitis B surface antigen, indicates a poor prognosis.
- HbsAG:HAA (hepatitis B surface antigen)—Indicates active hepatitis B either acute or chronic; is early indicator and can be present before clinical symptoms; if present with hepatitis B surface antigen, it indicates a poor prognosis.

Hepatitis C markers
- Anti-HCV (hepatitis C antibody)—Identifies total antibodies of the IgG close to the hepatitis C virus.

Hepatitis D markers
- HDAg (hepatitis delta antibody)—Identifies total antibodies of the IgG close to the hepatitis D virus; this virus requires the presence of HBsAg to express itself.

Hepatitis E markers
- IGM anti-HVE—Antibodies to hepatitis E virus.
- LFTs (Liver enzymes/liver function panel)—Panel usually consists of AST, ALT, alkaline phosphatase, bilirubin, and albumin; other tests are also included here.
- ALT (alanine aminotransferase)—Intracellular enzyme involved in amino acid metabolism; found in large concentrations in the liver and smaller concentrations in heart muscle and kidney; released with tissue damage; used to diagnose liver disease and to monitor course of hepatitis, cirrhosis, and drug therapy; helps differentiate between hemolytic jaundice and jaundice due to liver disease.
- AST (aspartate aminotransferase)—Intracellular enzyme involved in amino acid metabolism; found in large concentrations in the liver, skeletal muscle, heart, brain, and RBCs; released into blood when tissue, especially liver, is damaged.
- LDH (lactate dehydrogenase)—Intracellular enzyme found in almost all body tissues; is released after tissue damage but is not specific as to site.
- ALP (alkaline phosphatase)—Enzyme found in bone, liver, intestine, and placenta; rises during periods of bone growth, liver disease, or bile duct obstruction.
- GGT/GTTP (gamma glutamyltransferase/transpeptidase)—A biliary excretory enzyme that assists in transferring amino acids and peptides across cellular membranes; used to evaluate liver disease and hepatic metastasis and screen for alcoholism.
- Albumin—Major component of plasma proteins; influenced by nutritional state and hepatic functioning; gives indication of severity in chronic liver disease; low levels occur because of decreased hepatic synthesis.
- Bilirubin is produced in the liver, spleen, and bone marrow; is a by-product of hemoglobin metabolism; total bilirubin is broken down into direct (conjugated) normally excreted from the gastrointestinal (GI) tract; and indirect (free) bilirubin circulating in the blood; total bilirubin rises with any kind of jaundice; direct rises with obstructive or hepatic jaundice and is excreted by the kidneys; indirect bilirubin rises in hemolytic jaundice with increased amount of present in the blood.
- 5'-Nucleotide—A plasma membrane enzyme found in hepatic parenchyma and bile duct cells; will be elevated in liver cancer; when occurs with accompaning elevation in alkaline phosphatase indicates liver metastasis.
- OCT (ornithine carbamoyltransferase)—A liver enzyme involved in urea metabolism, elevations are specific and sensitive to liver cell disease.
- LAP (leucine aminopeptidase)—Enzyme found in liver, bile, and urine; helps with differential diagnosis when client presents with elevated alkaline phosphatase as it will be normal in bone disease.
- Amylase—Enzyme produced in pancreas and salivary glands that aids in digestion of complex carbohydrates; elevated in blood 2 to 3 days following acute pancreatitis attack; stays elevated in urine for 7 to 10 days.
- Lipase—Pancreatic enzyme that digests fats and triglycerides; elevated in association with amylase but is more specific than amylase.

eases like hepatitis or cirrhosis. Because bile does not reach the duodenum, stools are light colored, and because the bilirubin loaded blood is filtered by the kidneys, the urine becomes very dark. Without bile aiding digestion, digestion of fats is compromised and fat soluble vitamins are not absorbed.

Hemolytic jaundice is very different and develops in the presence of hemolytic anemias in which RBCs are hemolyzed with excessive amounts of bilirubin released. Physiological jaundice in newborns may develop shortly after birth because the liver is too immature to manage the bilirubin already in the blood. Normally, this condition only lasts a few days and is not usually serious.

54 Hepatitis

Viral Hepatitis: Important Characteristics

Characteristic	Type A	Type B	Type C	Type D	Type E
Mode of transmission	Waterborne Fecal-oral Venereal	Perinatal Blood/skin Venereal	Venereal Blood/skin	Venereal Blood	Waterborne Fecal-oral
Incubation period (range in days)	15 to 42	42 to 160	14 to 160	28 to 49	14 to 56
average	30	90	50	35	40
Onset	Abrupt	Insidious	Insidious	Insidious	Abrupt
Symptoms					
Fever	Common	Uncommon	Uncommon	Common	Common
Nausea/vomiting	Common	Common	Common	Common	Common
Jaundice	More common in adults than children	Occasionally	Uncommon	Common	Common
Outcome					
Severity	Mild	Moderate	Mild	Moderate to severe	Severe
Fulminating hepatitis	<.5%	<1%	Rare	3% to 4% with coinfection with hepatitis B	.3% to 3% 20% in pregnant women
Mortality rate	Low (<1%)	Low (1% to 3%)	Low (2%)	High (5%)	Moderate; high with pregnancy
Chronic hepatitis	No	Yes (5% to 10%)	Yes (80%)	<5% with coinfection 80% with superinfection	No
Carrier state	No	Yes (1 million in United States)	Yes	Yes	No
Relapse	Yes	Yes	Persistent	Unknown	Unknown
Carcinoma	No	Yes (25% to 40%)	Yes (20% to 30%)	No increase above that for hepatitis B	Unknown but but likely
Develop cirrhosis	No	40%	30%	Yes, with superinfection	No

Hepatitis may be caused by a viral infection or result from sensitivity to a hepatotoxic drug or chemical or from chronic, excessive alcohol intake. Hepatitis and its sequela affect more than 500 million people worldwide. Both sexes and all age groups are equally affected. Hepatitis may occur as an acute or chronic disease, be mild or fulminating, and be active or dormant. Once infected an individual can act as a carrier of the illness without having active symptoms. Hepatitis can cause cirrhosis or liver cancer and is the underlying basis for the majority of liver transplants.

Acute hepatitis is usually caused by one of the hepatotropic viruses (see above). These viruses specifically affect hepatocyte cells, causing the cell membrane to rupture and contents to leak out. Macrophages consume the destroyed cells. Cell necrosis can occur in isolated clusters with large regions developing as clusters enlarge and connect with each other, disrupting the normal architecture of the area. Cell damage can extend into the parenchyma, causing inflammation, disrupting the bile channel structure, and resulting in the pooling of bile and engorgement of the liver.

Acute hepatitis has four distinct periods: period of incubation, symptomatic preicteric period, symptomatic period with jaundice and sclera icterus, and period of convalescence. The individual is most infective during the last days of incubation and early days of acute symptoms. The symptomatic preicteric period is marked by nonspecific constitutional changes common to most viral syndromes (i.e., malaise, fatigue, anorexia, low grade fever, and muscle aches). Some patients with hepatitis B also experience rash, fever, and arthralgias. Jaundice does not occur with every type of hepatitis but is common in adults with hepatitis A and about half of those with hepatitis B. Hepatitis C does not generally produce jaundice. When jaundice develops, it is caused by conjugated hyperbilirubinemia and results in dark-colored urine, light-colored stools, and puritis as bile salts are retained. It can take weeks to months for jaundice and other symptoms to resolve.

Hepatoviruses

Hepatitis A is typically acquired as part of a local epidemic associated with shellfish harvested from contaminated water. Individuals are usually asymptomatic or only mildly ill. It may go unrecognized in children. About 50% of adults in the United States are seropositive for hepatitis A, many never realizing they have ever had it. Peak titers of IgM anti-HAV occur during the first week of clinical disease and usually disappear within 3 to 6 months. Titers of IgG anti-HAV peak 1 month and may persist for years. Recovery without complications is common; lifelong immunity to hepatitis A is conferred by one episode. Management is symptom supportive.

Hepatitis B, one of most serious hepatoviruses, is present in all body fluids except stool. Most individuals are infected during passage through the birth canal of an infected mother. More than 90% of those infected as children become hepatitis B carriers, with many going on to develop cirrhosis or hepatocellular carcinoma.

Infected hepatocytes synthesize and secrete massive quantities of a noninfective surface protein that appears in cells and serum as HBeAg. This indicates the disease is present. HBeAg appears shortly thereafter, indicating that active viral replication is taking place, infectivity is high, and progression to a chronic hepatitis state is likely. Management is aimed chiefly at prevention by vaccination against the disease. Hepatitis B immunoglobulin may be protective if given in large doses within 7 days of exposure and if followed by initiation of the hepatitis B vaccine series. Viral replication can be diminished in about 30% of cases by interferon therapy continued for at least 4 months. Other treatment is aimed at symptom management.

Hepatitis C often goes unnoticed and is discovered by following-up on routine blood tests that initially show elevated alanine aminotransferase (ALT)/aspartate aminotransferase (AST). Originally part of a viral group known as non-A-non-B hepatitis, hepatitis C is now thought to be responsible for 80% to 90% of these viruses. The mode of transmission often cannot be identified but it is thought that about 50% of cases have a past history of intravenous (IV) drug use. Recent data suggest that as many as 1 in 3 people with tattoos have been infected with the virus by that process. Persistent infection and chronic hepatitis are common. Cirrhosis can be present at the time of diagnosis or develop within 5 to 10 years. Because hepatitis C mutates at a rapid rate it is expected that a vaccine against it will not be found. Interferon, which boosts the body's immune response, cures about 25% of patients. Other treatment is supportive.

Hepatitis D exists and is able to persist only in the presence of hepatitis B. It can occur either as a coinfection or as a superinfection and is managed by managing the hepatitis B.

Hepatitis E is thought to be transmitted via contaminated drinking water and is found in almost half of adults in third world countries. It is usually a self-limiting illness resulting in neither chronicity nor carrier state. In pregnant women, however, it can result in fulminating hepatitis with a 20% mortality rate.

Cases of non-A-non-B hepatitis have resulted in the identification of other hepatitis viruses, most notably C and D, but also others about which little is known. A single case of hepatitis F suggests that the virus may not even exist. Hepatitis G has been seen with blood transfusions and causes cirrhosis as documented by liver biopsy.

Chronic hepatitis is diagnosed by symptomatic, serological, or histological evidence of continuing or relapsing hepatic disease lasting more than 6 months. It may be caused by either a hepatovirus (usually B or C), alcoholism, or drugs. Outcome is determined by the histological pattern that develops rather than the etiology of the disease. An individual may have only elevated enzyme; a single complaint, usually fatigue; or severe systemic symptoms associated with cirrhosis or hepatic failure. With mild or slowly progressing disease, the liver architecture is usually well preserved and function remains essentially intact. More severe or rapidly progressing disease results in more serious changes. Coalescing areas of necrosis extending into the parenchyma cause disruption of hepatic structures and functioning. Irreversible liver damage is characterized by deposits of fibrous tissue first in the portal tracts, later in the adjacent tissues, and finally enveloping whole lobules. Cirrhosis develops with large irregularly shaped nodules and broad bands of scarring. The individual can live for years with chronic hepatitis; however, when architectural changes, fibrous scars, and cellular death make even minimal liver functioning impossible, transplantation is the only option.

Fulminating hepatitis is a rapidly progressive form of the disease that can end with hepatic encephalopathy or death within 2 to 3 weeks. Uncommon but extremely serious, it is usually caused by superinfection of hepatitis D in a person with existing chronic hepatitis B or as a complication of hepatitis E in pregnant women. It may also result from drugs or chemicals, such as acetaminophen, isoniazid, halothane, or toxic mushrooms. Rapid and massive loss of liver tissue occurs. Surviving more than 1 week may allow hepatocytes to regenerate with the outcome determined by the pattern of destruction. Survivors are generally left with some degree of cirrhosis.

A *carrier* is an individual who has been infected by a hepatovirus but is either symptom free of the disease or has chronic liver damage but is currently without symptoms. In both states the individual harbors the hepatitis virus and is able to transmit it to others. Up to 95% of those affected with hepatitis B at birth become carriers. Most persons with hepatitis C are carriers.

55 Cirrhosis

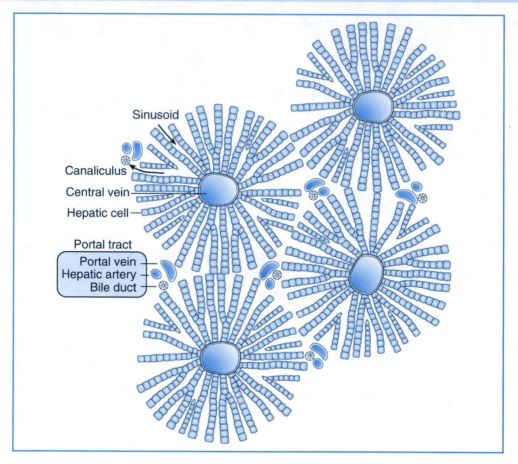

Sinusoid

Canaliculus

Central vein

Hepatic cell

Portal tract
  Portal vein
  Hepatic artery
  Bile duct

Cross section of a liver lobule showing the direction of blood flow in sinusoids toward the central vein and of bile toward the bile duct.

Overview

Cirrhosis is a condition of chronic, progressive, irreversible damage to the liver resulting in compromised hepatic functioning. The seventh leading cause of death in the United States, it affects about 11 million Americans. While caused by many different conditions, cirrhosis in the United States is most often caused by chronic alcohol consumption. In third world and developing countries, it usually results from chronic hepatitis, either B, C, or D. Symptoms are similar regardless of the cause. Fifty percent with an established diagnosis of cirrhosis survive for 2 years; 35% survive 5 years. About 40% of cases are discovered on autopsy.

Pathophysiology

The architecture of the liver is precisely arranged with each cell and structure having a specific function to perform. If only small areas are affected, the liver can maintain vital functions, but as larger sections are destroyed, its abilities are taxed beyond repair. Damaged liver cells are replaced by tissue that is thick, rigid, inflexible, and incapable of performing any of the functions of healthy hepatocytes. This scar tissue contracts, shrinking the organ, producing a nodular, bumpy appearance, and interfering with the normal vascular and bile pathways. Pressure gradients are affected, compromising blood flow in and out of the organ and backing up the bile. Bile stasis irritates and inflames hepatocytes, causing additional damage. Symptoms develop as the liver is first compromised, then fails.

Portal Hypertension

When the intrahepatic branches of the hepatic artery and portal vein are constricted by scar tissue, high pressure develops in the blood vessels leading to the liver. Veins swell, producing varices especially in the abdomen and esophagus. Organs connected to the liver via circulation (i.e., the spleen, pancreas, and stomach) swell as pressure rises. Collateral circulatory pathways develop to shunt as much blood as possible around the obstruction and back into the systemic circulation. Anastomosis develops to shunt blood from high pressure portal veins to lower pressure systemic vessels. However, veins of the systemic system are not structurally equipped to deal with the volume of diverted blood nor blood arriving under such high pressure. They dilate and form varicosities.

Hemorrhage, or a slow persistent bleed, is possible anywhere along the circulatory pathway. The vessels in the esophagus are particularly vulnerable as they are thin walled and especially prone to rupture. There is a 70% risk of death from a single esophageal bleed. Recurrence is common within 2 weeks of the first episode. Anastomosing varicosities in the abdominal cavity produce a temporary reduction of pressure in the portal system but cause changes that are not always obvious until it is too late to rectify them. Superficial abdominal varicosities are common.

Ascites

Ascites is the accumulation of fluid in the peritoneal cavity. First it occurs because high pressure within the obstructed portal system forces fluids to back up into the abdominal cavity. Secondly, the damaged liver is unable to produce a sufficient supply of albumin, a protein responsible for maintaining normal osmotic pressure and holding fluid in the capillaries. Without albumin, fluid leaks out of the capillaries, collecting in the abdomen. A similar process results in edema, particularly of the lower extremities.

Jaundice

Changes in liver structure impair its ability to manufacture and move bile. Surviving cells continue to produce bile but cannot move it through the collecting system. Bile accumulates in the liver, causing inflammation and necrosis. Some gets into the blood stream causing jaundice. Without bile, fats cannot be digested nor fat soluble vitamins absorbed. Stools become clay colored. Excess bile in the blood is excreted by the kidneys, producing dark urine.

Gynecomastia

Small amounts of estrogen are normally secreted by the adrenal gland in both sexes. A normal liver inactivates it but a cirrhotic liver cannot. The hormone builds up, producing feminine characteristics in the male (i.e., feminine distribution of body hair, testicles atrophy, and impotence). Females experience irregular menses.

Hepatic Encephalopathy

Severely damaged hepatic cells cannot detoxify blood; numerous poisons accumulate. One of them, ammonia, produces neurological manifestations, including confusion, disorientation, and a characteristic hand tremor called *liver flap*. A gastrointestinal (GI) tract bleed can significantly increase protein levels, causing the rapid onset of encephalopathy. Excessive protein ingestion, infection, or renal failure can also increase protein levels. Death is common.

Metabolic Dysfunction

Hepatocyte destruction produces metabolic dysfunction. Changes in protein metabolism result in decreased production of protein clotting factors, muscle wasting, hyperlipidemia, and hypoalbuminemia. Impaired metabolism of glucose results in either hyperglycemia or hypoglycemia. Reduced bile salts make absorption of fat-soluble vitamins from the GI tract difficult. Osteomalacia develops from lack of vitamin D and bleeding tendencies from lack of vitamin K. Without hepatocytes the liver cannot metabolize and/or clear substances like drugs and toxins.

Management

Liver damage is irreversible, but its progression can be delayed or halted. Management depends on the cause and is aimed at preventing further dysfunction and treating complications. Hepatitis-related disease may involve the use of interferon for viral hepatitis and corticosteroids for autoimmune hepatitis. Alcohol- or drug-induced cirrhosis requires complete abstinence. Nutritional management is essential to correct imbalances, manage complications, and promote health. Portal hypertension is treated with surgical intervention to position shunts where needed commonly: hepatorenal, transjugular, or peritovenous. Ascites/edema is treated with fluid restriction, low sodium diet, diuretics, and paracentesis, if needed. Esophageal varices are

Normal liver tissue.

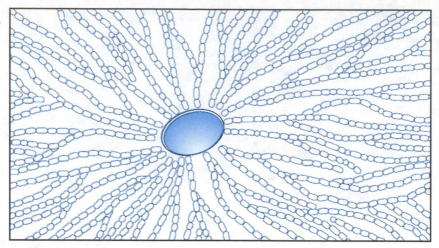

Cirrhotic liver. Note the bands of fibrous tissue and regenerating parenchyma.

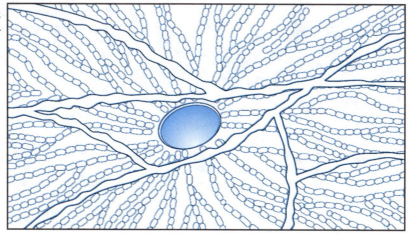

treated with endoscopy to band, shunt, or sclerose and are then used in combination with octreotide, a somatostatin.

Encephalopathy treatment seeks to find and eliminate the underlying cause. Dietary proteins are eliminated and the colon is evacuated to eliminate sources of protein breakdown. Antibiotics are given to suppress intestinal flora and decrease endogenous sources of ammonia production. Lactulose promotes the excretion of ammonia in the stool.

Transplantation is an option for some patients with severe cirrhosis, but wait time is long and not all patients are candidates. Alcoholics, who are not considered good candidates, must refrain from any drinking for at least 6 months to be eligible. Patients with hepatitis often have a return of their infectious disease after transplant. Individuals with any evidence of malignancy are not considered candidates for transplantation.

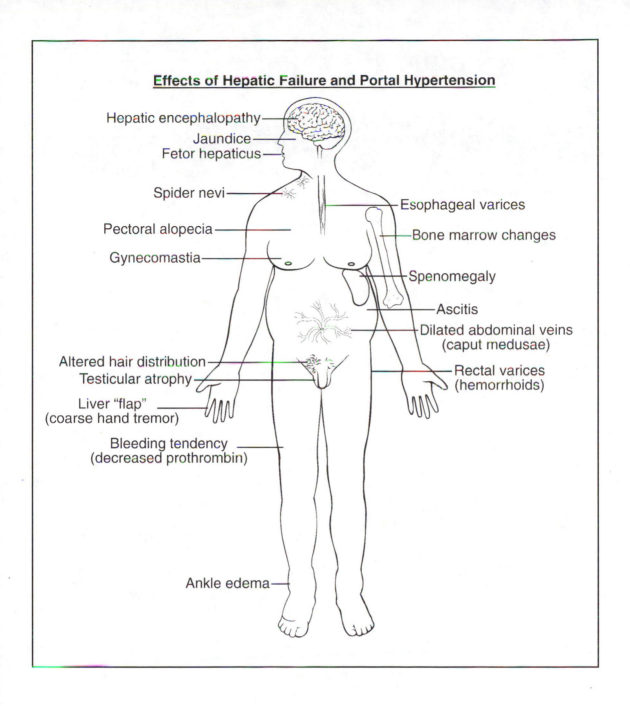

Effects of Hepatic Failure and Portal Hypertension

Hepatic encephalopathy

Jaundice

Fetor hepaticus

Spider nevi

Pectoral alopecia

Gynecomastia

Esophageal varices

Bone marrow changes

Spenomegaly

Ascitis

Dilated abdominal veins
(caput medusae)

Altered hair distribution

Testicular atrophy

Liver "flap"
(coarse hand tremor)

Bleeding tendency
(decreased prothrombin)

Rectal varices
(hemorrhoids)

Ankle edema

56 Pancreatitis and Gallbladder Diseases

Major Etiologies of Acute Pancreatitis
- Metabolic
- Alcohol consumption
- Hyperlipoproteinemia
- Hypercalcemia
- Mechanical
- Gallstones
- Trauma
- Vascular
- Shock
- Atheroembolism

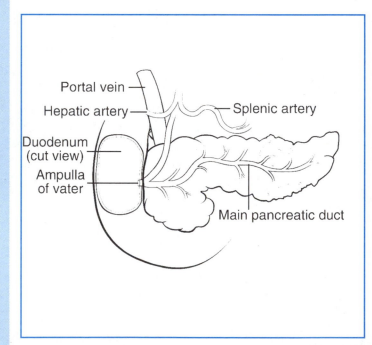

Portal vein

Hepatic artery

Splenic artery

Duodenum
(cut view)

Ampulla
of vater

Main pancreatic duct

Carcinoma of the tail of the pancreas. Most pancreatic tumors arise in the pancreatic ducts. Although small carcinomas of the head of the pancreas usually obstruct the internal pancreatic ducts so that the parenchyma of the exocrine pancreas then undergoes atrophy distal to the obstruction. Carcinomas of the body/tail are larger lesions that quickly invade adjacent organs (i.e., the spleen, colon, and adrenals) and metastasize to regional lymph nodes. Hepatic metastasis follows once the spleen is invaded.

Pancreatitis

Pancreatitis is more common in men than women and usually occurs after age 40. It may be acute or chronic. Acute pancreatitis usually results from a gallstone (>6.5 mm diameter) causing an obstruction of the pancreatic duct at its entrance to the duodenum.

As the common bile duct and the common pancreatic duct enter into the duodenum through a common channel (i.e., the ampulla of Vater), a stone lodged in the ampulla causes pancreatic juices to back up. Eventually, the pressure in the pancreatic ducts results in their rupture and pancreatic enzymes "escape" into the surrounding pancreatic tissues. The enzymes cause autodigestion, inflammation, edema, and necrosis of pancreatic cells. A second cause is excessive alcohol consumption. Alcohol forms plugs in the pancreatic ducts, causing edema and spasm of the pancreatic sphincter in the ampulla of Vater. It also activates the release of proteolytic enzymes. The obstruction of the duct and the excessive production of enzymes has the same result as above. Together gallstones and alcohol account for about 80% of acute pancreatic attacks. Other causes include infection, hyperlipidemia (when triglycerides >1,000), trauma, as a idiosyncratic reaction to drugs, and from heredity causes. Regardless of the cause, patients experience abrupt onset of deep epigastric pain that often radiates to the back, nausea, vomiting that does not improve, sweating, and weakness.

Eighty percent of patients with chronic pancreatitis are alcoholics, but only 5% to 10% of alcoholics develop chronic pancreatitis. Alcohol causes insoluble pancreatic proteins to be released, which calcify and occlude the large pancreatic duct. Recurrent episodes of acute pancreatitis produce inflammation and scarring, damage to the ductal system, and high blood pressure. It becomes a self-perpetuating disease with repeated episodes of acute pancreatitis eventually leading to endocrine and exocrine insufficiency. Without lipid enzymes, fats cannot be digested. Foul smelling, greasy stools and vitamin B_{12} malabsorption develop because undigested fats and fat soluble vitamins cannot be absorbed. Patients present with recurrent epigastric pain radiating to the back and weight loss due to maldigestion. The persistent severe pain not uncommonly leads to an addiction to narcotics.

Pancreatic Cancer

Adenocarcinoma of the pancreas is found more often in males, is relatively common, and has a high mortality rate. About 75% of cases involve the head of the pancreas, which is defined as the ampulla of Vater; the distal common bile duct; and the duodenum. This gives rise to symptoms that occur earlier than cancer of the body or tail of the pancreas, which can be well advanced before being detected. Cancer of the head of the pancreas causes obstructive jaundice and impairs digestion due to the inability of the bile and digestive enzymes to enter into the duodenum. Patients are unable to digest fats, leading to malabsorption of nutrients and weight loss. Lack of bile produces clay-colored stools. Cancer of the body or tail generally presents as diffuse, vague epigastric pain radiating to the back and diarrhea due to the malabsorption. It has a poor prognosis.

Cholelithiasis

Biliary calculi, also known as *gallstones*, are very common in both sexes and all races with their incidence increasing with age. They occur in about 20% of the population and are found in about one third of those with sickle cell anemia because of the repeated episodes of hemolysis. Women and the obese both have a greater incidence, as each excretes more cholesterol in their bile than do males and people of normal weight. Women with a history of multiple pregnancies are more likely to have stones because of the excessive amounts of estrogen produced by the placenta. Those on oral contraceptives are also prone because the synthetic estrogen saturates the gallbladder, increasing cholesterol production in the bile.

Gallstones are classified according to their chemical composition. In the United States and Europe, most are cholesterol stones. Eighty percent to 90% of the solids in bile consist of conjugated bile salts, lecithin, and cholesterol. Both cholesterol and lecithin are insoluble in water, but the presence of bile salts with lecithin enables the cholesterol to become soluble. When this process fails cholesterol microcrystals form and eventually become gallstones. The stones do not in and of themselves cause symptoms, and the condition can be entirely asymptomatic and detected only on radiograph or incidental to surgery or autopsy. It is when they move into the cystic duct or common bile duct and become impacted that they cause symptoms. They cause the smooth muscle of the duct to contract in an attempt to forcefully dislodge the stone. This produces a characteristic severe right upper quadrant (RUQ) abdominal pain called *biliary colic*. The gallbladder can contain one or many stones with each being large or small. If a stone blocks the common bile duct, bile can no longer be excreted into the duodenum and accumulates in the blood, causing obstructive jaundice.

Cholecystitis

This is an inflammation of the gallbladder and is usually caused by an obstruction, either gallstone or tumor, which makes it impossible for bile to leave the gallbladder. The bile becomes increasingly concentrated, irritating the lining and causing inflammation. The gallbladder becomes edematous and pain is felt in the RUQ radiating to the shoulder and/or through to the back. The client develops symptoms of infection with fever, chills, nausea, and vomiting. Treatment includes having the patient take nothing by mouth (NPO) to stop the release of bile and using intravenous (IV) fluids to maintain hydration, analgesics for pain, and antibiotics for the infection. Treatment is surgical intervention to remove the obstruction. While this can be accomplished during the acute attack, it is generally preferable to wait until the inflammation subsides before intervening surgically.

Complications of acute cholecystitis occur depending on where the obstruction occurs. Tissues die and gangrene develops without blood flow. An inflamed gallbladder can rupture, causing peritonitis. Bile can accu-

Types of Gallstones

Cholesterol

- Can be small or large, single or multiple, with small ones likely to enter the biliary tree, causing obstruction, pain (biliary colic), and jaundice
- More common in women >20 and men <60
- Strong association with female hormones (i.e., increased incidence with female gender, pregnancy, use of oral contraceptives)
- Increased incidence with obesity, those on crash diets, and those with hyperlipidemia syndromes

Bilirubin (Pigmented)

- Usually multiple, small, black stones that pass through the cystic duct into the common bile duct
- More common in Asians and those with chronic illnesses such as hemolytic syndromes, cystic fibrosis, and Crohn's disease

Mixed

- The most common type; usually found in large numbers
- Layers of stones form with a bilirubin nucleus surrounded by cholesterol and calcium deposits, which add on one at a time so that the size of the stone reveals something about its age

Gallstones. Note those in the gallbladder itself, the common bile duct, and at the ampule of Vater.

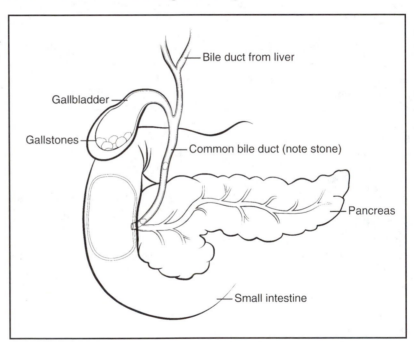

mulate in the liver ducts, damaging liver cells and producing biliary cirrhosis.

Individuals with chronic cholecystitis have nausea and indigestion after eating fatty foods. Fat in the duodenum stimulates the gallbladder to contract and release the bile, which produces the pain described previously. Treatment is dietary to control symptoms, but surgical intervention is needed for permanent relief. Once the gallbladder is removed bile flows directly from the liver into the duodenum with the flow increasing when fatty foods are digested.

PART VIII QUESTIONS

1. Where are nutrients primarily absorbed?

(A) Stomach

(B) Small intestine

(C) Large intestine

(D) They are absorbed in each of these sites.

2. Gastric secretions include all of the following except:

(A) Bicarbonate

(B) Pepsin

(C) Hydrochloric acid

(D) Mucous

3. What is the most common cause of chronic gastritis?

(A) Excessive alcohol intake

(B) Stress response

(C) *H. pylori*

(D) Pernicious anemia

4. Treatment for acute gastritis associated with stress response includes which of the following?

(A) Antacids

(B) Sucralfate

(C) Beta blockers

(D) Foods containing lactose

5. What is the most significant factor in the development of gastric ulcers?

(A) NSAIDs

(B) *H. pylori*

(C) Excess gastric acid

(D) Spicy foods

6. Factors that protect the gastric mucosa include all of the following except:

(A) Mucous

(B) Prostaglandins

(C) Pepsin

(D) Bicarbonate

7. How does *H. pylori*, a bacteria, cause ulcers?

(A) It increases production of gastric acid.

(B) It causes an inflammatory response that destroys tissue.

(C) It directly erodes sites in the mucosal wall.

(D) All of the above

8. What is the underlying pathology experienced by people with irritable bowel syndrome?

(A) Changes in mucous cell structure

(B) Excessive gastric secretions

(C) Hypersensitive responses to ordinary stimuli

(D) Impaired colonic reflexes

9. Which of the following statements about the relationship of IBS and psychiatric disorders is correct?

(A) People with IBS have poor coping skills.

(B) Women who have been sexually or physically abused may also have IBS.

(C) Anxiety and depression cause IBS.

(D) People with IBS often have psychiatric histories.

10. Jane S., 24, comes to the emergency room complaining of abdominal pain and bloody stools since yesterday afternoon. This has never happened to her before and she is very alarmed. While talking with her, she remembers that her aunt and grandmother both had similar complaints at times. She says neither of them ever ate fresh fruit for that reason. She has no fever but complains that she constantly feels as if she is going to have a bowel movement regardless of how often she goes. What do you suspect she has?

(A) Ulcerative colitis

(B) Irritable bowel disease

(C) Crohn's disease

(D) Infectious diarrhea

11. Pharmacological management of Crohn's disease may include the use of which of the following?

(A) Steroids

(B) Antibiotics

(C) Antidiarrheals

(D) All of the above

12. What is thought to cause diverticulitis?

(A) Genetics

(B) Infection

(C) Environmental factors

(D) Diet

13. Which of the following is a complication of diverticulitis?

(A) Abscess formation

(B) Peritonitis

(C) Local inflammation

(D) All of the above

14. An intestinal obstruction usually results in which of the following?

(A) Massive fluid and electrolyte imbalances

(B) Life-threatening peritonitis

(C) Bowel infarction

(D) All of the above

15. Which of the following is not associated with a bacterial gastroenteritis?

(A) Others who have shared the same food and water source are ill with similar symptoms.

(B) The source of contamination is unwashed surfaces or undercooked food.

(C) Individuals become ill within 12 hours of ingesting the contaminated product.

(D) It is highly contagious and spreads rapidly among children and the elderly.

16. Diarrhea is always accompanied by an increase in the water content of the stools. All of the following are responsible for this except:

(A) Increased fluid ingestion

(B) Increased fluid secretion

(C) Decreased fluid absorption

(D) Alteration in bowel motility

17. Adenocarcinoma of the esophagus is associated with which of the following?

(A) Gastritis

(B) Iron excess

(C) Alcoholism

(D) Barrett's esophagus

18. From what do colorectal cancers most often arise?

(A) Ulcerated tissue

(B) Adenomas

(C) Lipomas

(D) Diverticula

19. The liver receives blood from two sources, each with a different pressure gradient. This becomes important when the liver is not functioning properly. Which of the following is correct?

(A) Hepatic artery under high pressure; portal vein under low pressure

(B) Hepatic artery under moderately high pressure; portal vein under low pressure

(C) Mesenteric artery under high pressure; mesenteric vein under low pressure

(D) Mesenteric artery under moderately high pressure; mesenteric vein under low pressure

20. What do ALT and AST measure?

(A) Pancreatic damage

(B) Hepatic damage

(C) Hepatitis antibodies

(D) Gallstones

21. Jeanette tells you that several friends with whom she shared a beach house for 2 weeks a month ago have recently been diagnosed with hepatitis. She says she has been vaccinated against hepatitis and was not sexually active with anyone in this group. She asks if she is likely to get hepatitis too. How do you respond?

(A) No, the vaccination will protect you.

(B) No, not if you did not have unprotected sex.

(C) Possibly, the source may be from shellfish or poor handwashing.

(D) Possibly, but it has been a month and if you have not contracted it already, it's unlikely that you will.

22. Anitha and Vivic are a married couple. Both have hepatitis B and are now carriers of the disease. Which of the following statements about hepatitis B is true?

(A) Carriers cannot infect others if they are not having symptoms themselves.

(B) They probably infected each other.

(C) Their children will not be affected by their illness.

(D) They are both at risk for developing cirrhosis and carcinoma of the liver.

23. Cirrhosis may be caused by which of the following?

(A) Alcohol

(B) Hepatitis

(C) Obstruction

(D) All of the above

24. Esophageal varicosities are a result of which of the following?

(A) Ascites

(B) Portal hypertension

(C) Hepatic encephalopathy

(D) Metabolic dysfunction

25. Elevated levels of which substance produce hepatic encephalopathy?

(A) Nitrates

(B) Glucose

(C) Ammonia

(D) Albumin

26. Pancreatitis is commonly associated with which chronic disease?

(A) Multiple sclerosis

(B) Alcoholism

(C) Rheumatoid arthritis

(D) Diabetes

27. How are fatty foods digested following surgical resection for cholecystitis?

(A) By bile flowing directly from the liver into the duodenum

(B) By bile stored in the pancreatic ducts into the duodenum

(C) Fatty foods must be avoided to remain comfortable

(D) By dietary supplements or bile enzymes taken by mouth to digest fatty foods

1. The correct answer is B.

Most nutrients are absorbed in the small intestine. The stomach helps prepare food for digestion by the action of its enzymes. The food then passes into the small intestine where it undergoes further digestion and is absorbed by the microvilli. Water and electrolytes are absorbed by the large intestine.

2. The correct answer is A.

The stomach is very acidic as it works to initiate digestion of proteins, fats, and carbohydrates. Bicarbonate neutralizes acid and would work against this process if it were in the stomach.

3. The correct answer is C.

This pathogen is responsible for most chronic gastritis, PUD, and ultimately stomach cancers. It infects almost half of the population but is asymptomatic in most individuals and does not manifest itself until about age 60 in those who do develop symptoms.

4. The correct answer is B.

This is a complex salt of sucrose sulfate and aluminum hydroxide. In the acid environment of the stomach it becomes a gel-like substance that binds to both defective and normal mucosa and acts as a physical barrier to acid, pepsin, and bile acids. It also increases prostaglandin and mucous production. It has few side effects and is well tolerated.

5. The correct answer is A.

Gastric ulcers are more common in people >55 and most common in the group >75; these individuals frequently take large amounts of NSAIDs to control arthritis pain, making it the primary cause of ulcers. *H. pylori* is associated with PUD and in 90% of cases affects the duodenum. An imbalance of protective and aggressive factors, not excess stomach acid, is associated with the development of gastric ulcers. Spicy foods do not cause ulcers.

6. The correct answer is C.

Pepsin is an enzyme that causes mucosal injury in the intestine; all of the other choices protect the mucosa.

7. The correct answer is B.

The exact mechanism is not known, but it is thought that *H. pylori* releases toxins that produce an inflammatory response. This in turn damages tissues, allowing ulcer formation to occur.

8. The correct answer is C.

The etiology of IBS is not known, but studies have consistently shown that those with the syndrome respond to low levels of stimuli. The response produces increased motility, spasms, bloating, and discomfort.

9. The correct answer is B.

There is no causal relationship between psychiatric disorders and IBS. However, the CNS when stimulated by fear, sadness, anger, etc., will produce a variety of GI symptoms such as nausea, vomiting, diarrhea, and pain. People who experience panic attacks, have high anxiety, or are sad or fearful will have their CNSs overstimulated for long periods of time and, as a result, are likely to have such symptoms. If they have a hypersensitive gut, they can have a recurrent and prolonged response and IBS symptoms. Women who have been assaulted have been found to have a higher incidence of IBS than does the general population. This is probably due to the long term psychological trauma caused by such assaults. This places continued stress on the CNS and all other body systems.

10. The correct answer is A.

Ulcerative colitis is characterized by abrupt onset and bloody diarrhea plus abdominal pain. There is a familial tendency to develop the disease. *Tenesmus* is the term for discomfort caused by inflammation of the rectum, producing a feeling of incomplete emptying of the bowel. Some people with UC find that eating fresh fruits and vegetables exacerbates the symptoms.

11. The correct answer is D.

Management of Crohn's disease includes all of those listed plus antispasmodics, immunosuppressive, and bulk agents depending upon the type and severity of symptoms.

12. The correct answer is D.

The exact cause in unknown, but it is believed that diverticula develop in individuals with chronic constipation due to a lack of dietary fiber; hard stools require extra effort and higher intraluminal pressures for passage. This encourages a weak abdominal wall to pouch out, forming a diverticula.

13. The correct answer is D.

Any of these complications can happen depending on the size of the infection and whether or not it ruptures as a result of the inflammatory process.

14. The correct answer is A.

Failure to move abdominal contents along results in vomiting and the inability of fluids to reach the colon where fluid absorption occurs. Some fluids are lost through vomiting and more from inability of the body to absorb it.

15. The correct answer is D.

Bacterial AGE is not contagious as it is an ingested toxin and only those consuming contaminated food or water will become ill.

16. The correct answer is A.

The other choices are real factors in the increased water content of diarrheal stools. Patients with diarrhea may ingest fluid, but this does not cause the problem. Eating/drinking often triggers additional bowel movements.

17. The correct answer is D.

The rapid rise in esophageal cancer is due to Barrett's esophagus, which is a complication of chronic gastric esophagitis. The other choices are not associated with the development of adenocarcinoma of the esophagus.

18. The correct answer is B.

Adenoma polyps are considered to be the precursors of colorectal cancer. The association between the two is very strong so that screening exams routinely excise any colon polyps as they will progress to a cancerous state within 10 years if left in place. The other choices are not generally associated with the development of colorectal cancers although inflammatory bowel disease, particularly ulcerative colitis, is.

19. The correct answer is A.

The liver is supplied with one third of its blood from the hepatic artery delivered under high pressure and two thirds from the portal vein delivered under low pressure. The mesenteric artery and vein are concerned with the blood supply for the intestines, not the liver.

20. The correct answer is B.

These enzymes are contained in many types of tissue, including hepatic cells. They are released into the blood when hepatic tissue is injured.

21. The correct answer is C.

Hepatitis B is the only one of the viral hepatoviruses that has a vaccine to protect people from contracting it. Hepatitis D needs hepatitis B to exist and if she can not get hepatitis B, she will not get hepatitis D. Hepatitis A is transmitted by a fecal-oral route either from poor hand-washing or from contaminated foods, often shellfish. The average incubation period for getting hepatitis A is 30 days and for hepatitis C and E is longer. It is possible that this virus is responsible for her friends illnesses and she may come down with it too. Symptoms may be so mild that she may not realize she is sick at all, just tired. She should go to her health care provider and be tested.

22. The correct answer is B.

Hepatitis B is passed by sexual contact and contact with body fluid, especially blood, from infected people. It is frequently passed at birth from mother to child and that route produces most hepatitis B carriers. Both could have been infected as infants. Even though they are not experiencing symptoms they can infect others and there is a great risk they will infect children born to them.

23. The correct answer is D.

Each of these conditions can produce cirrhosis although by different mechanisms. Each results in the death of hepatocytes and changed liver architecture with the end result being severely impaired liver function.

24. The correct answer is B.

Esophageal varicosities are produced when the pressure increases within the GI system. Collateral circulation develops to deal with blood flow. Esophageal varices are one type of collateral vessel.

25. The correct answer is C.

Ammonia develops from the breakdown of urea and protein in the gut and the liver's inability to excrete them.

26. The correct answer is B.

Alcohol forms plugs in the pancreatic ducts, causing edema, spasm, and the release of other enzymes. There is no association between pancreatitis and multiple sclerosis or rheumatoid arthritis. Diabetes does not cause pancreatitis, but repeated bouts of chronic pancreatitis can exacerbate diabetes.

27. The correct answer is A.

Bile continues to be produced in the liver and flows directly into the duodenum in the presence of fats. Bile is not stored in the pancreatic ducts. Patients can eat fats in moderation. Neither dietary supplements nor bile enzymes are needed.

PART IX
Renal System
Bernadette R. Madara, EdD, APRN-CS

57 Anatomy and Physiology of the Renal System

Renal Function Tests

Test	Related Physiology
BUN (blood urea nitrogen)	The end product of protein metabolism is urea, which is excreted entirely by the kidneys; therefore, the BUN is an indication of liver and kidney function
Serum creatinine	When creatinine phosphate is used in skeletal muscle contractions creatinine is formed, which is entirely excreted by the kidneys; therefore, the serum creatinine level is an indication of renal function. The creatinine level is not affected by hepatic function so it is a more precise indication of renal function than is the BUN. A 50% reduction in glomerular filtration rate (GRF) doubles the creatinine level
24-hour urine collection for creatinine clearance	Measures GFR and is dependent upon renal artery perfusion and glomerular filtration (GF)
Urinalysis	Cloudy, foul smelling, white blood cells (WBCs) ➡ urinary tract infection (UTI) Dark yellow ➡ dehydration Acetone odor ➡ diabetic ketoacidosis Presence of protein ➡ injured glomerular membrane Glucose ➡ diabetes mellitus Ketones ➡ fatty acid metabolism Crystals ➡ renal stone formation possible Many hyaline casts ➡ proteinuria Cellular casts ➡ nephrotic syndrome
Intravenous pyelogram (IVP)	IV-administered, radiopaque dye allows the visualization of the kidneys, renal pelvis, ureters, and bladder
PSA (prostatic specific antigen)	PSA is a glycoprotein found in all prostatic epithelial cells. An increase may be indicative of prostatic enlargement, thus this test is used to screen for prostatic cancer and as an indicator of treatment success/failure

The regulation of fluid volume, blood pressure, and excretion of metabolic waste products and drug metabolites are the primary functions of the renal system. The kidneys are also responsible for conversion of vitamin D to its active form, serum pH regulation, and synthesis of hormones, such as atrial natriuretic peptide (APN), erythropoietin, and renin.

ANP, a hormone discovered in 1981, is released from muscle cells in the atria when the atrial walls are stretched. This hormone causes the vasodilation of afferent arterioles that lead into the glomerulus and efferent arterioles that lead out of the glomerulus, resulting in an increased glomerular filtration rate (GFR). ANP also inhibits aldosterone secretion and sodium reabsorption from the collecting tubules. All of these actions result in increased urine production and reduced blood volume.

The hormone erythropoietin stimulates the bone marrow to produce red blood cells (RBCs) in response to hypoxia from conditions such as anemia or from cardiac and/or pulmonary disease. If iron stores are adequate, an increase in RBCs results in added oxygen carrying capacity and reduced tissue hypoxia. As renal insufficiency progresses to renal failure, the kidneys' ability to produce erythropoietin declines, causing one form of anemia.

Blood pressure and blood volume are partially under the control of the renin-angiotensin-aldosterone regulatory cascade. A drop in renal blood flow stimulates the kidneys to release renin, which in turn converts angiotensinogen to angiotensin I. Angiotensin I enters the blood stream and circulates through lung tissue where the angiotensin-converting enzyme converts angiotensin I to angiotensin II, a powerful vasoconstrictor. Angiotensin II also causes the kidneys to reduce sodium and water excretion and stimulates aldosterone release, which increases sodium retention. These actions increase blood pressure, blood volume, and renal blood flow.

Vitamin D, in an inactive form, is either produced by the action of ultraviolet rays on cholesterol in the skin or ingested. The inactive form of vitamin D is converted to the active form by the kidneys. Active vitamin D, necessary for calcium and phosphate absorption from the small intestine, helps maintain strong bone formation. People with renal disease cannot convert vitamin D to its active form.

The kidneys either conserve bicarbonate, a base, or eliminate hydrogen ions, an acid, from the blood to help maintain serum pH. Buffers in the urine, which combine with hydrogen ions so that they can be eliminated, include bicarbonate, phosphate, and ammonia.

Renal Perfusion

The renal blood flow rate averages 20% to 25% of cardiac output or about 1,000 ml to 1,300 ml each minute, 600 to 700 cc of which is plasma, the remainder being composed of cells. Adequate blood flow to the kidneys is required to produce a sufficient GFR and urine production. When the sympathetic nervous system is stimulated, such as occurs in a stress response, both the afferent and efferent renal arterioles constrict, producing a decrease in renal blood flow. Constriction of the afferent arteriole alone produces a reduction in renal blood flow, glomerular filtration pressure, and GFR, while constriction of the efferent arteriole produces an increased resistance to glomerular outflow and increases the glomerular pressure and filtration rate.

Glomerular Filtration

The GFR is approximately 125 ml per minute. The fluid that is not returned to the circulation becomes a component of urine. Daily urine production is approximately 1.5 L. Nephrons are the functional units of the kidneys, and each kidney has approximately 1.2 million nephrons. In each tubular-shaped nephron is a plasma filtering capillary tuft created by the efferent and afferent arterioles called a *glomerulus*, which deposits its filtrate into a thin double-walled capsule called *Bowman's capsule*. From Bowman's capsule the filtrate travels through the proximal convoluted tubule, the loop of Henle, the distal convoluted tubule, and finally the collecting tubule. The collecting tubules empty into the renal pelvis, which is drained by the ureters. The ureters then empty into the bladder.

The role of the glomerulus is to filter plasma, and this filtering capability is controlled by capillary pressure, colloidal osmotic pressure, and capillary permeability. Approximately 125 ml of filtrate is processed each minute, although this GFR can vary from a few ml to a high of 200 ml per minute. The proximal convoluted tubules are responsible for approximately 65% of the reabsorption and secretion functions of the tubular system. In the proximal tubules reabsorption of essential substances such as Na, Cl, HCO_3, phosphate, glucose, amino acids, and water and the secretion of H+ ions and waste products including drug metabolites takes place. The loop of Henle is primarily concerned with reabsorbing water, some Na and Cl, and calcium. The distal convoluted tubule reabsorbs Na, K, Cl, bicarbonate, urea, and water, while secreting H+ ions and K. The collecting duct either reabsorbs or secretes Na, K, H+ ions, and ammonia depending upon the body's requirements.

An increased protein load or glucose load in the blood results in an increase in renal blood flow and GFR. This increased GFR allows urea, a waste product of protein metabolism, to be excreted in a timely manner. In persons with uncontrolled diabetes mellitus, the increase in GFR results in polyuria and polydipsia.

Urinary Tract Infection

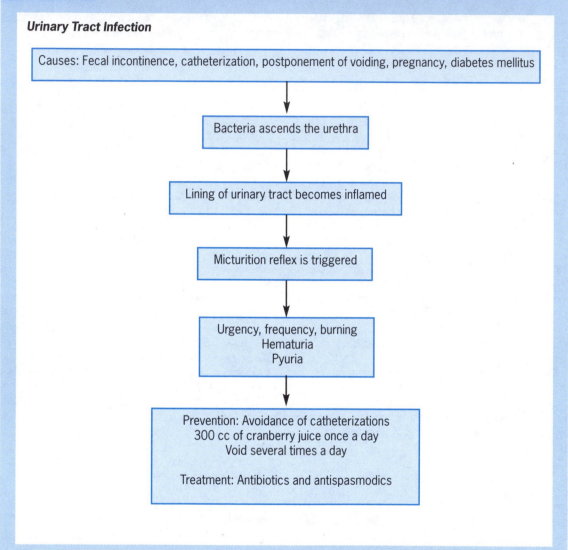

Causes: Fecal incontinence, catheterization, postponement of voiding, pregnancy, diabetes mellitus

↓

Bacteria ascends the urethra

↓

Lining of urinary tract becomes inflamed

↓

Micturition reflex is triggered

↓

Urgency, frequency, burning
Hematuria
Pyuria

↓

Prevention: Avoidance of catheterizations
300 cc of cranberry juice once a day
Void several times a day

Treatment: Antibiotics and antispasmodics

Introduction

This chapter discusses infections that affect the renal system either directly (i.e., urinary tract infection [UTI]) or indirectly (i.e., hemolytic uremic syndrome [HUS]). Pyelonephritis is classified as a tubulointerstitial disorder and is discussed in Chapter 63.

Urinary Tract Infections

Overview

UTIs are classified as lower or upper tract infections. Upper UTIs involve the ureters and kidneys, while lower UTIs involve the urethra and bladder. Lower UTIs are the second most common bacterial infections seen by doctors. It is estimated that 7 million people per year in the United States develop a UTI.

Generally, UTIs are caused by gram-negative bacteria common to the intestine (most commonly *Escherichia coli*) and are classified by the primary site affected. Urethritis involves inflammation of the urethra, while cystitis indicates inflammation of the bladder. It has been estimated than 43% of women, 12% of men, 15% to 25% of the elderly living in a nursing home, and 5% to 20% of the elderly living at home will have a UTI sometime during their lifetime. Despite a long urethra, the incidence of UTI in men increases greatly with age as prostatic hypertrophy increases urinary retention and lessened bacteriostatic prostatic secretions lower the body's defense mechanisms against infection.

Pathophysiology

Normally, a UTI is prevented by acidic urine, complete bladder emptying, a competent ureterovesical junction to prevent urine backflow, and bacteriostatic properties of the urethra and bladder. Ordinarily, the urinary tract above the urethra is sterile; therefore, if bacteria ascends the urethra and colonizes in the bladder, an inflammatory process is initiated. The process of voiding routinely cleanses the bladder and urethra. Thus, anything that interferes with this process, such as outflow obstruction, postponement of voiding, pregnancy, or diabetes mellitus, increases the risk of a UTI. Use of a spermicide or diaphragms, fecal incontinence, and catheterization have also been implicated as UTI risk factors. Approximately 1% of adults who have a straight catheterization and almost 100% of patients who have an indwelling catheter will develop a UTI within 3 to 4 days of catheter placement.

Bacteria are introduced into the bladder during the catheterization procedure. The process of catheterization also causes irritation and minute scraping of the urethra, creating a portal for bacterial entry. Additionally, an indwelling catheter prevents normal flushing of the urethra by urine, and bacteria may travel to the bladder through the catheter itself or via the exudate that collects between the outside of the catheter and the urethral walls. As bacteria adhere to the catheter, they produce a protective film that covers the surface of the catheter and protects the bacteria against antibiotic action, making eradication of the infection difficult.

A UTI during pregnancy occurs for several reasons. During pregnancy the renal calices, pelves, and ureters dilate while peristaltic activity of the ureters decreases. These changes are thought to occur because of the muscle-relaxing effects of progesterone-like hormones. The enlarging uterus also causes ureteral and bladder displacement.

Signs and symptoms of a UTI commonly include lower abdominal pain, urgency, frequency, burning on urination, microscopic hematuria, offensive urine odor, and cloudy urine (i.e., pyuria). Frequency, urgency, and burning upon voiding occur because the inflamed lining of the urinary tract creates irritation, which triggers the micturition reflex.

Cystitis in the elderly may be manifested as confusion, malaise, incontinence, nocturia, lethargy, and anorexia instead of the classic signs of a UTI. Diagnostic tests that confirm a UTI include urinalysis and urine culture for bacteriuria. Over 100,000 bacterial organisms per 1 cc of blood is the benchmark for a UTI. White blood cells in the urine also signal an infection.

Management

Reduction of controllable risk factors is the primary way to prevent UTIs. Antibiotics, forcing fluids, and urinary antispasmodics are frequently employed as treatments. Cranberry juice or blueberry juice has been used as a home remedy for UTIs for many years. The benefit of drinking cranberry juice lies in its ability to acidify urine, which decreases the bacteria's ability to adhere to bladder walls. Drinking 300 cc of cranberry juice daily has been shown to lessen the risk of incurring a UTI. Increasing fluid intake prior to sexual activity can also lessen a UTI in a woman because voiding after intercourse removes bacteria from the bladder outlet. Screening for bacteriuria during the first prenatal visit will allow for timely treatment of a UTI related to pregnancy. An untreated UTI may progress to pyelonephritis.

Hemolytic Uremic Syndrome

HUS, which causes endothelial damage and coagulopathy of the kidneys, gastrointestinal (GI) system, and central nervous system (CNS), is the most common cause of acute renal failure (ARF) in children younger than 5 years. Nonepidemic HUS is associated with pregnancy or nephrotoxic drugs or it may be inherited, although the exact cause is often unclear. In contrast to noninfectious HUS, the epidemic form of HUS has an infectious etiology and is transmitted through food and person-to-person contact. Although *Salmonella typhimurium*, *Shigella dysenteriae*, and *Campylobacter* are associated with HUS, the most common causative organism related to HUS outbreaks is *E. coli*, which is usually transmitted via contaminated ground beef or unpasteurized milk or cheese.

The toxin produced by the offending bacteria binds to cells on the renal, GI, and central nervous systems. Once the toxin gains access to the inside of the cells it prevents protein synthesis, leading to cellular death. Lipopolysaccharides produced by *E. coli* also activate the coagulation cascade, using up available platelets and putting down a fibrin network in the kidneys. As red blood cells (RBCs) pass through this fibrin network, they are hemolyzed. Signs and symptoms of HUS include diarrhea, which may be bloody; hemolytic anemia; renal failure; seizures; and fluid overload.

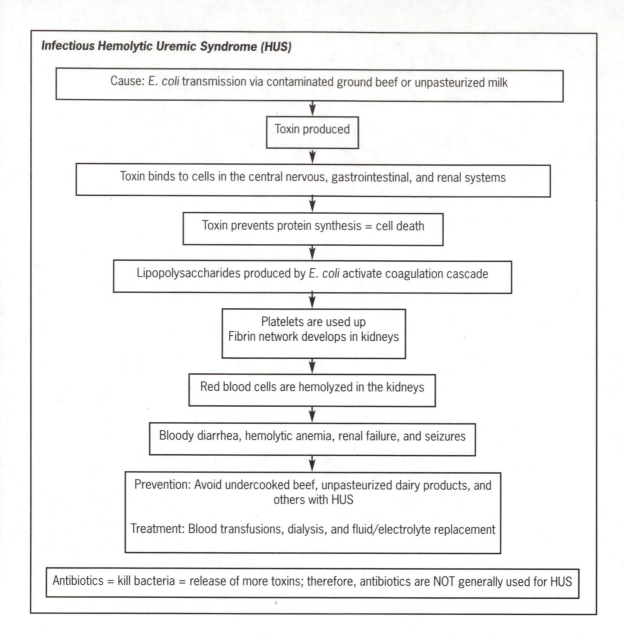

Infectious Hemolytic Uremic Syndrome (HUS)

Cause: *E. coli* transmission via contaminated ground beef or unpasteurized milk

↓

Toxin produced

↓

Toxin binds to cells in the central nervous, gastrointestinal, and renal systems

↓

Toxin prevents protein synthesis = cell death

↓

Lipopolysaccharides produced by *E. coli* activate coagulation cascade

↓

Platelets are used up
Fibrin network develops in kidneys

↓

Red blood cells are hemolyzed in the kidneys

↓

Bloody diarrhea, hemolytic anemia, renal failure, and seizures

↓

Prevention: Avoid undercooked beef, unpasteurized dairy products, and others with HUS

Treatment: Blood transfusions, dialysis, and fluid/electrolyte replacement

Antibiotics = kill bacteria = release of more toxins; therefore, antibiotics are NOT generally used for HUS

Management

Avoidance of undercooked beef, unpasteurized dairy products, and those with HUS is the primary mode of prevention. Treatment includes blood transfusions, fluid and electrolytes, and dialysis, if needed. Antibiotics that cause *E. coli* cell death result in an additional release of toxins and may, therefore, not be used.

Glomerulonephritis

59

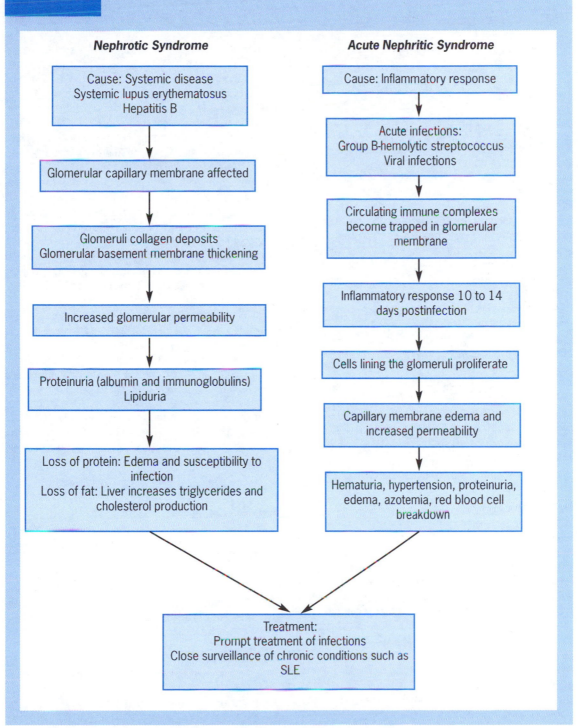

Nephrotic Syndrome

Cause: Systemic disease
Systemic lupus erythematosus
Hepatitis B

↓

Glomerular capillary membrane affected

↓

Glomeruli collagen deposits
Glomerular basement membrane thickening

↓

Increased glomerular permeability

↓

Proteinuria (albumin and immunoglobulins)
Lipiduria

↓

Loss of protein: Edema and susceptibility to
infection
Loss of fat: Liver increases triglycerides and
cholesterol production

Acute Nephritic Syndrome

Cause: Inflammatory response

↓

Acute infections:
Group B-hemolytic streptococcus
Viral infections

↓

Circulating immune complexes
become trapped in glomerular
membrane

↓

Inflammatory response 10 to 14
days postinfection

↓

Cells lining the glomeruli proliferate

↓

Capillary membrane edema and
increased permeability

↓

Hematuria, hypertension, proteinuria,
edema, azotemia, red blood cell
breakdown

Treatment:
Prompt treatment of infections
Close surveillance of chronic conditions such as
SLE

Overview

Glomerulonephritis, classified as either nephrotic syndrome or nephritic syndrome, affects males more often than females and is the leading cause of chronic renal failure in the United States. Inflammatory injury to the glomeruli (nephritic syndrome) can occur as a result of antibodies interacting with normally occurring antigens in the glomeruli or as a result of antibody-antigen complexes which become lodged in the glomerular membrane (nephrotic syndrome). Chronic glomerulonephritis (CG) is the end-stage of many types of glomerulonephritis but it can also develop without a history of prior renal disease. In CG the kidneys are small and the glomeruli are sclerosed, leading to renal failure.

Nephrotic Syndrome

Pathophysiology

Nephrotic syndrome is caused by systemic diseases such as systemic lupus erythematosus and hepatitis B, as a reaction to gold therapy, and idiopathically. This syndrome affects the glomerular capillary membrane, leading to increased glomerular permeability, secondary to collagen deposits in glomeruli and thickening of the glomerular basement membrane. Proteinuria, including loss of albumin and immunoglobulins, equal to or exceeding 3.5 grams per day, lipiduria (i.e., fat in the urine), low serum albumin, generalized edema due to low serum colloidal osmotic pressure, and hyperlipidemia are characteristics of nephrotic syndrome. Loss of immunoglobulins increases the chance of developing infections. As a compensatory reaction to proteinuria, the body increases albumin production and the liver increases triglycerides and cholesterol production. This puts a person with nephrotic syndrome at risk for atherosclerosis. Hypercoagulability with resultant venous clot formation, especially in the renal veins, is thought to occur because of the loss of clot inhibiting factors from the urine.

Nephritic Syndrome

Pathophysiology

Nephritic syndrome is caused by diseases such as infections that initiate an inflammatory response of the cells of the glomerulus. Signs and symptoms of nephritic syndrome include hematuria, urinary casts and leukocytes, low glomerular filtration rate (GFR), azotemia, oliguria (i.e., urine output less than 400 mL/day), and hypertension. Red blood cells spill into the urine as the glomerular capillary walls are damaged by the inflammatory process. A low GFR develops as a result of the change in hemodynamic pressure caused by the loss of red blood cells (RBCs). As the GFR drops, so does renal function, leading to azotemia, oliguria, and hypertension caused by water retention.

Acute glomerulonephritis (AG), a type of nephritic syndrome, may follow an infection caused by group B-hemolytic streptococci. Up to 8% of children who have a streptococcal infection, such as impetigo or pharyngitis, develop AG. Viral infectious agents, which cause chicken pox, mumps, and measles, may also cause AG. In AG generalized infections result in circulating immune complexes that become trapped in the glomerular membrane and cause an inflammatory response 10 to 14 days after the initial infection. As the cells lining the glomeruli proliferate in response to the inflammatory process, the capillary membrane swells and becomes permeable. Signs and symptoms of AG include hematuria, hypertension, proteinuria, edema, azotemia, and coffee-colored urine produced by RBC breakdown. Most children with AG recover completely, while 40% of adults with AG will have permanent impaired renal function and possibly renal failure.

The most common cause of primary nephritic syndrome in the United States is Buerger's disease, also called *IgA nephropathy*. In this type of AG, IgA and IgG immune complexes are deposited in the mesangial cells of the glomerulus. The mesangial cells are found between the capillary tufts and provide structural support for the glomerulus. IgA nephropathy may present as a single occurrence 50% of the time or may develop into a slowly progressing disease over several decades. Signs and symptoms of IgA nephropathy include hematuria lasting 2 to 6 days and mild proteinuria.

Rapidly progressive glomerular nephritis (RPGN) associated with systemic diseases such as systemic lupus erythematosus, vasculitis, and acute infections begins abruptly but rarely resolves spontaneously. In RPGN, glomerular cells proliferate, macrophages are activated, and crescent-shaped structures are formed that block Bowman's capsule in the nephron. Approximately 70% of the glomeruli are affected, leading to a rapid decline in renal function. About half of the people with RPGN will require dialysis and most of these people develop renal failure.

Diabetes-Related Nephrotic Syndrome

Pathophysiology

Approximately 30% of people with type I diabetes mellitus will develop diabetic nephropathy (DN), which mainly affects the glomerulus, eventually producing nonnephrotic proteinuria, nephrotic syndrome, and renal failure. In DN the glomerular capillary membrane thickens probably due to hypertension and hyperglycemia, mesangial cells proliferate and block the capillary lumen, thereby reducing the area for glomerular filtration.

DN occurs in five stages. Stage 1 is indicated by enlarged kidneys and increased intraglomerular pressure. Renal function begins to decline during stage 2. Hypertension develops and microalbuminuria is detected during stage 3. Stage 4 signals increased protein spilling in the urine and a further drop in renal function. Because the kidneys are failing, hypertension worsens. Dialysis and/or transplant is required in stage 5. Unfortunately, people with type II diabetes may already be in stage 3 by the time a diagnosis of diabetes is made.

Management

Tight control of serum glucose and use of angiotensin-converting enzyme inhibitors can reverse early glomerular changes in CN and prevent chronic renal failure. Prompt treatment of streptococcal infections with antibiotics can prevent acute glomerulonephritis.

Once glomerulonephritis has occurred pharmacological interventions are used to manage the symptoms. Systemic steroids are given to reduce inflammation, angiotensin enzyme inhibitors prevent protein loss and slow the progression of renal failure, broad spectrum antibiotics prevent a lingering infection, and antihypertensives maintain blood pressure at desired levels. Sodium is restricted until edema and hypertension resolve. Plasmapheresis has been used experimentally to remove serum immune complexes as a treatment for immune-mediated forms of glomerulonephritis.

60 Micturition and Incontinence

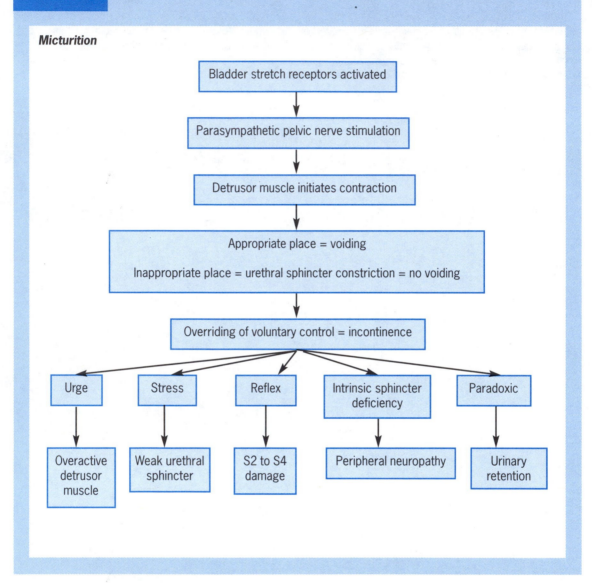

Micturition

Bladder stretch receptors activated

↓

Parasympathetic pelvic nerve stimulation

↓

Detrusor muscle initiates contraction

↓

Appropriate place = voiding

Inappropriate place = urethral sphincter constriction = no voiding

↓

Overriding of voluntary control = incontinence

Urge	Stress	Reflex	Intrinsic sphincter deficiency	Paradoxic
Overactive detrusor muscle	Weak urethral sphincter	S2 to S4 damage	Peripheral neuropathy	Urinary retention

Overview

Functional incontinence occurs in infants and young children when the bladder reaches a certain fullness. By the age of 2 or 3, a child learns to recognize the signals indicating the urge to void and bladder training can begin. Enuresis, or bed wetting, may last until late childhood. Children who sleep deeply may not notice the urge to void, and bedwetting occurs. Elders with cognitive impairment may have functional incontinence.

Pathophysiology

As the bladder fills to between 150 cc and 300 cc, stretch receptors in the bladder walls are activated, creating the sensation of the need to void. Parasympathetic pelvic nerves transmit this signal to the detrusor muscle, initiating bladder contractions. The higher the amount of urine in the bladder, the stronger the impulse to micturate. Sympathetic nerve innervation of the detrusor muscle and internal sphincter prevents premature parasympathetic stimulation and maintains the muscle tone of the internal sphincter. Higher-level motor impulses inhibit the voiding reflex by constricting the urethral sphincter and delaying voiding. Generally, ignoring the urge to void prevents release of the external sphincter, and neuron fatigue delays further stimulation of the voiding reflex arc for a few minutes to 1 hour. If the urge to void continues to be ignored, bladder reflex contractions eventually take over and cause involuntary voiding. Although micturition is generally under voluntary control, an overfilled or irritated bladder will result in incontinence or the involuntary passage of urine.

Incontinence

Overview

Approximately 13 million adults over the age of 60 have either transient or chronic urinary incontinence. Complications of urinary incontinence include skin breakdown, depression, caregiver and personal stress, social isolation, and economic hardship caused by the cost of incontinence-related supplies. It is estimated that 50% of institutionalized elderly and 11% to 55% of community-dwelling elderly experience urinary incontinence. As a person ages, bladder capacity, sphincter tone, sensation, and the ability to inhibit detrusor contractions decrease, causing the involuntary passage of urine while the person is awake or, in some instances, asleep.

Pathophysiology

Transient incontinence can be caused by medications such as beta blockers, alcohol, caffeine, and diuretics or by a urinary tract infection, which causes bladder and urethral irritation. Delirium and restricted mobility can also cause transient incontinence. Chronic incontinence occurs when the bladder loses its ability to store urine or empty urine effectively.

Urge incontinence, which is also called *instability incontinence* or *detrusor hyperreflexia*, is a type of chronic incontinence that is caused by inappropriate, repetitive, strong contraction of the detrusor muscle which eventually overcomes urethral sphincter control. This type of incontinence has numerous etiologies such as central nervous system disease or damage from a brain attack (e.g., cerebrovascular accident [CVA]), dementia, Parkinson's disease, and frontal lobe or cerebellum brain tumors. In urge incontinence the detrusor muscle becomes overactive, the bladder contracts when the urge to void is felt, and the ability to postpone voiding is lost. A feeling of urgency precedes the passage of large amounts of urine, thus the name *urge incontinence*.

Reflex incontinence is caused by trauma or damage to the nervous system as seen in spinal cord injury above S2 to S4, multiple sclerosis, and diabetes mellitus. Detrusor hyperreflexia occurs even though there is no sensation of the need to void. These conditions do not result in a feeling of urgency prior to the incontinence.

Urinary retention causes overflow incontinence (i.e., paradoxic incontinence) and involves a deficient detrusor muscle or bladder outlet obstruction. In this type of incontinence the bladder does not empty completely because of detrusor muscle malfunction as occurs with polio and multiple sclerosis or from blockage of the bladder outlet from conditions such as prostatic enlargement and urethral stricture. Pelvic surgery and diabetes mellitus may result in overflow incontinence because of damage to the parasympathetic innervation of the detrusor muscle. Chronic overdistention, also called *nurse's bladder* or *teacher's bladder*, occurs because of a perceived inability to interrupt work in order to void. This chronic avoidance to empty the bladder results in detrusor muscle areflexia and overflow incontinence. Symptoms associated with overflow incontinence may include urgency, frequency, nocturia, dribbling and an intermittent urinary stream, or a lack of urgency if nerve damage is present.

Stress incontinence involves a weak urethral sphincter in contrast to urge incontinence and overflow incontinence, which involve the detrusor muscle. A person with stress incontinence will experience leakage of small amounts of urine with any activity that increases intra-abdominal pressure, such as coughing, sneezing, or exercising. Pelvic floor relaxation, which results in the descent of pelvic organs and is associated with aging, vaginal childbirth, and obesity, has been implicated as a cause of stress incontinence. Pelvic floor relaxation causes the urethra to move out of its normal position. As a result, the urethral sphincter does not sense the sudden increase in intra-abdominal pressure, thus when bladder pressure exceeds urethral closure pressure, the urethral sphincter does not close and leaking of urine occurs.

Intrinsic sphincter deficiency (ISD) is another cause of stress incontinence. ISD occurs when there is damage to the neuromuscular components of the proximal urethra or pelvic floor muscles. Conditions such as peripheral neuropathy associated with diabetes mellitus and nerve damage resulting from radical prostatectomy or transurethral resection of the prostate may result in ISD.

Diagnostic studies that identify the cause of incontinence include voiding cystourethrogram, urodynamic testing, cystoscopy, and urine culture.

Management

Prevention of incontinence is sometimes possible. Tight control of diabetes mellitus, for example, may prevent incontinence associated with diabetic neuropathy, not routinely delaying voiding will prevent some cases of overflow incontinence, and treatment of a urinary tract infection will reverse incontinence associated with bladder wall and urethral irritation.

Other causes of incontinence cannot be avoided, but bladder retraining may be possible. Techniques used to correct incontinence include biofeedback to teach pelvic floor muscle exercises (e.g., Kegel exercises); timed voiding and habit training, which involves establishing a routine voiding schedule; and dietary modifications to reduce caffeine and alcohol, which act as diuretics.

Estrogen replacement in postmenopausal women may reduce stress incontinence. Anticholinergics and bladder smooth muscle relaxants, such as propantheline bromide and oxybutynin chloride, are used to reduce urge incontinence because they inhibit detrusor muscle contractions and increase bladder capacity.

Drugs such as Sudafed (Pfizer, New York, NY) cause smooth muscle contractions of the bladder neck and help reduce stress incontinence. Urecholine (Odyssey Pharmaceuticals, East Hanover, NJ), a cholinergic receptor stimulator, increases detrusor muscle tone and is used to treat urinary retention and overflow incontinence. Doxazosin mesylate and finasteride are used to treat urinary retention caused by prostatic hypertrophy. Desmopressin acetate nasal spray, a form of vasopressin, is used to treat enuresis because it reduces urine volume by promoting water reabsorption.

Overflow incontinence can be relieved with intermittent self-catheterization. Surgical treatment of incontinence includes repairing of pelvic floor muscles, removing of the prostate gland to correct outflow obstruction (although this may result in incontinence if nerves are damaged), or implanting an artificial urethral sphincter.

61 Renal Calculi and Benign Prostatic Hypertrophy

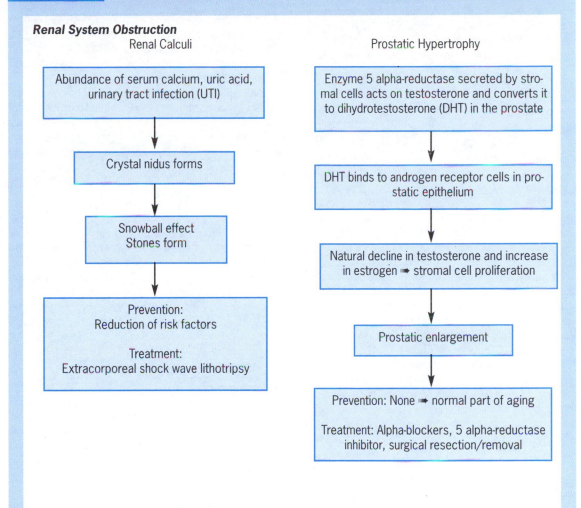

Renal System Obstruction

Renal Calculi

| Abundance of serum calcium, uric acid, urinary tract infection (UTI) |
↓
| Crystal nidus forms |
↓
| Snowball effect
Stones form |
↓
| Prevention:
Reduction of risk factors

Treatment:
Extracorporeal shock wave lithotripsy |

Prostatic Hypertrophy

| Enzyme 5 alpha-reductase secreted by stromal cells acts on testosterone and converts it to dihydrotestosterone (DHT) in the prostate |
↓
| DHT binds to androgen receptor cells in prostatic epithelium |
↓
| Natural decline in testosterone and increase in estrogen ➡ stromal cell proliferation |
↓
| Prostatic enlargement |
↓
| Prevention: None ➡ normal part of aging

Treatment: Alpha-blockers, 5 alpha-reductase inhibitor, surgical resection/removal |

Introduction

This chapter discusses two causes of renal system obstruction: renal calculi and prostatic hyperplasia.

Renal Calculi

Overview

The presence of renal calculi (i.e., masses of crystals), which can range in size from microscopic to several centimeters in diameter, is the most common cause of renal system obstruction. Calculi are more common in men than in women, are more likely in Caucasians than in African Americans, and develop most frequently between the ages of 20 and 40. The most common sites for stone formation are the renal pelvis, ureters, and bladder.

Approximately 10% to 15% of individuals will have renal calculi during their lifetime, with people living in the southern and midwestern United States at greatest risk for calculi development. Each year approximately 1 million people are hospitalized because of renal calculi and another 1 million are treated for this condition on an out patient basis.

Pathophysiology

Renal calculi form either because of metabolic abnormalities, an urinary tract infection (UTI), or an aberrant urine pH. Normally, we are protected from calculi development by calculi-inhibitors including citrate, magnesium, and pyrophosphate and endogenous compounds secreted by renal tubular cells, specifically nephrocalcin, uropontin, and Tamm-Horsfall protein.

When a nucleus (i.e., nidus) of crystals or organic material forms in the urinary tract and ions precipitate out of the urine and stick to the nucleus, a stone forms, much like a snowball that when rolled in the snow forms a larger and larger mass. Approximately 75% of renal calculi are calcium based, 10% are uric acid based, and 14% have a magnesium ammonium phosphate (i.e., struvite) base formed by urea-splitting bacteria associated with a UTI.

Radiopaque calcium stones form because of an abundance of calcium in the blood as the result of excessive bone reabsorption secondary to immobility, bone disease, or renal tubular acidosis. Uric acid stones develop in acidic urine secondary to conditions such as gout, thiazide diuretic use, or a high-purine diet. Unlike calcium stones they are not radiopaque, and thus do not show up on x-ray.

Struvite stones are composed of magnesium ammonium phosphate and form in alkaline urine when a UTI is present. Urease, an enzyme from the bacteria, splits urea into ammonia and carbon dioxide. As the ammonia takes up a hydrogen ion, an ammonium ion is formed, which creates alkaline urine and results in an increase in urine phosphate levels. Phosphate, magnesium, and the ammonium ions then combine to form a stone, usually in the renal pelvis, and are often called *staghorn stones* because of their shape.

Small stones may not cause any signs and symptoms; however, large stones can block the renal pelvis or ureters. Ureteral spasms (i.e., colic), which are intensely painful, occur when the body tries to move stones out of the ureters or urethra. Renal calculi in the renal pelvis may be asymptomatic or can cause hydronephrosis when the stone prevents the downward flow of urine into the bladder. Other signs and symptoms of renal calculi include hematuria as the result of trauma caused by sharp-edged stones, decreased urine output, and sediment or actual stones in the urine.

Management

General risk factors leading to calculi development are stasis of urine, high serum calcium or uric acid levels, vegetarian diet (changes urinary pH), high protein diet, UTI, abnormal urinary pH, deficiency of crystal-inhibiting factors, and low urine output. A urinary pH below 5.5 is a risk factor for uric acid stone formation, while a urinary pH above 7.5 is a risk factor for struvite stone formation. Dietary changes may be utilized to prevent the concentration of stone-forming crystals in the urine. A person with stones composed of calcium oxalate, for example, will be encouraged to limit the intake of high oxalate foods such as spinach and chocolate. Regardless of the chemical composition of the calculi, the most effective way to prevent stone formation is to increase fluid intake to 2.5 to 3.5 liters spaced throughout the day.

Small stones (under 5 mm) usually pass spontaneously, while larger stones may require extracorporeal shock wave lithotripsy during which high frequency sound waves are directed at the stone in order to pulverize it. Occasionally, lithotomy (i.e., surgical removal) may be necessary.

Prostatic Hyperplasia

Overview

It is estimated that over 50% of men over the age of 50 and 80% of men over the age of 70 will develop benign prostatic hyperplasia (BPH), a nonmalignant enlargement of the prostate gland and a significant cause of UTI in men. This condition accounts for approximately 4 million office visits per year in the United States. Men living in Japan have the lowest incidence of BPH and this is thought to be due to a diet high in natural estrogen. The only risk factor thus far identified as relating to BPH is aging.

Pathophysiology

The exact cause of BPH is unknown, but two theories have emerged, both of which focus on the proliferation of prostatic stromal cells. One theory focuses on a hormonal cause associated with aging and the other on programmed cell death. As a man ages, the normal hormonal balance of androgens and estrogen changes as the testicular production of testosterone declines, leading to a relative increase of estrogen. In the prostate, circulating testosterone is converted to dihydrotestosterone (DHT) under the influence of an enzyme 5 alpha-reductase secreted by stromal cells. DHT then binds to androgen receptors in prostatic epithelium and promotes tissue growth. It is postulated that a naturally occurring decline in testosterone coupled with an increase in estrogen causes stromal cells proliferation which in turn causes prostatic tissue growth. Prior to middle age, the balance between prostatic growth-inhibiting factors and growth-promoting factors is fairly constant. An imbalance in the factors may occur with aging, accounting for hyperplasia of the prostate gland. Regardless of the etiology, as the prostate enlarges, it compresses the urethra, leading to outflow obstruction, stasis of urine, and UTI.

Typically, a man with BPH will complain of hesitancy, a weak urinary stream, frequency, dribbling, and a feeling of a full bladder. Because the bladder is constantly distended, overflow incontinence is common. Rectal exam reveals a large, palpable prostate with a rubbery surface. A uroflowmetry that records a urinary flow rate of less than 10 ml per second indicates outlet obstruction. Urinalysis will show white blood cells (WBCs) and microscopic WBCs if inflammation and infection are present. Prostate size correlates poorly with symptoms. Some men with a seemingly normal-sized prostate gland will have marked symptoms, while others with a very large prostate gland will be asymptomatic.

Management

Prevention of BPH is not possible, although the risk for developing BPH increases if the man's father also had BPH in his 50's. Treatment is aimed at relieving bladder outlet obstruction and preserving renal function. Medications that can relieve the symptoms of BPH include alpha-blockers, such as terazosin and prazosin, which relax smooth muscle cells of the prostate and bladder neck (enhancing bladder emptying) and finasteride, a 5 alpha-reductase inhibitor, which blocks the conversion of testosterone to DHT (reducing prostate size). Treatment with finasteride can reduce the size of a prostate gland by 20% to 50%.

Surgical treatment includes newer, less invasive procedures such as interstitial laser therapy, transurethral laser ablation, balloon dilatation, as well as standard transurethral resection.

62

Renal Failure

Renal Failure

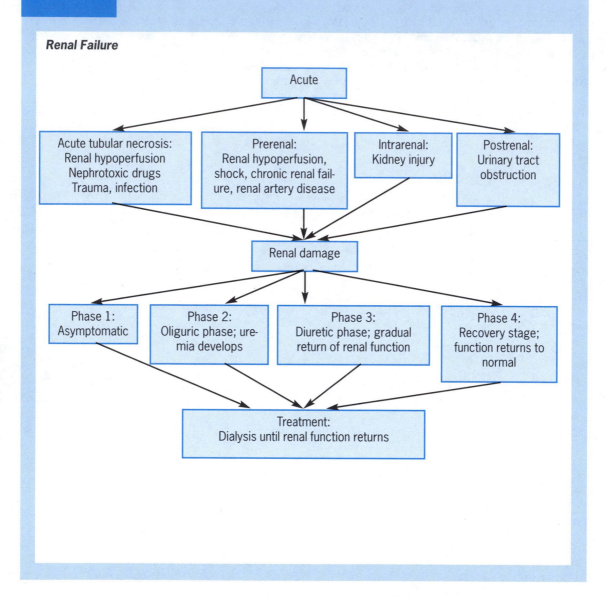

Overview

Renal failure is classified as acute or chronic. Acute renal failure (ARF) has a mortality rate of 10% to 60%, begins abruptly, and is generally reversible, whereas chronic renal failure (CRF) has an eventual mortality rate of 100% (without dialysis and/or renal transplantation), is irreversible, and results in a slow, steady decline of renal function.

Prevention of ARF depends in part on limiting one's exposure to nephrotoxic agents and prevention and prompt treatment of shock, especially in the elderly and people with renal insufficiency. CRF can be avoided with tight control of hypertension and diabetes; genetic counseling for persons with polycystic renal disease, which is an inheritable cause of renal failure; and prompt treatment of ARF.

Acute Renal Failure

Pathophysiology

Approximately 10,000 people develop ARF each year. It has been estimated that 5% of hospitalized clients and 30% of clients in critical care units develop this syndrome.

Acute tubular necrosis (ATN) is one cause of ARF. ATN occurs because of renal hypoperfusion or in response to nephrotoxic drugs such as aminoglycosides and chemicals such as radiologic dyes, which set up an inflammatory process leading to tubular edema, obstruction, and ischemia. Up to 12% of patients exposed to radiocontrast agents develop ATN. Other causes of ATN are major trauma; systemic infections; and muscle breakdown, which produces myoglobin, a substance that clogs renal tubules. Damaged tubules result in a decreased ability to maintain homeostasis. ATN usually resolves in about 8 weeks.

Prerenal factors (i.e., factors causing ARF that occur prior to blood being filtered by the kidneys) are caused by renal hypoperfusion and account for approximately 55% of ARF cases per year. Prerenal factors include shock, congestive heart failure, volume depletion from vomiting, or renal artery disease. In prerenal ARF, urine osmolality is high and urine sodium is low because, although renal perfusion is greatly decreased, renal tubular function is normal.

Intrarenal ARF results from injury to the kidney itself from emboli or ATN. Sodium cannot be conserved and urine cannot be concentrated because of glomerular damage. Postrenal or obstructive ARF results from urinary tract obstruction by renal calculi or prostatic enlargement, thus urine osmolarity and sodium levels are usually unaffected.

ARF has four phases. In the initial phase, the patient may be asymptomatic although renal damage is occurring. During the oliguric phase, which lasts a few days to a few weeks, impaired glomerular filtration causes solute and water reabsorption, urine output declines to 400 cc or less per day, and serum waste products cannot be removed. As the patient becomes symptomatic, a condition known as uremia (i.e., urine in the blood) develops. Neurotoxicity from uremia causes an altered mental status and altered peripheral sensation. Electrolyte imbalance causes dysrhythmias, water retention may lead to congestive heart failure and hypertension, and metabolic acidosis may develop because of the kidney's ability to excrete hydrogen ions. In addition to anemia caused by decreased erythropoietin production, blood loss may be caused by gastrointestinal (GI) bleeding secondary to platelet and protein anticoagulant dysfunction.

During the third phase, or the diuretic phase, which lasts days to weeks, there is a gradual return of renal function due to cellular regeneration and healing. Excessive urine output leading to dehydration and electrolyte imbalance may occur during this stage as a result of incompetent tubular transport of water and solutes. The fourth and final stage is the recovery stage during which glomerular function gradually returns to normal. The recovery stage may take 3 to 12 months.

Chronic Renal Failure

Pathophysiology

In CRF, renal function steadily declines as nephrons are replaced with scar tissue. Renal insufficiency denotes a 20% to 50% reduction in the glomerular filtration rate (GFR). When renal function in each kidney is reduced by 50%, signs and symptoms of mild azotemia (i.e., build up of nitrogenous waste products in the blood), polyuria, nocturia, hypertension, and anemia become apparent. The term *renal failure* is used when the GFR drops to 20% to 25% of normal. During renal failure, uremia (symptom complex indicating multiple organ system dysfunction) is apparent along with fluid and electrolyte imbalances. When the GFR drops from a normal level of 125 ml a minute to less than 10 ml a minute the kidney's loss of ability to maintain its homeostatic functions occurs, denoting the destruction of 90% of the nephrons and the onset of end-stage renal disease (ESRD).

Approximately 500,000 people in the United States have ESRD, with men, African Americans, and Native Americans affected more often than women and Caucasians. Diabetes causes 36% of ESRD cases, while hypertension is responsible for 30% of ESRD cases. Other major causes of ESRD include sickle cell disease, glomerulonephritis, and polycystic kidney disease.

ESRD is the result of glomerulosclerosis, tubulointerstitial injury, and/or vascular injury. Glomerulosclerosis is the progressive hardening of the glomerular capillaries. This process of epithelial and endothelial injury results in protein spilling into the urine. Tubulointerstitial injury causes the loss of tubular transport functions as the tubules become inflamed, edematous, and necrotic. Vascular injury to renal blood vessels causes ischemia and damage to renal tissue.

Clinical signs and symptoms of CRF are similar to those of ARF, but include additional effects of long-term uremia such as renal osteodystrophy, malnutrition, pruritus, peripheral neuropathy, and altered reproductive functioning. Renal osteodystrophy, or demineralization of bone, has three major causes. First, the kidneys loose their ability to activate vitamin D, which results in decreased absorption of calcium from food. Second, there is a decreased excretion of parathyroid hormone, which leads to demineralization of bones and teeth. Third, there is retention of phosphate, which leads to increased renal excretion of calcium.

Malnutrition occurs because of anorexia, malaise, dietary protein restriction, and proteinuria. Dietary protein is restricted in an attempt to reduce the protein load on the kidneys. Hypoalbuminemia causes fragile capillaries, poor wound healing, and decreased immune system function, which increases susceptibility to infections.

Retained serum toxins cause a dermal inflammatory process and pruritus. The skin may have a grayish-yellowish cast because of the build up of urinary pigments. Uremic frost occurs when the body attempts to rid itself of uric acid and other toxins through sweat.

Restless leg syndrome (i.e., spontaneous movement of the feet and legs), altered sensation, weakness, and diminished deep tendon reflexes occur because of neurotoxicity caused by uremia. An alteration in hormone levels causes a lack of ovulation and menstruation, the inability to carry a fetus to term, impotence, and decreased sperm counts.

Management

Treatment for ARF is through dialysis until renal function returns. CRF is treated by conservative management of renal insufficiency and then by dialysis or renal transplantation as needed. Conservative management aimed at retaining as much renal function as possible includes utilization of a protein restricted diet and control of hypertension. Anemia has been successfully treated with recombinant human erythropoietin (i.e., Epogen [Amgen Inc., Thousand Oaks, CA]). Dietary restriction of phosphates, the administration of phosphate-binding antacids, and activated vitamin D and calcium have been shown to reduce osteodystrophy. Metabolic acidosis is treated with sodium bicarbonate. Salt and water restriction, along with antihypertensives, may be necessary to control hypertension.

63 Tubulointerstitial Disorders

Renal Tubular Acidosis

Proximal tubule defects:
Loss of bicarbonate and sodium
Hypovolemia
Increased aldosterone secretion
Hypokalemia

Distal tubule defects:
Inability to excrete hydrogen ions
Loss of sodium and bicarbonate
Hypovolemia
Increased aldosterone secretion
Hypokalemia
Increased parathyroid production
Osteomalacia
Renal calculi
Growth retardation

Prevention: Prompt diagnosis of urinary tract infection (UTI)

Treatment: Replacement of bicarbonate reverses the other electrolyte losses

Overview

Renal disorders that affect the proximal and distal tubules and sometimes the tissue surrounding the tubules are termed *tubulointerstitial disorders* (TD) and include renal tubular acidosis, pyelonephritis, and drug-related nephropathies. These disorders may be acute or chronic. Acute disease produces an abrupt onset of signs and symptoms, while chronic disorders result in fibrosis and atrophy of nephrons. Early signs of TD include signs and symptoms of fluid and electrolyte imbalance such as nocturia, polyuria, and metabolic acidosis.

Renal Tubular Acidosis

Pathophysiology

Proximal tubular defects hinder bicarbonate reabsorption, while distal tubular defects result in a reduction of the secretion of metabolic acids both of which lead to metabolic acidosis, bone disease, renal calculi, and growth retardation in children.

Because the proximal tubules are where 90% to 95% of filtered bicarbonate is reabsorbed, defects affecting this area result in a loss of bicarbonate and sodium into the urine. Associated with the loss of bicarbonate and sodium is a reduction of serum bicarbonate levels, hypovolemia, increased aldosterone secretion, and hypokalemia. The distal tubules continue to function and excrete metabolic acids. Eventually, the proximal tubules regain enough function to reabsorb a small amount of bicarbonate.

Distal tubular defects, in contrast, result in a decreased ability to excrete hydrogen ions into the urine with a concomitant loss of sodium and bicarbonate. As in proximal tubular defects, hypovolemia results, leading to increased aldosterone secretion and hypokalemia. In an attempt to buffer the rising serum hydrogen ions, calcium is leeched from the bones. As calcium is excreted in the urine, the production of parathyroid hormone occurs, leading to osteomalacia, bone pain, renal calculi, and impaired growth in children.

Management

Prompt treatment of an urinary tract infection (UTI) may help prevent tubular defects. Treatment of proximal and distal tubular defects is focused on replacement of bicarbonate, which then leads to a return of Na and K balance.

Pyelonephritis

Pathophysiology

Pyelonephritis, an upper UTI and inflammatory disorder of the renal pelvis and parenchyma classified as a TD, can be acute or chronic. Females over the age of 50 are more likely to develop pyelonephritis. Risk factors such as renal calculi; presence of an indwelling urinary catheter; diabetes mellitus, which lowers resistance to infection; or catheterization are common causes of this syndrome. In children a condition called *vesicoureteral reflux*, which moves urine from the bladder back to the kidneys, is associated with pyelonephritis. In adults a risk factor for developing pyelonephritis is bladder outflow obstruction resulting from calculi, tumors, or prostatic hypertrophy.

Acute pyelonephritis is caused by a bacterial infection that travels from the urethra to the kidney or from bloodborne bacteria. It generally involves patchy foci of infection and sometimes small areas of localized abscess formation; however, the glomeruli are spared from major damage. Gram-negative bacteria and enterococci, which normally inhabit the intestine, are usually responsible for causing acute pyelonephritis.

Signs and symptoms of acute pyelonephritis include abrupt onset of dull, constant flank pain or back pain, fever and chills, and other signs of infection such as malaise and headache. Symptoms of bladder irritation such as urgency, frequency, and burning are common. Urinalysis may reveal casts, which are clumps of cells that form in the collecting tubules and are shed in the urine, because they are indicative of an inflammatory process. Bacteria in the urine above 100,000 per ml indicates infection as does an elevated serum neutrophil count.

In contrast to acute pyelonephritis, chronic pyelonephritis is a progressive process. Chronic pyelonephritis is associated with recurring acute bacterial or nonbacterial infections or most commonly an autoimmune process involving the kidneys. Inflammation, fibrosis, and scarring of the tubules occur, which results in renal tissue destruction. Approximately 11% to 20% of end-stage renal disease is caused by chronic pyelonephritis.

A person with pyelonephritis may be asymptomatic or have some of the signs and symptoms associated with acute pyelonephritis. Polyuria and nocturia occur as the kidneys lose their ability to concentrate urine. Hypertension may develop as the disease progresses. An intravenous pyelogram will detect a change in kidney size and function.

Management

Prevention of acute pyelonephritis can be accomplished by avoiding the risk factors associated with its development. Of primary importance is prevention of lower UTIs. In women, wiping from front to back after a bowel movement will prevent spread of fecal bacteria to the urinary tract. Therapy for acute pyelonephritis includes antibiotics, hydration, and urinary analgesics. The treatment of chronic pyelonephritis is aimed at removing the underlying cause in order to prevent renal damage. Surgery to correct structural defects associated with outflow problems is indicated.

Drug-Related Nephropathies

Pathophysiology

Several classes of drugs can cause functional and structural changes in the kidneys, especially in the elderly. Tubulointerstitial nephritis (TN) is caused by a hypersensitivity reaction to commonly prescribed drugs such as sulfonamides, methicillin and other synthetic antibiotics, Lasix, and thiazide diuretics. It takes from 2 to 40 days after exposure to the offending drug for signs and symptoms of nephritis, including fever, hematuria, mild proteinuria, rash, and eosinophilia, to appear. Half of the people with TN will develop acute renal failure. Most people fully recover once the drug is stopped.

Prostaglandins help to regulate tubular blood flow. Nonsteroidal anti-inflammatory drugs (NSAIDs) inhibit prostaglandin synthesis and, thus, cause renal damage in some individuals. The elderly, people with renal insufficiency and/or disease, and those who are dehydrated are at greatest risk from developing NSAID-related renal damage.

Management

Avoidance of drugs known to cause renal damage, especially in the elderly and those with renal insufficiency, and adequate hydration are ways to prevent drug-induced renal pathology.

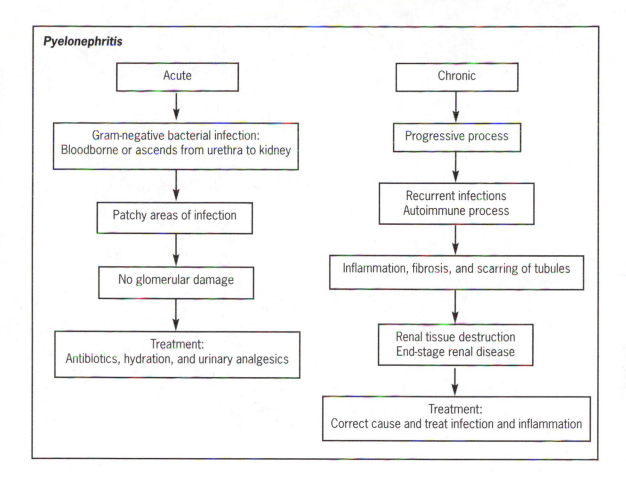

Pyelonephritis

Acute

↓

Gram-negative bacterial infection:
Bloodborne or ascends from urethra to kidney

↓

Patchy areas of infection

↓

No glomerular damage

↓

Treatment:
Antibiotics, hydration, and urinary analgesics

Chronic

↓

Progressive process

↓

Recurrent infections
Autoimmune process

↓

Inflammation, fibrosis, and scarring of tubules

↓

Renal tissue destruction
End-stage renal disease

↓

Treatment:
Correct cause and treat infection and inflammation

PART IX QUESTIONS

1. Which of the following is a major function of the kidneys?

(A) Converting vitamin D to the active form

(B) The proliferation of leukocytes

(C) Converting angiotensin I to angiotensin II

(D) Producing antibodies

2. What is the most sensitive indicator of renal function?

(A) BUN

(B) Serum creatinine

(C) Urinalysis

(D) RBC count

3. Which of the following statements about urinary tract infections (UTIS) is true?

(A) UTIs are more common in men than in women.

(B) UTIs frequently result from highly acidic urine.

(C) UTIs are prevented by voiding.

(D) UTIs occur in 70% of patients with an indwelling catheter.

4. A nurse explains hemolytic uremic syndrome (HUS) to the parents of a child with the disorder. Which of the following statements is true?

(A) Antibiotics are the treatment of choice for HUS.

(B) Seizure activity is a symptom of HUS.

(C) HUS is spread by the use of all dairy products.

(D) HUS is caused by streptococci alternans.

5. The pathology of the nephrotic syndrome includes which of the following?

(A) Thickening of the basement membrane and glomeruli collagen deposits

(B) Glomeruli damage by group B hemolytic streptococci

(C) IgA hyperactivity

(D) Glomerular proliferation

6. The treatment plan for a patient with glomerulonephritis includes which of the following?

(A) Blood transfusions to correct anemia

(B) A high protein diet to restore albumin levels

(C) Potassium restriction to correct electrolyte imbalance

(D) Systemic steroids to reduce inflammation

7. Stretch receptors in the bladder are initially stimulated when the bladder fills to:

(A) 150 cc

(B) 400 cc

(C) 550 cc

(D) 600 cc

8. Which of the following causes urge incontinence?

(A) Damage to the spinal cord at the level of S2 to S4

(B) Urinary retention

(C) An overactive detrusor muscle

(D) A weak urethral sphincter

9. Which of the following statements about struvite renal calculi is true?

(A) Struvite calculi are caused by an abundance of calcium in the blood.

(B) Struvite calculi may result from a UTI.

(C) Struvite calculi are more common when the urine is acidic.

(D) Struvite calculi are frequently composed of uric acid.

10. When explaining finasteride to a patient, the nurse stresses which of the following?

(A) It can reduce the size of the prostate gland by 50% to 75%.

(B) It is an estrogen supplement associated with reduction in prostate size.

(C) It causes the proliferation of stromal cells in the prostate.

(D) It blocks the conversion of testosterone to DHT, thereby reducing prostate size.

11. Which of the following is true about acute renal failure (ARF)?

(A) It usually progresses to chronic renal failure.

(B) It initially produces profuse urine with a low specific gravity.

(C) It may take 1 year to resolve.

(D) It is commonly caused by radiologic dyes.

12. Renal insufficiency develops when the glomerular filtration rates drop by which of the following?

(A) 10%

(B) 30%

(C) 60%

(D) 90%

13. Renal tubular acidosis results in which of the following?

(A) An imbalance of bicarbonate levels

(B) Hyperglycemia

(C) Fluid retention

(D) Hypernatremia

14. Signs and symptoms of drug-related nephropathy include which of the following?

(A) Cardiac dysrhythmia

(B) Subnormal body temperature

(C) Bradycardia

(D) Rash

1. The correct answer is A.

Inactive vitamin D is converted to the active form by the kidneys.

2. The correct answer is B.

Creatinine is cleared from the blood by the kidneys. Unlike the BUN, it does not rise or fall in response to fluid balance.

3. The correct answer is C.

Voiding removes bacteria from the bladder and urethra.

4. The correct answer is B.

Seizure activity, bloody diarrhea, anemia, and renal failure are symptoms of HUS.

5. The correct answer is A.

The nephrotic syndrome causes increased glomerular capillary membrane permeability and basement membrane thickening as a result of collagen deposits in the glomeruli.

6. The correct answer is D.

Systemic steroids help reduce inflammation, while a low protein diet slows the progression to renal failure.

7. The correct answer is A.

Parasympathetic pelvic nerves are stimulated when the bladder fills to between 150 cc and 300 cc.

8. The correct answer is C.

An overactive detrusor muscle causes repetitive, strong contractions of the muscle, which overcomes urethral sphincter control.

9. The correct answer is B.

The bacteria that causes a UTI produces an enzyme that splits urea into ammonia and carbon dioxide, creating an alkaline urine and increased phosphate, which combines with magnesium and ammonium to form a calculi.

10. The correct answer is D.

Lowering the level of DHT results in less prostatic tissue growth. The prostate normally converts testosterone to DHT.

11. The correct answer is C.

The resolution stage of acute renal failure may take 3 to 12 months.

12. The correct answer is B.

The term renal insufficiency is used when the GFR drops between 20% and 50%.

13. The correct answer is A.

When either the distal or proximal tubules are damaged, bicarbonate is excreted.

14. The correct answer is D.

Signs and symptoms of drug-related nephropathy include fever, hematuria, proteinuria, rash, and an elevated eosinophil count.

PART X

Orthopedics

Suzanne MacAvoy, EdD, APRN-C

64 Bone Physiology

Age-Related Changes in Bone
- Decreased bone mass
- Decreased bone strength
- Decreased calcium absorption
- Increased demineralization

Types of Fractures
- Simple (closed)—Skin intact
- Compound (open)—Skin broken, bone exposed
- Displaced—Bone continuity disrupted
- Nondisplaced—Fractured bone remains in alignment
- Incomplete—Portion of the bone remains intact
- Comminuted—Three or more bone fragments
- Impacted—One fragment imbedded in another
- Depressed—Fractured bone driven inward (skull)
- Pathological—Associated with disease/disorder
- Avulsion—Fragment torn off due to twisting/pulling
- Compression—Crushed
- Stress—Minute fracture related to repetitive stress

Bone consists of an organic matrix upon which mineral salts are deposited. Protein, vitamin A, and vitamin C are needed for its formation by fibroblasts. Calcium, phosphorus, and vitamin D are needed to form the inorganic compounds. Bone serves as a reservoir for calcium, phosphorus, and other minerals. Cancellous or trabecular bone is made up of thin plates, is spongy, and contains marrow. It is formed in response to stress and is found in bones such as vertebrae and skull as well as the ends of long bones. The interlacing structure of these plates provides tensile strength and structural support for compact bone. Compact bone is found primarily in the long bones and in the outer layers of all bones. It is firm, dense, and resistant to compression and shearing.

Collagen is the basic building block of bone matrix. It provides resilience or tensile strength. Without the collagen matrix, bone would be too hard and brittle. Calcium and other minerals lend strength and rigidity and provide compressive strength to bone. Ground substance consisting of protein polysaccharides or glycosaminoglycans serves as an adhesive between the layers of collagen matrix. It serves as a medium for diffusion of nutrients, oxygen, waste products, electrolytes, and minerals between bone tissue and blood vessels and influences calcium deposition and calcification. Vitamins A and C are also needed for its formation.

Osteoblasts and osteoclasts work synergistically to form and maintain bone. Osteoblasts synthesize osteoid, which forms the organic protein of the matrix. Osteocytes are calcified osteoblasts. Osteoblasts lay down bone and osteoclasts cause its' resorption and removal. It is this constant process of breakdown and buildup of bone, termed *remodeling*, that repairs damage and keeps bones strong in response to environmental stressors. Bone is laid down where it is needed and reabsorbed where it is not needed. A small percentage of bone is undergoing remodeling at any given time. The remodeling process takes approximately 4 months to complete one cycle. Bone turnover is dependent upon many factors, such as amounts of various hormones, amount of stress on the bones, nutritional status, adequacy of circulation, age, and overall health. Physical stress on bone leads to deposition of additional bone at the site of increased stress. This is the principle underlying weight-bearing exercise for menopausal women and ambulation in the latter stages of bone healing after fractures.

The basic unit of cortical bone is the haversian system. It is the channels within this system that allow nutrients from the blood to reach the osteocytes. Circulation within compact bone is supplied by one or more arteries and veins, which pierce the bone and enter the marrow. Blood then enters the haversian system to nourish the bone. Necrosis of the bone can occur if this blood supply is obstructed or obliterated. Cancellous bone lacks the haversian system. Circulation in cancellous bone takes place within the trabeculae, which are filled with red marrow.

Periosteum is a tough fibrous membrane that covers the bone. It is very vascular, contains pain receptors, and is responsible for osteogenesis. It supplies blood to the bones via Volkmann's canals. The inner portion of the long bones is referred to as the *medullary canal*. The medullary cavity and trabecular spaces are lined by the endosteum that contains osteogenic cells and the bone marrow. Intact periosteum is necessary for healthy bone; if disrupted by trauma or disease, it leads to the death of the bone because of interference with the blood supply.

Additional substances also play a critical role in bone metabolism. Vitamin D is a fat soluble vitamin that controls the absorption of calcium from the intestine and increases calcium reabsorption in the kidneys. Parathyroid hormone promotes the formation of osteoclasts and retards production of osteoblasts, thereby enhancing bone breakdown. Calcitonin, a thyroid hormone, decreases osteoclastic activity and increases osteoblastic activity, thereby reducing bone breakdown and enhancing its formation. Estrogen enhances the osteoblastic activity in women; testosterone increases bone length and density in men.

Longitudinal and circumferential bone growth occurs via growth of cartilaginous tissue, which gradually ossifies into bone. This ossification is accelerated during puberty. Longitudinal growth of long bones takes place at the growth plate at the ends of long bones. Good nutrition, physical activity, and exercise from childhood onward are essential for the development and maintenance of healthy bones. Calcium and/or vitamin D should be supplemented during periods of increased need (e.g., rapid growth, pregnancy) through dietary means, if at all possible. Oral calcium supplements are available. Calcium carbonate contains the highest amount of elemental calcium, while calcium citrate is best absorbed.

Fractures and Bone Healing

A local inflammatory process is necessary for bone healing to occur, as with healing of any other tissue. The edges of the fracture site become necrotic, are reabsorbed, and are eventually replaced by new bone. Bone healing begins with formation of a hematoma and granulation tissue, which gradually transforms into callus. It takes 2 to 6 weeks for callus formation. Callus, which is osteoid tissue, binds the bone but is initially neither stable nor strong. As calcium deposits within the callus, it is transformed into bone tissue. This process of ossification can take from 3 weeks to several months; however, bone healing ordinarily takes 4 to 6 weeks. It is dependent upon a variety of factors such as age, nutrition, blood supply, type, and location of the fracture and others. Compact bone develops callus both externally and internally. The external callus often forms a palpable lump at the site of the fracture, which gradually will become smaller as ossification occurs, although it may not disappear entirely. Cancellous bone develops internal callus, and healing is ordinarily faster in this type of bone. The remodeling phase of bone healing may take as long as a year depending on the degree and type of fracture, as well as other factors. It is during this phase that the bone reshapes to meet the mechanical requirements placed upon it. Delayed union, malunion, or nonunion may occur due to poor nutrition, poor circulation, malalignment, premature weight bearing, and/or other factors. Ossification occurs more quickly in children and more slowly in the elderly.

The growth plate is a site of common fracture in children and has the potential to lead to limb length discrepancies. These fractures may not always be visible on x-ray. Cancellous bone is more susceptible to compression fractures and is a common site of postmenopausal fractures and other osteoporotic fractures.

Fractures are often accompanied by extensive soft tissue damage, depending upon the site, the cause, and the degree of injury. Compartment syndrome is a serious complication that results from an increase in pressure in the given compartment. The pressure impinges on the nerves and blood vessels contained within it and can compromise the distal extremity if not identified and treated promptly. Infection is also a serious complication that can lead to osteomyelitis.

Management

Rest, immobilization, compression, and elevation (RICE) is the mainstay of initial treatment of orthopedic injuries. Immobilization of fractures until callus forms and ossification begins is critical. Partial weight bearing is prescribed once ossification has begun as determined by x-ray. Full weight bearing without external support is prescribed once ossification is complete.

Bleeding, inflammation, and possible contamination need to be considered in management. Pain management with pharmacologic and nonpharmacologic measures and prevention of complications of immobility are also very important.

Haversian system.

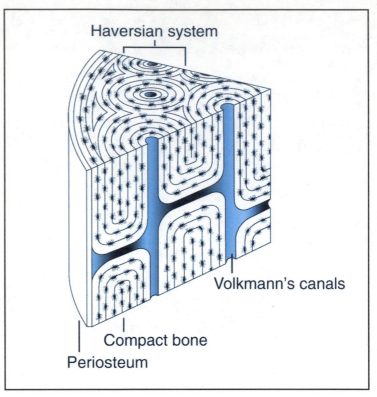

Haversian system

Volkmann's canals

Compact bone

Periosteum

Long bone structures.

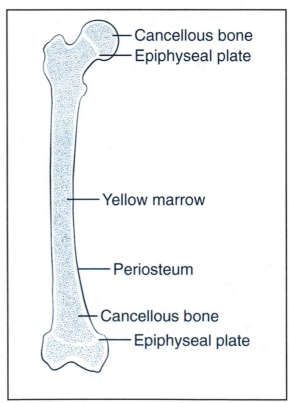

Cancellous bone
Epiphyseal plate

Yellow marrow

Periosteum

Cancellous bone
Epiphyseal plate

65 Osteoporosis

Risk Factors for Osteoporosis

Caucasian or Asian	Female	Early menopause
Scandinavian	Fair, blonde	Late menarche
Small frame	Physical inactivity	Postmenopausal
Excessive nicotine	Excessive alcohol intake	Family history
Internal fixation with a metal implant		

Red Flags for Osteoporosis

- Presence of risk factors
- Kyphosis
- Fracture with slight or no trauma
- Hip fracture preceding a fall
- Loss of height >2 inches of adult height

Common Diagnostic Tests

- MRI, CT, bone scan
- Bone density tests—DEXA (safest and most reliable)
- Blood work—Ca, PO_4, vitamin D, parathyroid, alkaline phosphatase

Drugs and Health Problems Associated with Osteoporosis

Drugs	Health Problems
Thyroid replacement	Thyrotoxicosis
Glucocorticoids	Cushing's disease
Heparin	Type I diabetes
Lithium	Malabsorption
Chemotherapy	Rheumatoid arthritis
Anticonvulsants	Hemolytic anemia
Tetracyclines	Anorexia nervosa
Selected diuretics	Hepatobiliary dysfunction
Phenothiazines	
Cyclosporine	
Selected antacids	

Osteoporosis occurs when the rate of bone resorption exceeds the rate of bone formation. There are two types of primary osteoporosis: type I is associated with postmenopausal estrogen loss and type II is associated with aging. Secondary, or type II, osteoporosis is due to some underlying disease or pathology. Osteoporosis can be due to either a decrease in activity of the osteoblasts, which are responsible for bone formation, or an increase in activity of the osteoclasts, which are responsible for bone breakdown. It can be either regional or generalized. Early osteoporosis is asymptomatic and considerable bone loss (30% to 50%) can occur before it is detectable on x-ray.

Osteoporosis is more common in women than in men with the peak incidence in women beginning within 5 years of menopause. In men, demineralization begins around the age of 65 to 70 and is due to a decrease in testosterone and other factors. Osteoporosis in males has less clinical significance because their bones are larger and more dense than those of women. The bone loss during menopause is due to an increase in osteoclastic activity, while that occurring with aging is mediated by a decrease in osteoblastic activity.

Cancellous or trabecular bone is more susceptible to osteoporosis associated with the decrease in estrogen with menopause (e.g., vertebrae, distal wrist). Osteoporosis associated with aging occurs in both genders and involves both cancellous and cortical bone. The cortical bone becomes thinner, and there is a reduction in the number and size of trabeculae in cancellous bone. Fractures in type II osteoporosis frequently occur in the femoral neck, proximal humerus, and proximal tibia. The effect of osteoporosis is most significant in cancellous bone, which results in a decrease in the resilience or tensile strength of the bone and a decrease in the amount of internal support it affords surrounding compact or cortical bone.

The bone remodeling cycle in persons with osteoporosis may take up to 2 years versus the normal time of 4 months. If circulation to the bone is impaired, the remodeling process is hindered, further contributing to the development of osteoporosis and likelihood of fractures. There is a very high morbidity and mortality rate following hip fracture in the elderly so every effort should be made to prevent osteoporosis and reduce fall risk in this population. Fifty percent die within 1 year of presentation. Most of those who survive have a significant reduction in independence and functional ability.

Factors that contribute to bone loss include genetic predisposition; hormonal imbalance; nutritional deficits, especially protein, calcium, and vitamins C and D; age; use of certain medications; as well as certain diseases. Excessive coffee, tobacco, and alcohol use can also contribute. The osteoporosis due to medications is termed *iatrogenic osteoporosis*. Steroids interfere with glucose utilization and cause breakdown of protein, which forms the matrix of bone. They also depress osteoblastic activity. Long-term heparin use increases collagen breakdown. Other medications that can contribute to osteoporosis include anticonvulsants, barbiturates, thyroid hormones, and, possibly, loop diuretics.

Disuse osteoporosis occurs with prolonged immobility and is due to lack of stress on long bones. This results in a decrease in osteoblastic activity and an increase in osteoclastic activity, with an overall decrease in bone mass. It is thought that muscular activity plays a role in enhancing circulation to the bone and in stimulating osteoblastic activity. In addition, stress on bones alters electrical charges on the surface of the bone, which stimulates new bone formation.

Metastatic bone tumors result in osteoporotic changes in bone tissue, particularly in older adults. This can be particularly painful because of the pressure exerted upon the periosteum from the proliferating cell mass. If the tumor causes elevation of the periosteum, new bone formation becomes erratic or impaired. *Pathological fractures* can occur as a consequence of osteoporosis, bone metastasis, or other causes.

Paget's disease is a disease of chronic bone inflammation that results in softening and bowing of the long bones. In widespread disease it can involve most bones. There is an increase in osteoclastic activity with a compensatory increase in osteoblastic activity. The new formed bone exceeds that broken down; however, it is structurally abnormal, resulting in bone that is porous and soft. The long bones are bowed and other bones are often misshapen. Fractures are common. This may be a very painful condition if accompanied by fractures and/or compression of nerves. Other more common causes of *secondary osteoporosis* include hyperthyroidism, hyperparathyroidism, Cushing's disease, diabetes mellitus, and chronic renal failure.

Management

Prevention is key with osteoporosis. Good nutrition in women is particularly important from childhood through the age of 30, as those are the years when maximum bone formation takes place. The recommended intake of calcium in children and adolescents is 1,800 mg/day. Premenopausal and postmenopausal women on hormone replacement therapy and adult men need 1,000 mg of elemental calcium daily; postmenopausal women without hormone replacement therapy need 1,500 mg of elemental calcium daily. Calcium carbonate contains the highest amount of elemental calcium; however, calcium citrate is better absorbed. In addition to calcium, phosphorus and vitamin D are needed for adequate mineralization, and protein and vitamins A and C are needed for formation of bone matrix. Weight-bearing exercise and calcium and vitamin d supplementation have an important role in long-term management.

Once osteoporosis is present, the goal of management is to slow the rate of calcium and bone loss and stop progression of the disease. Medications are available to either increase bone formation or osteoblastic activity or to decrease osteoclastic activity or bone loss. Estrogen replacement therapy in postmenopausal women does not increase bone mass, but it does halt further progression and is ordinarily recommended unless contraindicated. Weight-bearing exercise and calcium and vitamin D supplementation have an important place in long-term management. Management of secondary osteoporosis lies in correcting or ameliorating the underlying cause when possible.

Osteomyelitis

Osteomyelitis is an infection of the bone that results in some of the same structural abnormalities as osteoporosis (i.e., destruction of cortical and cancellous

Types of Osteoporosis

Postmenopausal	Senile	Secondary
55 to 70 years	75 to 90 years	Variable
F 20:1	F 2:1	F 1:1
Vertebrae	Vertebrae, hip, pelvis, and humerus	Vertebrae and hip

Bone Remodeling

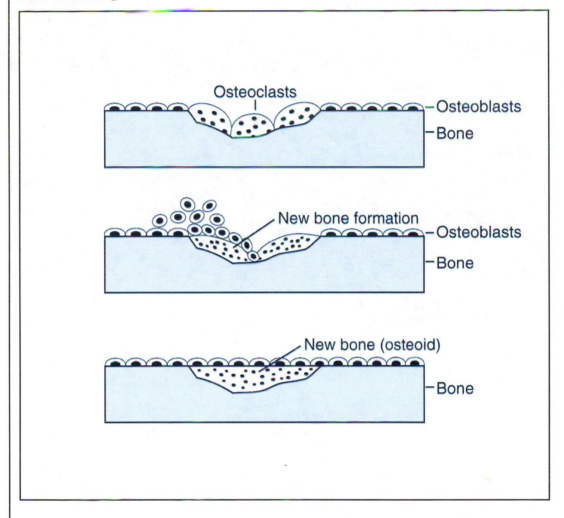

bone and propensity to fracture). Osteomyelitis can be severe and is a very serious problem because of the difficulty of eradicating the infection once it is present. Therefore, meticulous attention is paid to prevention.

Pathogenic gram-positive or gram-negative organisms can reach the body via the blood adjacent soft tissue or be introduced directly with trauma or during or after surgery. The nature of circulation to and within bone makes it difficult for antibiotics to reach involved tissue in sufficient concentrations to eradicate the organisms. It also contributes to the difficulty of removal of waste products of the inflammation/immune response and necrotic tissue. Organisms can remain sequestered within the bony tissue, and infection can reactivate at a later time if the person becomes immunosuppressed or after trauma. Osteomyelitis can also become chronic, especially if initial treatment was insufficient. Aggressive antibiotic therapy is the mainstay of treatment. Sometimes surgical debridement and/or replacement of orthopedic appliances is necessary.

66 Arthritis

Types of Joints
- Synarthrosis—Immovable (e.g., cranial sutures)
- Fibrous—Rigid surface (e.g., cranial)
- Amphiarthrosis—Partially moveable (e.g., symphysis)
- Cartilaginous—Slightly moveable (e.g., ribs, sternum)
- Diarthrosis—Freely moveable (e.g., hip, knees)
- Synovial—Considerable movement (e.g., fingers, elbow)

Types of Cartilage
- Elastic—Most flexible (e.g., ear, epiglottis)
- Hyaline—Most common (e.g., most joints, nose)
- Fibrous—Most rigid (e.g., pelvis, intervertebral discs)

Definitions
- Tendons—Attach muscle to bone
- Ligaments—Attach bone to bone

Common Diagnostic Tests with Gout
- Joint aspiration
- Serum uric acid
- ESR
- WBC

Common Diagnostic Tests with Rheumatoid Arthritis

Rh factor titer	Urinalysis
Complete blood count with differential	FOBT
Sedimentation rate	Joint aspiration
Chem.	X-ray
LFT	ANA if indicated

Three major forms of arthritis are osteoarthritis, rheumatoid arthritis, and gout. All three of these diseases involve the entire joint structure, including the synovial membrane, articular cartilage, tendons, ligaments, adjacent bone, and joint spaces. X-ray is used to confirm diagnosis and monitor progression. Blood work is done only if indicated.

Collagen is the primary building block of cartilage. It is continuously being renewed and remodeled by chondrocytes. Cartilage does not possess a blood supply or nerve endings; therefore, it requires long periods of time to heal. It is nourished by diffusion of nutrients from surrounding capillaries. Its function is to absorb shock, reduce friction, and distribute weight bearing. Tendons have pain receptors but a limited blood supply, so they also take a long time to heal. Joint spaces are filled with synovial fluid, which lubricates, nourishes, cushions, and facilitates movement.

Osteoarthritis

Introduction

Osteoarthritis is a progressive, degenerative joint disease affecting primarily peripheral and central weight-bearing joints and fingers. Primary or idiopathic osteoarthritis is associated with aging, while secondary osteoarthritis is related to some other condition or process and is often a result of repeated or severe joint stress or trauma. Osteoarthritis has an asymmetrical distribution and is a local disease. It is the most common form of arthritis with degenerative changes often beginning between the ages of 40 to 50. Early symptoms are often mild and frequently ignored or compensated for by those who have them. The incidence is higher in males.

Pathophysiology

Osteoarthritis is characterized by progressive erosion of articular cartilage, which results from the breakdown of protein and collagen by enzymes. Increased water is absorbed because of disruption in pumping action, so the cartilage becomes less able to tolerate weight bearing and loses some of its tensile strength. As osteoarthritis progresses, bits of articular cartilage flake off and longitudinal fissures develop. The cartilage becomes thin or absent, leaving the bone unprotected. Subchondral bone becomes thick and sclerotic and can develop cysts. Osteophytes (bone spurs) develop at the joint margin, which can also break off, causing synovitis and joint effusion. The joint capsule becomes thickened and may adhere to underlying structures. Knees, hips, vertebrae, and fingers are the most common sites. Pain associated with osteoarthritis arises from a combination of articular distension, inflammation, and fibrosis.

Management

Osteoarthritis is managed by a combination of rest and exercise, including range of motion exercises to maintain joint mobility. Weight reduction is important if indicated. Ambulation aids may be necessary to reduce stress on weight-bearing joints. Pain management with acetaminophen and other nonsteroidal anti-inflammatory drugs (NSAIDs) is usually sufficient. Patient education is important in the management of this chronic condition. Surgery and joint replacement is sometimes indicated.

Rheumatoid Arthritis

Introduction

Rheumatoid arthritis is a systemic, inflammatory disease of connective tissue. For many, there is a strong autoimmune component; a genetic predisposition is also possible. The joints most commonly involved are the hands, wrists, knees, feet, and upper cervical spine. In adults, joint involvement is symmetrical.

Rheumatoid arthritis is characterized by inflammatory damage or destruction of the synovial membrane and articular cartilage. It eventually involves the joint capsule, ligaments, and tendons, resulting in pain, joint deformity, and loss of function. It is also accompanied by systemic inflammatory symptoms and nonarticular pathologic manifestations in other body systems such as cardiac, pulmonary, or ophthalmic.

Rheumatoid arthritis is more common in women and generally occurs in young or middle-aged adults. It is characterized by remissions and exacerbations and can progress to severe debilitation with significant loss of functional ability.

Pathophysiology

Rheumatoid factor has been found in most people with rheumatoid arthritis and 60% to 80% have the B lymphocyte alloantigen HLA-DR4. The stimulus for the abnormal immune reaction is not known but several theories have been postulated, including injury, stress, autonomic changes, and physical activity.

The immune complexes formed between rheumatoid factor and IgG activate the complement system and leukocyte release of lysosomal enzymes. These initiate and enhance the inflammatory response. Immune complexes are deposited on synovial membranes and phagocytized by macrophages. The enzymes that are released degrade synovial tissue and articular cartilage. This continued inflammatory response results in hypertrophy, which impairs local circulation and invades local joint structures. Granulation tissue forms, which covers the articular cartilage leading to pannus formation. Pannus is vascularized scar tissue that erodes and destroys articular cartilage, leading to bone erosion, cysts, fissures, and bone spurs. As the pannus becomes more fibrotic, it causes tendons and ligaments to shorten. Secondary muscle atrophy, fibrosis, and the inflammatory destruction that follows it contributes to laxity of ligaments and tendons, causing joint instability, subluxation, and contractures. The characteristic ulnar deviation and swan-neck deformity of the hands are easily recognized. Subcutaneous nodules comprised of inflammatory cells and cellular debris may present over extensor surfaces of elbows and fingers as well as other areas.

Management

The goals of management are to decrease pain, prevent deformity, and maintain functional ability. Local joint rest and periodic daily systemic rest, as well as exercise, are mainstays of management. Physical measures include use of heat, cold, and other physical therapy techniques. Pain relief is very important. Acetylsalicylic acid and NSAIDs are used, as well as a variety of other medications, with more advanced dis-

Synovial joint.

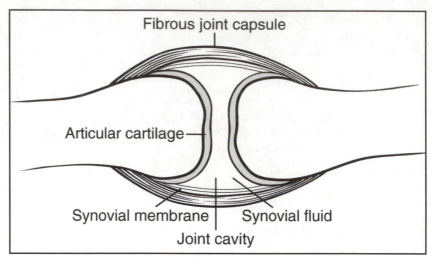

Fibrous joint capsule

Articular cartilage

Synovial membrane

Synovial fluid

Joint cavity

Cross-section of knee joint.

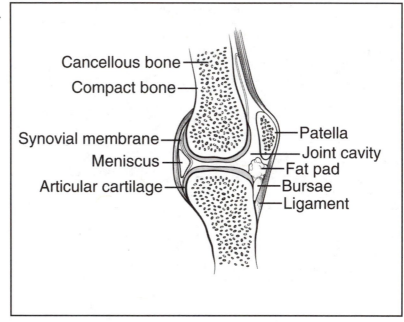

Cancellous bone

Compact bone

Synovial membrane

Meniscus

Articular cartilage

Patella

Joint cavity

Fat pad

Bursae

Ligament

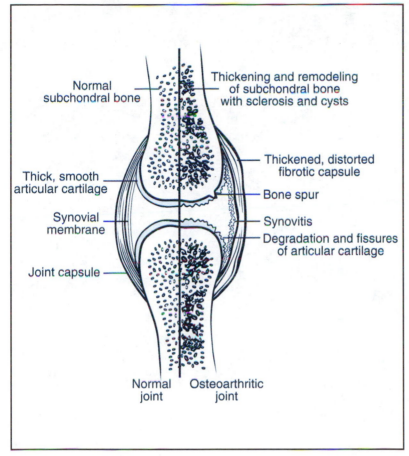

Osteoarthritis.

Normal subchondral bone

Thickening and remodeling of subchondral bone with sclerosis and cysts

Thick, smooth articular cartilage

Thickened, distorted fibrotic capsule

Bone spur

Synovial membrane

Synovitis

Degradation and fissures of articular cartilage

Joint capsule

Normal joint

Osteoarthritic joint

ease. Surgery may be done to correct deformity, improve function, and decrease pain.

Gout

Introduction

Gout, which is asymptomatic in the early phase, is a disorder characterized by disturbances of uric acid metabolism that lead to hyperuricemia and deposition of urate salts in articular, periarticular, and subcutaneous tissue, which initiates an inflammatory response. Renal stones are a common sequelae. Gout is most frequently found in middle-aged men and postmenopausal women. It involves weight-bearing joints of the lower extremities, particularly the great toe.

Pathophysiology

Uric acid is a breakdown product of purines. An increase in uric acid can result from either an increased breakdown or production of purine. Two other mechanisms are an increased turnover of nucleic acids, which are necessary for various intracellular processes, and a lack of uricase, an enzyme that oxidizes uric acid to a soluble compound. The resultant hyperuricemia and deposition of urate crystals are accompanied by an acute local inflammatory response and severe pain. An acute attack, which last 3 to 10 days, is often triggered by trauma, stress, or use of alcohol or drugs. Asymptomatic periods between attacks are termed intercritical periods. As the disease progresses, urate crystals in subcutaneous tissue and joints cause the formation of nodules called tophi. This is the chronic phase of the disease. The tophi can erode and drain through the skin. The chronic inflammation caused by the tophi can lead to deforming arthritis. Uric acid is excreted by the kidneys. If its excretion is impaired or its reabsorption is increased, uric acid levels become elevated.

Management

The goals of management are to control pain, prevent acute attacks, prevent or reverse complications, and prevent renal calculi. NSAIDs are used for pain management. Medications are also used to reduce hyperuricemia by either increasing the excretion of uric acid or decreasing its formation. Additional measures during an acute attack include decreased weight bearing, elevation, and ice. Dietary measures include a low purine diet and increased fluid intake. Intra-articular steroid injections may be indicated.

Low Back Pain

Changes with Aging
- Dehydration of intervertebral discs
- Narrowing of disc spaces
- Decreased height, kyphosis
- Decreased flexibility of lumbar curve and flattening of lumbar curve

Definitions
- Tendons—Attach muscle to bone
- Ligaments—Attach bone to bone

Grades of Strains/Sprains

Grade 1
- Minimal tearing and edema
- Local tenderness
- No change in muscle mass

Grade 2
- Moderate tearing
- Moderate pain, edema
- Muscular defect may be palpable

Grade 3
- Severe or complete tear
- Severe pain and edema
- Large palpable defect

Common Diagnostic Tests and PE Maneuvers
- Lumbosacral x-ray
- Magnetic resonance imaging (MRI)/computed tomography (CT)
- Electromyogram (EMG)
- Neurological exam
- Straight leg raise test

Introduction

Low back pain of musculoskeletal origin is one of the most common causes of pain in adults and results in significant loss of work hours. Although it is sometimes caused by acute injury, it is commonly chronic and often caused by soft tissue strain, sprain, or overuse due to muscle weakness, deconditioning, obesity, poor body mechanics, or poor posture. It may be accompanied by sciatica in which pain occurs along the distribution of one or both sciatic nerves. Other musculoskeletal or neurological conditions can also cause low back pain such as degenerative disc disease, arthritis, herniated nucleus pulposus, fibromyalgia, bursitis, radiculitis, fibrosis, stenosis, and vertebral fracture. Ninety percent of acute low back problems will resolve spontaneously within 4 weeks.

The vertebral column is supported by a complex group of strong, serially arranged muscles, fascia, and ligaments that extend from the pelvis to the skull. Functionally, these serve as a single muscle and maintain extension of the vertebral column. These structures work in conjunction with those of the abdomen, thorax, pelvis, neck, and head to afford the trunk full range of motion. The muscles of the abdomen are particularly important in providing additional support to the back. If they have poor tone or strength, weight bearing is transferred from the anterior spine to the posterior spine, causing muscle spasm and low back pain.

Vertebral joints are classified as amphiarthroses or partially moveable joints. The intervertebral discs are pad-like structures between the vertebrae that help stabilize them and act as shock absorbers between them. The outer layer of the disc is a tough fibrous layer referred to as the *annular layer*. The inner portion is more viscid and is called the *nucleus pulposus*. It lies close to the posterior portion of the disc. The nucleus pulposus changes shape with spinal movement, causing bulging of the annulus. The discs are strongly attached to adjacent vertebral bodies. Because of their high water content, the discs are subject to dehydration as people age, resulting in thinning of the discs, a decrease in shock absorbency, less spinal stability, and less ability to tolerate stress and strain. They also help to maintain the normal spinal curvatures.

Pathophysiology

The pain associated with low back pain may be due to a variety of mechanisms, and consideration of the underlying pathophysiology will direct the selection of the most appropriate treatment options. Direct tissue injury, as well as inflammation and spasm, all contribute to the degree of pain experienced. Vertebral malalignment and disc degeneration can likewise result in low back pain. Pain from other sites may also be referred to the low back, such as renal and aortic. Inflammation commonly accompanies low back pain, regardless of the cause. Compression, inflammation, and edema of nerve roots can also contribute to back pain of musculoskeletal origin. Muscle spasm, which is a compensatory or protective mechanism associated with trauma, can be exceedingly painful.

Muscular changes with aging that can predispose to or exacerbate low back pain include a decrease in size and number of muscle cells and capillaries, a decrease in muscle fiber diameter, and a decrease in muscle mass. There is also increased fat deposition, decreased elastic tissue, and increased collagen. Muscle cells are less responsive to neurotransmitters, which contributes to a decrease in response to stimulation by the nervous system. These cellular changes result in decreased muscle tone, strength, endurance, and elastic tissue. Over time, these changes result in a functional decrease in muscle strength of 30% to 50%. However, this process can be slowed by good nutrition and regular active exercise as one ages.

Herniated nucleus pulposis (HNP), referred to by lay persons as a *slipped disc*, is a protrusion of the posterior portion of the nucleus pulposus through the fibrous annular capsule. The nucleus pulposus may also protrude into the annulus and cause bulging of the disc without an actual herniation. Both protrusion of the nucleus pulposus and bulging of the annulus can cause compression of adjacent nerve roots and pain. Actual rupture of the disc is relatively uncommon.

Disc problems are most common between L3 to L4 to L5 to S1, which is the most flexible portion of the vertebral column. The precise location of the defect or injury can be assessed by examination of the distribution of the lumbosacral nerves and appropriate reflexes. Herniations at C5 to C7 also occur but are less frequent. Ligamentous injury frequently occurs in conjunction with a herniated nucleus pulposus and significant muscle spasm is often present.

Pain caused by pressure of a protruding disc on adjacent nerve roots or spinal nerves is referred to as *radicular pain*. In addition to pain, paresthesias, weakness, and decreased reflexes may also accompany nerve root compression or irritation. With appropriate management and self-care, these will often resolve fairly rapidly.

Degenerative disc disease results from a fibrosis and thinning of the nucleus pulposus which is associated with aging. This narrowing can result in vertebral instability, spinal stenosis, or rupture of the disc.

Spinal stenosis, which occurs primarily in middle-aged and older adults, is the narrowing of the spinal canal by soft tissue (i.e., fibrosis) or bony tissue. Pressure on nerve roots results in pain and neurogenic claudication, which is relieved by sitting or flexion of the lumbar spine.

Management

It is important that management be tailored to the pathophysiology involved (e.g., muscle relaxants for muscle spasm, nonsteroidal anti-inflammatory drugs [NSAIDs] for pain and inflammation). Bedrest reduces pressure on the discs, allowing water, which was forced out by compression, to re-enter and re-establish compressibility. Rest for 2 to 3 days is recommended if the injury is severe. Otherwise, normal activity may be maintained as tolerated. Prolonged bedrest is avoided because of the muscle weakness that accompanies immobility. Physical measures such as support, heat, ice, and other physical therapy techniques are an important part of treatment.

Dermatomes (lumbar/sacral nerve root innervation) (reprinted with permission from Jacobs, K., & Jacobs, L. [2001]. *Quick reference dictionary for occupational therapy* [3rd ed.]. Thorofare, NJ: SLACK Incorporated).

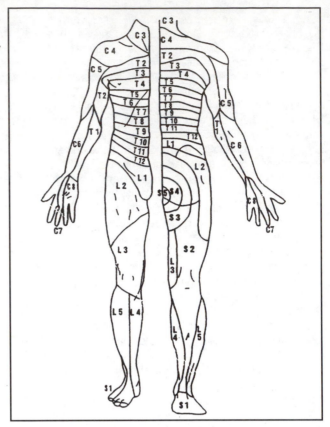

Vertebral segment.

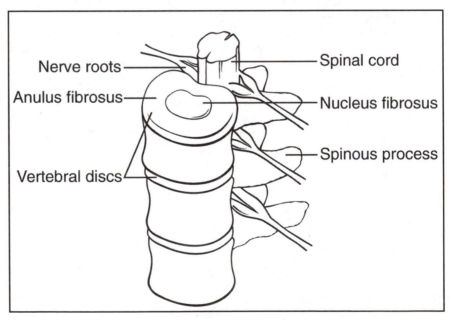

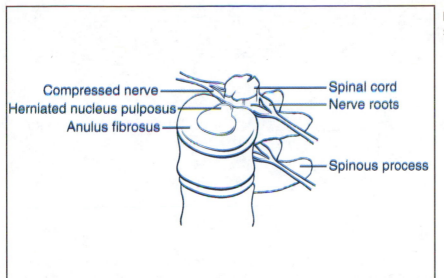

Herniated nucleus pulposus (HNP).

Compressed nerve
Herniated nucleus pulposus
Anulus fibrosus

Spinal cord
Nerve roots

Spinous process

Pain management is very important. Non-narcotic analgesics are the mainstay of pain management. NSAIDs, including acetaminophen, are the initial drugs of choice. Synthetic narcotic analgesics, such as oxycodone, are used for brief periods of time during acute attack, only in NSAIDs ineffective or contraindicated. Narcotics are avoided unless all other pharmacological and nonpharmacological measures have been exhausted and are a last resort for intractable pain. Care must be taken to avoid or compensate for side effects and avoid toxic effects of analgesic medications since some of these medications may be used for long periods of time, depending upon the particular disorder.

Patient education regarding body mechanics, stretching, and strengthening exercises (once the acute phase has passed) and techniques to reduce strain to back muscles is very important. Increasing flexibility and strength of the lower extremities and strength of the abdominal muscles is important as is regular exercise for overall musculoskeletal health. Occupational factors need to be considered and modified if indicated. Occasionally, surgery is necessary with certain conditions such as spinal stenosis, herniated nucleus pulposus, if there is severe compression or if more conservative management is unsuccessful.

1. Changes associated with aging that can contribute to low back pain include all of the following except?

(A) Muscle spasm

(B) Narrowing of disc spaces

(C) Decreased water content of intervertebral discs

(D) Decreased flexibility of lumbar curve

2. Mrs. L., your neighbor, is 62 years old, is 5' 3" tall, and weighs approximately 160 lbs. She is complaining of low back pain. She cannot identify any precipitating factor but she reports having had "back problems" off and on for years. It ordinarily goes away on its own if she "takes it easy." She reports sometimes taking acetaminophen or ibuprofen, which helps. This time, however, she says her back has been bothering her for the last 2 months and is present most of the time, although it gets worse when she's been more active. She mentions that she just took a week off and "stayed in bed the entire time." When she returned to her normal activity yesterday, her back pain came right back and may even be a little worse. What is the most appropriate response?

(A) "You probably have a slipped disc. You should make an appointment to be seen by your primary care provider to have some tests done."

(B) "Back pain is commonly associated with aging. You could try one of the nutritional supplements from the health food store."

(C) "Lots of times exercises and weight loss will help back problems. I'd recommend that you join a gym and try to lose 25 to 30 lbs."

(D) "Staying in bed for a week may have caused your muscles to become weaker. You should see your primary care provider to check your back and suggest some exercises and other things that can help you."

3. Most low back pain is due to which of the following?

(A) Vertebral fractures

(B) Herniated intervertebral discs

(C) Muscle sprain/strain

(D) Obesity

4. Degenerative disc disease commonly occurs in whom?

(A) Those with a poor dietary calcium intake.

(B) Those with a narrowing of the spinal canal.

(C) People as they age.

(D) In athletes, particularly African-American males.

5. What is the basic pathophysiology underlying osteoporosis?

(A) An imbalance between osteoclastic and osteoblastic activity

(B) An increase in osteoblastic activity

(C) A decrease in osteoclastic activity

(D) Impaired calcium absorption that leads to a decrease in osteoclastic activity

6. Which of the following would be an appropriate response for you to make to a 40-year-old woman who is interested in learning what she can do to decrease her risk for osteoporosis?

(A) "You should take hormones to replace estrogen once you reach menopause."

(B) "If you do not have risk factors in your history, you probably don't need to do anything special."

(C) "Weight-bearing exercises and an adequate intake of calcium and vitamin D are important factors in preventing osteoporosis."

(D) "Osteoporosis is inevitable, so there's nothing much you can do to prevent it."

7. Which of the following medications may contribute to iatrogenic osteoporosis?

(A) Steroids

(B) Thyroid hormones

(C) Heparin

(D) NSAIDs

8. Which of the following statements about osteoporosis in men is true?

(A) Osteoporosis is less significant in men because their bones are more dense.

(B) Demineralization in men begins in the late 70's or early 80's.

(C) Men do not get osteoporosis because it is an estrogen dependent disorder.

(D) Men have fewer vertebral compression fractures than women because they have less trabecular bone.

9. What provides tensile strength?

(A) Compact bone

(B) Trabecular bone

(C) Periosteum

(D) Haversian system

10. What portion of the bone contains pain receptors?

(A) Endosteum

(B) Marrow

(C) Haversian system

(D) Periosteum

11. The matrix of bone is made of which of the following?

(A) Bone marrow

(B) Collagen

(C) Calcium

(D) Cartilage

12. Callus formation at the site of a fracture takes 2 to 6 weeks. Which of the following statements about bone healing is true?

(A) The most important vitamin in bone healing is vitamin B.

(B) Callus is strong and stable.

(C) The palpable bump at the site of a fracture will gradually disappear as ossification takes place.

(D) Bone remodeling takes 6 to 8 weeks during which time it is important for the patient to avoid stress to the fracture site.

13. Which of the following statements best reflects the pathophysiology of osteoarthritis?

(A) It is characterized by thinning of the articular cartilage, commonly affects weight-bearing joints, and has an asymmetrical distribution.

(B) It is a systemic inflammatory disease that affects many joint structures in a symmetrical fashion and can also involve other body systems.

(C) It is a systemic disease with several phases and is accompanied by hyperuricemia with deposition of urate crystals in joints and other tissues.

(D) It is a disease of aging that ultimately results in profound disability. It commonly contributes to pathological fractures due to increased excretion of calcium and protein by the kidneys.

14. Mrs. T. has rheumatoid arthritis and has been told that she needs to do exercises regularly and that a plan will be worked out with her the next day. Which of the following statements indicates that she understands the rationale for exercise with this disease?

(A) "I know I have to do lots of exercises now so the inflammation in my joints will go away."

(B) "I understand that exercise of my joints is important to help prevent loss of motion."

(C) "Since exercise is so important, I plan to do as much as I can, regardless of whether it hurts or not—'no pain, no gain'."

(D) "They told me I needed to do regular exercise. I think they mean just of my hips and shoulders, because my knees and hands hurt too much."

15. Which of the following classifications of medications is commonly used with osteoarthritis, rheumatoid arthritis, and gout?

(A) Narcotics

(B) Steroids

(C) Uricosurics

(D) NSAIDs

16. What is involved in the pathophysiology of gout?

(A) A reduction of uric acid, which allows calcium to precipitate

(B) Inflammation resulting from intra-articular deposition of urate crystals

(C) Thinning of the articular cartilage, leading to splitting and fragmentation

(D) Formation of tophi in the kidneys, which impairs excretion of uric acid

PART X ANSWERS

1. The correct answer is A.

Muscle spasm is usually a consequence of strain, overuse, or injury.

2. The correct answer is D.

Postural muscles lose strength at approximately 3% per day with bedrest. A referral is indicated for appropriate diagnosis and treatment. The other options contain inappropriate suggestions or incorrect information.

3. The correct answer is C.

This is the most common cause, usually due to deconditioning or overuse. A and B are less common sources of back pain. D is sometimes a contributing factor.

4. The correct answer is C.

Degenerative disc disease results from fibrosis and thinning of the nucleus pulposus associated with aging.

5. The correct answer is A.

It is a disturbance in the balance between osteoclastic and osteoblastic activity, from a variety of causes, and results in osteoporosis. The other choices are incorrect or incomplete.

6. The correct answer is C.

Weight bearing helps increase osteoblastic activity. Vitamin D is needed for calcium absorption, which is necessary for new bone formation. The other choices are incorrect because estrogen replacement is not recommended for all women, and all older women are at some degree of risk and should modify their lifestyle and/or diet as indicated.

7. The correct answer is A.

Long-term use of glucocorticoid hormones can commonly cause osteoporosis; the others do not.

8. The correct answer is A

Bones in men are more dense and thicker than those of women. The other choices are incorrect because demineralization in men begins in the late 60's, and men do get osteoporosis and vertebral compression fractures.

9. The correct answer is B.

The mesh-like network provides the tensile strength. The other options include parts of bone structure but do not provide tensile strength.

10. The correct answer is D.

Because this is the only bone tissue that contains pain receptors any process that disrupts or results in pressure on the periosteum will cause pain.

11. The correct answer is B.

The matrix is collagen tissue. Minerals deposit on this tissue.

12. The correct answer is C.

Vitamins D and C are the most important for bone healing. The other choices are incorrect because callus is unstable and not as strong as bone tissue, and bone remodeling can take as much as a year, depending upon a number of factors.

13. The correct answer is A.

Osteoarthritis is caused by wear and tear and trauma and can occur in middle age as well as in the elderly. The other options describe other forms of arthritis.

14. The correct answer is B.

Individualized exercise plans are important in order to maintain as much joint function as possible, while at the same time preventing additional joint damage. (This is the rationale for why choice D is incorrect.) Choices A and C are incorrect because arthritis does not go away and exercise should not be done to the point of pain.

15. The correct answer is C.

These are anti-inflammatory medications used with all of these conditions. The other choices are incorrect because narcotics are not used for long-term treatment of arthritis; under certain circumstances, steroids are sometimes used with rheumatoid arthritis; and NSAIDs are used with gout.

16. The correct answer is B.

This is the only option that describes the pathology of gout.

REFERENCES

Part I

Bullock, B. A., & Henze, R. L. (2000). *Focus on pathophysiology*. Philadelphia, PA: Lippincott, Williams & Wilkins.

Copstead, L. E. C., & Banasik, J. L. (2000). *Pathophysiology: Biological and behavioral perspectives* (2nd ed.). Philadelphia, PA: W. B. Saunders.

McCance, K. L., & Huether, S. E. (1998). *Pathophysiology* (3rd ed.). St. Louis, MO: C. V. Mosby Co.

Metheny, N. M. (1996). *Fluid and electrolyte balance* (3rd ed.). Philadelphia, PA: Lippincott, Williams & Wilkins.

Uphold, C. R., & Graham, M. V. (1998). *Clinical guidelines in family practice*. Gainesville, FL: Barmarrae Books.

Part II

Dambro, M. R. (Ed.). (2001). *Griffith's 5-minute clinical consultant*. Philadelphia, PA: Lippincott, Williams & Wilkins.

Groer, M. W. (2001). *Advanced pathophysiology: Application to clinical practice*. Philadelphia, PA: Lippincott, Williams & Wilkins.

Hansen, M. (1998). *Pathophysiology: Foundations of disease and clinical interventions*. Philadelphia, PA: W. B. Saunders.

Huether, S. E., & McCance, K. L. (2000). *Understanding pathophysiology* (2nd ed.). St. Louis, MO: C. V. Mosby Co.

Langford, R. W., & Thompson, J. D. (2000). *Mosby's handbook of diseases* (2nd ed.). St. Louis, MO: C. V. Mosby Co.

LeMone, P., & Burke, K. M. (2000). *Medical surgical nursing: Critical thinking in client care* (2nd ed.). Upper Saddle River, NJ: Prentice Hall Health.

Pagana, K. D., & Pagana, T. J. (2001). *Mosby's diagnostic and laboratory test reference*. St. Louis, MO: C. V. Mosby Co.

Porth, C. M. (1998). *Pathophysiology: Concepts of altered health* (5th ed.). Philadelphia, PA: Lippincott, Williams & Wilkins.

Zollo, A. J. (1997). *Medical secrets* (2nd ed.). Philadelphia, PA: Hanley & Belfus, Inc.

Part III

Blackwell, S., & Hendrix, P. (2001). Common anemias. *Clinician Reviews, 11*, 3.

Crowley, L. V. (2001). *An introduction to human disease: Pathology and pathophysiology correlations* (5th ed.). Sudbury, MA: Jones and Bartlett Publishers.

Dambro, M. R. (Ed.). (1999). *Griffith's 5-minute clinical consult*. Philadelphia, PA: Lippincott, Williams & Wilkins.

Fischbach, F. (2000). *A manual of laboratory and diagnostic tests* (6th ed.). Philadelphia, PA: Lippincott, Williams & Wilkins.

Groer, M. W. (2001). *Advanced pathophysiology: Application to clinical practice*. Philadelphia, PA: Lippincott, Williams & Wilkins.

Kumar, V., Cotran, R. S., & Robbins, S. L. (1997). *Basic pathophysiology* (6th ed.). Philadelphia, PA: W. B. Saunders.

Mulvihill, M. L., Zenman, M., Holdaway, P., Tompary, E., & Turchany, J. (2001). *Human diseases: A systemic approach* (5th ed.). Upper Saddle River, NJ: Prentice Hall Health.

Nicoll, D., McPhee, S. J., Pignone, M., Detmer, W. M., & Chou, T. (2001). *Pocket guide to diagnostic tests* (3rd ed.). New York, NY: Lange Medical Books/McGraw-Hill.

Porth, C. M. (1998). *Pathophysiology: Concepts of altered health* (5th ed.). Philadelphia, PA: Lippincott, Williams & Wilkins.

Tierney, L. M. Jr., McPhee, S. J., & Papadakis, M. A. (2001). *Current medical diagnosis and treatment* (40th ed.). New York, NY: Lange Medical Books/McGraw-Hill.

Part IV

Lewis, S., Heitkemper, M., & Dirksen, S. (2000). *Medical surgical nursing* (5th ed.). St Louis, MO: C. V. Mosby Co.

McCance, K. L., & Huether, S. E. (1998). *Pathophysiology* (3rd ed.). St. Louis, MO: C. V. Mosby Co.

Moore, L., Crosby, L., & Hamilton, D. (1998). *Pharmacology for nursing care* (3rd ed.). Philadelphia, PA: W. B. Saunders.

Phipps, W., Sands, J., & Marek, J. (1999). *Medical surgical nursing* (6th ed.). St. Louis, MO: C. V. Mosby Co.

Smeltzer, S., & Bare, B. (2000). *Textbook of medical surgical nursing* (9th ed.). Philadelphia, PA: Lippincott, Williams & Wilkins.

Tierney, L. M. (Ed.). (1999). *Current medical diagnosis and treatment* (38th ed.). Stanford, CT: Appleton and Lange.

Totora, G., & Grabowski, S. (1996). *Principles of anatomy and physiology* (8th ed.). New York, NY: Harper and Collins.

Part V

Bullock, B. A., & Henze, R. L. (2000). *Focus on pathophysiology*. Philadelphia, PA: Lippincott, Williams & Wilkins.

Copstead, L. E. C., & Banasik, J. L. (2000). *Pathophysiology: Biological and behavioral perspectives* (2nd ed.). Philadelphia, PA: W. B. Saunders.

McCance, K. L., & Huether, S. E. (1998). *Pathophysiology* (3rd ed.). St. Louis, MO: C. V. Mosby Co.

Uphold, C. R., & Graham, M. V. (1998). *Clinical guidelines in family practice*. Gainesville, FL: Barmarrae Books.

Part VI

Dambro, M. R. (Ed.). (2001). *Griffith's 5-minute clinical consultant*. Philadelphia, PA: Lippincott, Williams & Wilkins.

Groer, M. W. (2001). *Advanced pathophysiology: Application to clinical practice*. Philadelphia, PA: Lippincott, Williams & Wilkins.

Hansen, M. (1998). *Pathophysiology: Foundations of disease and clinical interventions*. Philadelphia, PA: W. B. Saunders.

Huether, S. E., & McCance, K. L. (2000). *Understanding pathophysiology* (2nd ed.). St. Louis, MO: C. V. Mosby Co.

Langford, R. W., & Thompson, J. D. (2000). *Mosby's handbook of diseases* (2nd ed.). St. Louis, MO: C. V. Mosby Co.

LeMone, P., & Burke, K. M. (2000). *Medical surgical nursing: Critical thinking in client care* (2nd ed.). Upper Saddle River, NJ: Prentice Hall Health.

Pagana, K. D., & Pagana, T. J. (2001). *Mosby's diagnostic and laboratory test reference*. St. Louis, MO: C. V. Mosby Co.

Porth, C. M. (1998). *Pathophysiology: Concepts of altered health* (5th ed.). Philadelphia, PA: Lippincott, Williams & Wilkins.

Zollo, A. J. (1997). *Medical secrets* (2nd ed.). Philadelphia, PA: Hanley & Belfus, Inc.

Part VII

Lewis, S., Heitkemper, M., & Dirksen, S. (2000). *Medical surgical nursing* (5th ed.). St Louis, MO: C. V. Mosby Co.

McCance, K. L., & Huether, S. E. (1998). *Pathophysiology* (3rd ed.). St. Louis, MO: C. V. Mosby Co.

Moore, L., Crosby, L., & Hamilton, D. (1998). *Pharmacology for nursing care* (3rd ed.). Philadelphia, PA: W. B. Saunders.

Phipps, W., Sands, J., & Marek, J. (1999). *Medical surgical nursing* (6th ed.). St. Louis, MO: C. V. Mosby Co.

Smeltzer, S., & Bare, B. (2000). *Textbook of medical surgical nursing* (9th ed.). Philadelphia, PA: Lippincott, Williams & Wilkins.

Part VIII

Alderman, J. (1999). Managing irritable bowel syndrome. *Advance for Nurse Practitioners, 7*, 1.

Carlson, E. (1998). Irritable bowel syndrome. *The Nurse Practitioner Journal, 23*, 1.

Crowley, L. V. (2001). *An introduction to human disease: Pathology and pathophysiology correlations* (5th ed.). Sudbury, MA: Jones and Bartlett Publishers.

Dambro, M. R. (Ed.). (1999). *Griffith's 5-minute clinical consult*. Philadelphia, PA: Lippincott, Williams & Wilkins.

Fischbach, F. (2000). *A manual of laboratory and diagnostic tests* (6th ed.). Philadelphia, PA: Lippincott, Williams & Wilkins.

Groer, M. W. (2001). *Advanced pathophysiology: Application to clinical practice*. Philadelphia, PA: Lippincott, Williams & Wilkins.

Kumar, V., Cotran, R. S., & Robbins, S. L. (1997). *Basic pathophysiology* (6th ed.). Philadelphia, PA: W. B. Saunders.

Mulvihill, M. L., Zenman, M., Holdaway, P., Tompary, E., & Turchany, J. (2001). *Human diseases: A systemic approach* (5th ed.). Upper Saddle River, NJ: Prentice Hall Health.

Nicoll, D., McPhee, S. J., Pignone, M., Detmer, W. M., & Chou, T. (2001). *Pocket guide to diagnostic tests* (3rd ed.). New York, NY: Lange Medical Books/McGraw-Hill.

Norton, B. (1998). Crohn's disease. *Advance for Nurse Practitioners, 6*, 9.

Pardi, D. S., & Tremane, W. J. (1998). Inflammatory bowel disease: Keys to diagnosis and treatment. *Consultant, 38*, 1.

Porth, C. M. (1998). *Pathophysiology: Concepts of altered health* (5th ed.). Philadelphia, PA: Lippincott, Williams & Wilkins.

Rose, S. (1998). *Gastrointestinal and hepatobiliary pathophysiology*. Madison, CT: Fence Creek Publishing.

Seller, R. H. (2000). *Differential diagnosis of common complaints* (4th ed.). Philadelphia, PA: W. B. Saunders.

Tierney, L. M. Jr., McPhee, S. J., & Papadakis, M. A. (2001). *Current medical diagnosis and treatment* (40th ed.). New York, NY: Lange Medical Books/McGraw Hill.

Part IX

Dambro, M. R. (Ed). (2001). *Griffith's 5-minute clinical consultant*. Philadelphia, PA: Lippincott, Williams & Wilkins.

Groer, M. W. (2001). *Advanced pathophysiology: Application to clinical practice*. Philadelphia, PA: Lippincott, Williams & Wilkins.

Hansen, M. (1998). *Pathophysiology: Foundations of disease and clinical interventions*. Philadelphia, PA: W. B. Saunders.

Huether, S. E., & McCance, K. L. (2000). *Understanding pathophysiology* (2nd ed.). St. Louis, MO: C. V. Mosby Co.

Langford, R. W., & Thompson, J. D. (2000). *Mosby's handbook of diseases* (2nd ed.). St. Louis, MO: C. V. Mosby Co.

LeMone, P., & Burke, K. M. (2000). *Medical surgical nursing: Critical thinking in client care* (2nd ed.). Upper Saddle River, NJ: Prentice Hall Health.

Pagana, K. D., & Pagana, T. J. (2001). *Mosby's diagnostic and laboratory test reference.* St. Louis, MO: C. V. Mosby Co.

Porth, C. M. (1998). *Pathophysiology: Concepts of altered health* (5th ed.). Philadelphia, PA: Lippincott, Williams & Wilkins.

Zollo, A. J. (1997). *Medical secrets* (2nd ed.). Philadelphia, PA: Hanley & Belfus, Inc.

Part X

Bullock, B. A., & Henze, R. L. (2000). *Focus on pathophysiology.* Philadelphia, PA: Lippincott, Williams & Wilkins.

Copstead, L. E. C., & Banasik, J. L. (2000). *Pathophysiology: Biological and behavioral perspectives* (2nd ed.). Philadelphia, PA: W. B. Saunders.

McCance, K. L., & Huether, S. E. (1998). *Pathophysiology* (3rd ed.). St. Louis, MO: C. V. Mosby Co.

Uphold, C. R., & Graham, M. V. (1998). *Clinical guidelines in family practice.* Gainesville, FL: Barmarrae Books.

INDEX

iron deficiency anemia, 39–40
irritable bowel syndrome, 176–179, 193

jaundice, 202, 204, 209
joints
    anatomy and physiology of, 242, 254, 255
    inflammation of (arthritis), 252–255

kidney, 12–13, 222–223
    disorders of
        calculi, 233–234
        in diabetes mellitus, 90, 228–229
        drug-induced, 240
        failure, 236–238
        glomerulonephritis, 227–229
        hemolytic uremic syndrome, 225–226
        infections, 224–225, 240, 241
        nephritic syndrome, 227–228
        nephrotic syndrome, 227–229
        renal tubular acidosis, 239–240
        in systemic lupus erythematosus, 30
        tubulointerstitial, 239–241

large intestine. See colon
LDL (low density lipoprotein), 129
leukocytes, 24–25
lipids, blood, disorders of, 128–130
liver, 167, 201–211
    disorders of, 202, 204
        cancer, 199
        cirrhosis, 208–211
        fat accumulation in, 202
        inflammation (hepatitis), 201, 203, 205–207
        injury of, 202
        tests for, 201, 203
    transplantation of, 210
low back pain, 256–259
lung
    cancer of, 108–110
    injury of, in ARDS, 102–103
lupus, 29, 30
Lyme disease, 29–30
lymphatic system, 25
lymphocytes, 25

macrophages, 25
magnesium balance, 10
Manning criteria, for irritable bowel syndrome, 176
Mantoux test, for tuberculosis, 115
mast cells, 19
meningitis, 57–58
metabolic acidosis and alkalosis, 11–13
metabolic disorders
    in cirrhosis, 209
    diabetes mellitus, 87–90, 228–229
micturition, problems with, 230–232

mineralocorticoids, 85–86
mitral valve, 153–155
monocytes, 25
Monro-Kellie doctrine, 53
mouth, digestive function of, 164, 167
multiple sclerosis, 68–69
myelin, 49, 68–69
myocardial infarction, 132–134, 140
myocardium, 122–123
    cardiomyopathies of, 145–148
    inflammation of (myocarditis), 150–151

nausea and vomiting, 169, 194–196
negative feedback, in endocrine system, 76–77
nephritic syndrome, 227–228
nephrotic syndrome, 227–229
nerve root disorders, 257–259
nervous system, 48–69. See also brain
    anatomy and physiology of, 48–51
    disorders of
        cerebrovascular accident, 63–66, 136
        in cirrhosis, 209–210
        degenerative, 67–69
        in diabetes mellitus, 89–90
        infections, 57–58
        manifestations of, 48
        spinal cord, 49, 51, 60–62
        trauma, 59–62
neurotransmitters, 49–51, 67–68, 85, 86
neutrophils, 24–25
nonsteroidal anti-inflammatory drugs
    asthma due to, 100
    gastritis due to, 169–171
    nephropathy due to, 240
    peptic ulcer disease due to, 173–174
nosocomial infections, pneumonia, 112

obstruction
    gastric outlet, 175, 194
    intestinal, 184, 189–190
occlusive disease, arterial, 157
orthopedic conditions, 246–259
    arthritis, 252–255
    back pain, 256–259
    fractures, 246, 247
    gout, 255
    osteoarthritis, 253
    osteomyelitis, 250–251
    osteoporosis, 249–251
    physiologic considerations in, 246–248
    rheumatoid arthritis, 253, 255
osmolality, 2–3, 6–7
ossification, 247
osteoarthritis, 253
osteomyelitis, 250–251
osteoporosis, 249–251

superior vena cava syndrome, in lung cancer, 109
supraventricular dysrhythmias, 142–144
surfactant, pulmonary, 97
systemic lupus erythematosus, 29, 30
systole, 122–123
  blood pressure in, 135
  ventricular dysfunction during, 140

T_3 (triiodothyronine), 79–81
T_4 (thyroxine), 79–81
T cells, 26–27, 32
tachyarrhythmias, 142–144
thalassemia, 42, 43
thrombophlebitis, 157–158
thrombosis
  cerebrovascular accident in, 63–64
  coronary artery, 132
  pulmonary embolism in, 103–104
thyroid and thyroid hormones, 79–81
tick bites, Lyme disease from, 29–30
tonicity, 7
tophi, in gout, 255
transfusions, HIV transmission in, 33
transient ischemic attack, 64
transplantation, liver, 210
trauma
  head, 59–62
  spinal cord, 60–62
traveler's diarrhea, 193
tricuspid valve, 153–155
triglycerides, blood levels of, 129
triiodothyronine, 79–81
tuberculosis, 114–116
tubulointerstitial disorders, 239–241

ulcer(s)
  in Crohn's disease, 176, 178, 183–185
  peptic, 168–175
ulcerative colitis, 176, 178, 180–182
unconsciousness, 52–53
urinary tract, 222–241
  anatomy and physiology of, 222–223
  disorders of
    calculi, 233–234
    function tests for, 222

glomerulonephritis, 227–229
hemolytic uremic syndrome, 225–226
incontinence, 230–232
infections, 224–226, 240
kidney failure, 236–238
prostatic hyperplasia, 234–235
tubulointerstitial disorders, 239–241

valves, heart, 122–123, 150–155
varicose veins, 157–158
  esophageal, 209
vascular disorders. See cardiovascular system, disorders of
vegetative state, 53
veins
  anatomy of, 123
  chronic insufficiency of, 157–158
  thrombosis of, 103–104
  varicose, 157–158
ventilation, 97
ventilation/perfusion scan, 96
ventricles, 122–123
  disorders of
    aneurysms, 156–157
    cardiomyopathy, 145–148
    dysrhythmias, 142–144
    failure, 139–141
verbal deficits, in cerebrovascular accident, 64–65
vertebral joints, 257
viral infections, 21–23
  encephalitis, 58
  gastroenteritis, 191–196
  meningitis, 57
  pneumonia, 112
vitamin B_{12}, for pernicious anemia, 44, 169
vitamin D
  in bone metabolism, 246–247, 247
  for hypoparathyroidism, 83
VLDL (very low density lipoprotein), 129
volvulus, 190
vomiting, 169, 194–196

white blood cells (leukocytes), 24–25

Zollinger-Ellison syndrome, 173

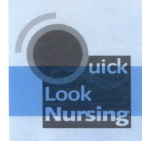

Expand Your Library
With These Exceptional Texts!

Other Exciting Books in the Quick Look Nursing *Series Include:*

Title	Book #	Price
❏ Quick Look Nursing: Growth and Development Through the Lifespan	25066	$21.95
❏ Quick Look Nursing: Legal and Ethical Issues in Nursing	25058	$21.95
❏ Quick Look Nursing: Pathophysiology	25651	$23.95
❏ Quick Look Nursing: Nutrition	25015	$17.95

Subtotal $____

NJ and CA Sales Tax* $____

Handling Charge $ 4.50

Total $____

Name: _____

Address: _____

City: _____ State: _____ Zip Code: _____

Phone: _____ Fax: _____

Charge my: ❏ [American Express] ❏ [MasterCard] ❏ [VISA] Account#:_____

Exp. date: _____ Signature: _____

Prices are subject to change. Shipping charges may apply.

*Purchases in NJ and CA are subject to tax. Please add applicable state and local taxes.

CODE: 2A556

Mail Order Form To: SLACK Incorporated
Professional Book Division
6900 Grove Road
Thorofare, NJ 08086-9864

Call: 800-257-8290 or 856-848-1000
Fax: 856-853-5991
Email: Orders@slackinc.com

Visit Our World Wide Web: www.slackbooks.com